IMMUNITY TO BLOOD PARASITES OF ANIMALS AND MAN

ADVANCES IN EXPERIMENTAL MEDICINE AND BIOLOGY

Recent Volumes in this Series

IMMUNITY TO BLOOD PARASITES OF ANIMALS AND MAN

Edited by

Louis H. Miller

National Institute of Allergy
 and Infectious Diseases
Bethesda, Maryland

and

John A. Pino and
John J. McKelvey, Jr.

The Rockefeller Foundation
New York, New York

PLENUM PRESS • NEW YORK AND LONDON

Library of Congress Cataloging in Publication Data

Main entry under title:

Immunity to blood parasites of animals and man.

(Advances in experimental medicine and biology; v. 93)
"Based on papers presented at the Rockefeller Foundation Study and Conference Center at Bellagio, Italy, September, 1975."
Includes indexes.
1. Medical parasitology—Immunological aspects—Congresses. 2. Veterinary parasitology—Immunological aspects—Congresses. 3. Vaccination—Congresses. 4. Vaccination of animals—Congresses. I. Miller, Louis H. II. Pino, John A. III. McKelvey, John J. IV. Series. [DNLM: 1. Antigens—Congresses. 2. Immunization—Congresses. 3. Parasitic diseases—Congresses. 4. Parasitic diseases—Veterinary—Congresses. W1 AD559 v. 93/WC695 I31 1975]
RC157.I45   616.9'6   77-16094
ISBN 0-306-32693-0

Based on papers presented at the Rockefeller Foundation Study
and Conference Center at Bellagio, Italy, September, 1975

© 1977 Plenum Press, New York
A Division of Plenum Publishing Corporation
227 West 17th Street, New York, N.Y. 10011

Printed in the United States of America

ACKNOWLEDGMENTS

In Chapter 1, Figures 1 and 2 are from Brown et al. (1968) "Immunity to malaria: the antibody response to antigenic variation in *Plasmodium knowlesi*," *Immunology* 14: 127-138, reproduced by permission of Blackwell Scientific Publications, Ltd., Oxford. Figure 3 is from Brown, K.N. (1973) "Antibody induced variation in malaria parasites," *Nature* 242: 49-50, reproduced by permission of Macmillan Journals, Ltd., London. Figure 7 is from Brown, K.N., and Hills, L.A. (1974) "Antigenic variation and immunity to *Plasmodium knowlesi*," *Transactions, Royal Society of Tropical Medicine and Hygiene* 68: 139-142, reproduced by permission of the Society.

In Chapter 6, Figure 1 is from Cohen, S., and Sadun, E.H., Eds. (1976) *Immunity to Parasitic Diseases*, reproduced by permission of Blackwell Scientific Publications, Ltd., Oxford. Figure 2 is from Bannister, L.H., et al. (1975) "Structure and behaviour of *Plasmodium knowlesi* merozoites *in vitro*," *Parasitology* 71: 483-491, reproduced by permission of Cambridge University Press, New York. Figure 3 is from Mitchell, G.H., et al. (1974) "A merozoite vaccine effective against *Plasmodium knowlesi* malaria," *Nature* 252: 311-313, reproduced by permission of Macmillan Journals, Ltd., London. Figures 4, 5, and 6 are from Dennis, E.D., et al. (1975) "*In vitro* isolation of *Plasmodium knowlesi* merozoites using polycarbonate sieves," *Parasitology* 71: 475-481, reproduced by permission of Cambridge University Press, New York. Table 1 is from Miller, L.H. (1975) "Transfusion malaria," in *Transmissable Disease and Blood Transfusion*, Greenwalt, T.J., and Jamieson, G.A., Eds., reproduced by permission of the publisher, Grune & Stratton, Inc., New York.

In Chapter 9, Figure 1 is from Ristic, M., et al. (1963) "Biochemical and biophysical characterization of soluble *Anaplasma* antigens," *American Journal of Veterinary Research* 24: 472-477, reproduced by permission of the American Veterinary Medical Association.

In Chapter 10, Tables 1 through 7 are from Radley, E., et al. (1975) "East Coast fever," *Veterinary Parasitology* 1: 35-60, reproduced by permission of Elsevier Scientific Publishing Company, Amsterdam.

PREFACE

Since the turn of the century, certain parasitic diseases of livestock have frustrated efforts to bring them under control by vaccination techniques; East Coast fever and trypanosomiasis are two such diseases. East Coast fever (ECF) kills a half million cattle annually; and 3 million are killed each year by trypanosomiasis, which is widely spread over tropical Africa. Together, these diseases have closed some 7 million square kilometers of land to livestock grazing—land that might otherwise support an additional 120 million head of cattle.

In 1970 W.A. Malmquist of the U.S. Department of Agriculture, in collaboration with K.N. Brown, M.P. Cunningham, and other associates at the East African Veterinary Research Organization in Kenya, succeeded in cultivating *in vitro* the protozoal organisms responsible for East Coast fever. This success, obtained utilizing tissue cultures, encouraged a number of organizations to support research on these parasites in an accelerated effort to develop field vaccines.

The International Laboratory for Research on Animal Diseases (ILRAD) was created in 1973. Its initial efforts have included the consolidation and advancement of methods for immunization against ECF of cattle and African trypanosomiasis of animals and man. Trypanosomiasis, a disease of much wider range than ECF, is even more intransigent in the face of efforts to control it by immunological techniques, although the recent success of Hirumi and associates at ILRAD in culturing African trypanosomes should afford new approaches to research in this field. At the same time, veterinarians and researchers from associated disciplines have made steady progress in acquiring the knowledge and developing the methodology that would lead to bringing other livestock diseases, anaplasmosis and babesiosis, under control by vaccination techniques. These two diseases are widespread not only in Africa and Latin America, but in the United States as well.

Of equal importance to development in the tropical world are the diseases of man. The drain from diseases such as malaria must be measured not only in terms of mortality and morbidity but also in the loss of productivity that indirectly affects the food supply. Technical and administrative problems have hampered the standard approach to the control of malaria, i.e., antimalarials and insecticide spraying of houses. However, recent advances in malaria research — the cultivation of *Plasmodium falciparum* by W. Trager and J. Jensen, and new approaches to vaccination in animals—have raised the hope that a human vaccine may be available in the near future.

Certain characteristics of blood-borne parasites are common to the disease process in both animals and man. For example, antigenic variation—a phenomenon that enables the parasite to survive successive waves of antibodies produced by the host—occurs in malaria, babesiosis, and trypanosomiasis.

A paramount need has existed to review antigenic variation and other possible mechanisms by which these parasites have been able to counteract the innate resistance and immunological defenses of their hosts. Accordingly, in September 1975, authorities on diseases of man (Chagas' disease, sleeping sickness, and malaria) and of livestock (trypanosomiasis, ECF, babesiosis, and anaplasmosis) convened at the Rockefeller Foundation Study and Conference Center at Bellagio, Italy, to report on the state of the art and science of immunological approaches for dealing with these diseases. Cellular biologists knowledgeable about antigenic variation per se also participated. The names and institutional affiliations of the participants are listed in Appendix A. Responding to the wishes of the conferees, Dr. Barry Bloom summarized the proceedings in the April 1, 1976, issue of *Nature*.

This volume, an outgrowth of the conference at Bellagio, is based on selected papers that have been revised, expanded, and updated for this publication. It is intended for the use of students, instructors, research workers, and practitioners concerned with blood-borne parasitic diseases. We hope that the information made available to them in this book will help speed the day when these diseases will be brought under control by immunological techniques similar to those which have long been successful against a wide range of pathogenic viruses and bacteria.

Dr. Ian McIntyre, then Dean of the Faculty of Veterinary Medicine, University of Glasgow, Scotland, bore major responsibility in organizing the Conference. His own group of associates has been especially active in research on trypano-tolerant cattle of West Africa and on the pathology of trypanosomiasis.

We extend our thanks to Dr. and Mrs. William Olson, Director and Assistant Director, respectively, of the Bellagio Study and Conference Center, for the warm, professional hospitality they gave. We also express our appreciation to Mr. Henry Rommey and his staff at The Rockefeller Foundation, and to Mr. Gilbert Tauber, for their editorial advice and assistance in the production of this book.

Louis H. Miller
John A. Pino
John J. McKelvey, Jr.

New York
June 1977

CONTENTS

INTRODUCTION

This book focuses on the potentialities and problems of developing effective vaccines against bloodstream parasites of man and his livestock. The parasites dealt with are a diverse group: trypanosomes, plasmodia, theilerias, anaplasmas, and babesias. All have arthropods as vectors during a portion of their complex life cycles. Tsetse flies transmit salivarian trypanosomes, which cause sleeping sickness in man and trypanosomiasis in cattle; reduviid "kissing" bugs transmit Chagas' disease; mosquitoes are the vectors of malarial parasites; and different species of ticks transmit East Coast fever (ECF), anaplasmosis, and babesiosis of cattle. These diseases are among the most devastating and economically costly of those of parasitic origin.

To be sure, the parasitic diseases discussed herein yield to methods other than immunoprophylaxis for their prevention and control. Often the vector is the vulnerable target. In Africa, the use of insecticides and the clearing of bush to eliminate tsetse flies have succeeded in controlling trypanosomiasis of livestock. But areas cleared of the fly readily become reinfested. Mosquito control and DDT spraying of houses have been standard procedure in campaigns against malaria. By this and supporting means, the World Health Organization (WHO) has been successful, over the past several decades, in eradicating or controlling malaria in many areas where it had been endemic. Yet 500 million people in 66 countries live in areas where eradication cannot be implemented. Malaria is resurgent in Pakistan, Bangladesh, Sri Lanka, and several provinces of India where it had once been brought under control. The prevention of Chagas' disease depends almost exclusively on proper housing that does not harbor the reduviid "assassin" or "kissing" bugs. Cattle dips to wipe out tick infestations have been standard preventive measures against ECF, anaplasmosis, and babesiosis, but they, too, become impractical under conditions of heavy tick infestation.

Drugs directed against the parasites themselves have helped to control some of the diseases in question, such as malaria. But these methods also have their shortcomings. In addition to the deleterious effects of such drugs on the host, drug-resistant strains of parasites may evolve. The chemotherapeutic agents tested against Chagas' disease have been disappointing. They reduce parasitemia, but to be effective they must be administered at dose levels that are poorly tolerated by humans. Drugs have also been used against the salivarian trypanosomes that afflict cattle in Africa, but in areas of very heavy "fly" infestation, the frequency of application becomes uneconomic and unacceptable.

1

Not only the shortcomings of drugs and vector control justify a search for effective immunoprophylaxis against parasitic diseases. The immune response is intrinsically efficient, and there is ample evidence that it can protect against these diseases.

In nature, humans and animals develop resistance to parasitic diseases; however, this resistance falls short of the immune response characteristic of many viral infections. For example, whereas a single viral infection may confer long-lasting immunity, resistance to malaria is conferred only after repeated challenge. Some strains of cattle possess a natural resistance to trypanosomiasis. There are indigenous breeds of cattle in Africa that display an immune response to salivarian trypanosomes and are able to survive under conditions of heavy challenge. The tick-borne diseases already yield to vaccines—routinely in the case of babesiosis and at least experimentally in the case of anaplasmosis and ECF.

The intricate life cycles of the parasites, their versatility in thwarting their hosts' defenses, and the complexity of immunity per se make the course ahead a formidable one. In research on trypanosomes, scientists have yet to develop a technique of immunization that will clearly confer protection on domestic animals grazing in endemic areas—to say nothing of immunizing human beings against the trypanosomes causing sleeping sickness. Research on the malarial organisms is advancing along two essential lines: one an attack on the sporozoite stage, the other on the merozoites. Immunity to the sporozoite stage occurs in mice, monkeys, and man, but is short-lived with available methods of vaccination. Merozoite immunity may be the more practical to achieve, as suggested by Miller (Chapter 7). Research on immunoprophylaxis against Chagas' disease must also advance along two lines: protection against the parasitemia of the acute phase, and protection in the chronic stage of the disease, when the parasites are not usually found in the blood. A crucial problem in the development of a vaccine against Chagas' disease is the possibility that the immune response itself may be responsible, at least in part, for the heart damage and intestinal enlargement associated with the chronic stage of the disease.

A major phenomenon that can thwart efforts to immunize man and livestock against disease is antigenic variation. This is a widely recognized characteristic of the salivarian trypanosomes that cause sleeping sickness in man and trypanosomiasis of cattle in Africa. Much less is known about antigenic variation among the trypanosomes responsible for Chagas' disease.

Striking similarities exist between antigenic variation in malaria and in the African trypanosomiases. In neither case is it known whether antigenic variation results from mutation or from the phenotypic expression of alternative genes triggered in some still unknown fashion, but the phenomenon appears to limit the effectiveness of vaccination against both. In malaria the phenotypic expression is on the surface of the infected erythrocytes and, possibly, merozoites;

in trypanosomiasis the expression is in the antigenic determinants on the surface coat of the trypanosomes. Recent advances in the test-tube cultivation of the erythrocytic cycle of *Plasmodium falciparum* and of the bloodstream form of the *brucei* group of trypanosomes enhance opportunities for more fruitful *in vitro* research on antigenic variation.

Among the tick-borne parasites, *Babesia argentina (=bovis)*, closely related to the malarial parasites, submits to immunoprophylaxis despite occurrence of antigenic variation. It is known, however, that this organism reverts to a fundamental antigenic type in its passage through its vector, *Boophilus* ticks. There is now evidence that this might also occur, at least to some extent, with salivarian trypanosomes.

Successful vaccinations have been achieved in babesiosis, theileriosis, and anaplasmosis. In each case, viable parasites were used, either as attenuated parasites (anaplasmosis), as infections modified by treatment (theileriosis), or as a low inoculum of reduced virulence (babesiosis in calves). In babesiosis and anaplasmosis, killed vaccines of erythrocytic origin combined with adjuvants caused hemolytic anemia on challenge with live organisms, and are of limited effectiveness. Vaccination with erythrocytic stages of the malarial parasites in adjuvant may present similar problems. The problems posed by killed vaccines in babesiosis and anaplasmosis indicate that research in veterinary parasitology may help those attempting to develop vaccines against malaria in man. Live vaccines, however, also cause problems, as outlined in Chapter 8 on babesiosis. In this case, veterinary science may profit from the experience with killed vaccines against malaria.

Acquired resistance may not always be demonstrated to depend on antibodies; cell-mediated immunity (CMI) may also provide a part of the defense against bloodstream parasites, and it is important that one have a thorough understanding of cellular immunity and the parasites. In Chapter 4, Dr. G.B. Mackaness outlines the criteria for evaluating the importance of CMI in host resistance to infection.

Among the 13 chapters in this book, the first three afford a comparision of antigenic variation as a phenomenon and as it affects immunoprophylaxis against malaria, babesiosis, and the salivarian trypanosomiases. Chapter 4 describes the role of cell-mediated immunity in the immune response. Chapters 5 through 8, devoted to the malarial parasite, enable one to compare the problems of approaching immunological control by an attack on the sporozoite stage and on the merozoite stage. The successes achieved in vaccination against tick-borne disease of cattle appear in Chapters 9 through 11. The status of attempts to invoke immunity for the control of Chagas' disease are presented in Chapters 12 and 13. Collectively, these reviews should be of great help to individual workers attempting to bear down on some of the most intractable and widespread infectious diseases known to man.

1

ANTIGENIC VARIATION IN MALARIA

K. N. Brown

Division of Parasitology
National Institute for Medical Research
Mill Hill, London NW7 IAA, England

INTRODUCTION

Like most protozoan infections malaria is usually chronic. Even in the absence of persistent exoerythrocytic infection parasites may remain in the blood for months after antiplasmodial antibody is detectable in the serum.

It is now known that antigenic variation analogous to that in trypanosomes occurs in chronic erythrocytic malaria. This was first indicated by the work of Cox (1959) and was unequivocally shown by the studies of Brown & Brown (1965) and Brown et al. (1968). Their observations have been confirmed and amplified by several subsequent studies (Voller & Rossan 1969a; Brown et al. 1970a, 1970b; Butcher & Cohen 1972 [on *Plasmodium knowlesi*]; Voller & Rossan 1969b [on *P. cynomolgi*]; Briggs & Wellde 1969 [on *P. berghei*]).

So far a detailed analysis has been possible only with *P. knowlesi* in rhesus monkeys. *Plasmodium knowlesi* infection is particularly suited for these studies, since all parasites in the blood tend to be in the same stage of the cell cycle at any given time, and erythrocytes infected with mature parasites can be readily separated from uninfected cells. The *P. knowlesi* studies will be discussed in detail in this chapter, and the results obtained will be related to experiments in which rodent malarias were used to study the role of lymphocyte subpopulations in protective immunity.

It should be emphasized that antigenic variation has yet to be demonstrated in the plasmodia that cause human malarias. Circumstantial evidence suggests that it is likely to occur, but until unequivocal proof is forthcoming the wider implications of this paper rest on the assumption that antigenic variation occurs in human malarias.

SCHIZONT-INFECTED CELL AGGLUTINATION TEST

This test was first described by Eaton (1938). He found that erythrocytes infected with *P. knowlesi* schizonts were agglutinated in serum from immune monkeys. Uninfected erythrocytes and erythrocytes infected with preschizont forms were not agglutinated. Using the schizont-infected cell agglutination (SICA) test, Brown & Brown (1965) and Brown et al. (1968) found that antigenic variation occurred repeatedly in chronic infections and that different *P. knowlesi* strains have different repertoires of variants (Figures 1 and 2). Variant-specific agglutinating antisera were raised by immunizing rhesus monkeys with one antigenic variant type, either by infection and drug cure or by incorporation of freeze-thawed schizont-infected cells in Freund's complete adjuvant (FCA) or incomplete adjuvant (FIA).

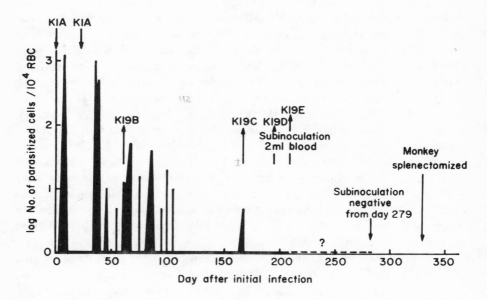

Figure 1. Parasitemia in monkey K19. The monkey was infected with stabilate KIA on day 0, and cured by drug therapy when the parasitemia was 12.5%. Ten days later it was reinfected with stabilate KIA. Parasites were isolated as stabilates at the times indicated by the upward arrows. Serum samples were also collected at frequent intervals. (From Brown et al. 1968.)

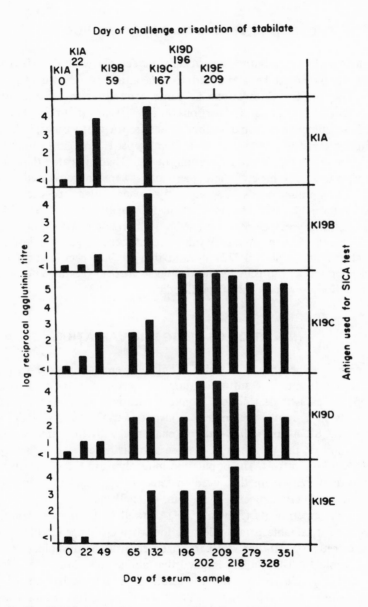

Figure 2. The SICA response, in serum samples collected from monkey K19, against stabilates isolated on the days indicated in Figure 1. (From Brown et al. 1968.)

PROTECTIVE VARIANT-SPECIFIC ANTIBODIES

Although antigenic variation was readily detectable with the SICA test, no protective action could be attributed to this antibody (Brown et al. 1970a, 1970b). However, the fluctuations in parasite numbers in chronic infections indicated that a substantial proportion of any given variant population was destroyed, presumably by some antibody specific for that variant, before a new population emerged with different variable antigens. Histological evidence (Taliaferro & Cannon 1936; Taliaferro & Mulligan 1937) had indicated that vast numbers of parasitized erythrocytes and merozoites were phagocytosed in animals going through immune crisis. Consequently, when variant-specific opsonizing antibodies were demonstrated (Brown et al. 1970b; Brown & Hills 1974) and it appeared that the presence of these antibodies correlated with protection, this suggested that variant-specific antibodies might control parasite levels. Other workers (Butcher & Cohen 1972) showed that variant-specific antibodies also inhibited infection of red cells by merozoites *in vitro*, suggesting another *in vivo* protective action by variant-specific antibodies.

INDUCTION OF ANTIGENIC VARIATION

In numerous experiments in which monkeys were immunized with known variants, it was found that antigenic variation occurred in the total absence of protection, i.e., parasite destruction. Monkeys sensitized with disrupted schizont-infected cells in Freund's incomplete adjuvant (FIA) produced high levels of variant-specific SICA antibodies, but on challenge with the same variant type used to immunize, the parasitemia in these animals developed at the same rate as in unsensitized controls. The population multiplying in these animals was of a different variant type from that used to sensitize and challenge, and gave no SICA reaction with sera collected at the time of challenge.

Subsequent experiments (Brown 1973) showed that variation could be induced without detectable parasite destruction when challenge infections were of the order of only 10, 10^2, or 10^3 parasitized cells of the homologous serotype (Figure 3, Table 1). This finding implied that antigenic variation in *P. knowlesi* was a phenotypic change and not the result of immunoselection of mutant forms, a conclusion in agreement with current thinking on trypanosome antigenic variation (Cross 1975). However, definitive proof that antigenic variation in malaria parasites is phenotypic must await development of suitable *in vitro* techniques.

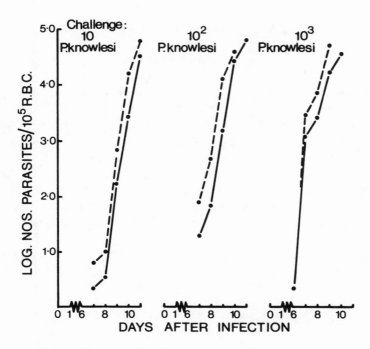

Figure 3. Parasitemia in monkeys sensitized with dead *P. knowlesi* schizont-infected cells and challenged intravenously with homologous parasites as indicated. (From Brown 1973.)

Table 1
Schizont-Infected Red Cell Agglutination Response

	SICA Test (log reciprocal titer)
Sensitizing stabilate[a]	> 5.83
Breakthrough stabilate[b]	< 1.0

[a] Parasites from the stabilate used to sensitize with schizont-infected cells in FIA.

[b] Parasites breaking through after homologous intravenous challenge with 10 ring-stage parasites.

ANTIGENIC VARIATION AND THE CELL CYCLE

Whether or not it is phenotypic, the evidence for antigenic variation in plasmodia now seems very difficult to refute. But the nature of the antigen is unresolved. So too, is the perplexing problem of the mechanism by which it appears on the surface of infected erythrocytes.

Erythrocytes infected with immature parasites (Figures 4 and 5) are not agglutinated, but this may be because they do not synthesize the relevant antigen or do not produce enough of it. Sections through parasitized erythrocytes show an increasing breakdown in red cell structure as the parasite matures, although the erythrocyte membrane appears to remain intact (Figure 6). Treatment of ^{51}Cr-label schizont-infected cells with anti-red-cell serum will release chromium, indicating that the membrane retains some functional integrity (Brown et al. 1970b).

So little is known, however, about interaction of the parasite and erythrocyte that it is difficult even to speculate about likely mechanisms. The extracellular merozoite is exposed to direct antibody action (Butcher & Cohen 1972; Miller et al. 1975), suggesting that it is at this stage that antigenic variation might be induced by nonlethal antibody. New techniques for isolating merozoites (Mitchell et al. 1973; Dennis et al. 1975) and for the *in vitro* cultivation of malaria parasites (Trager & Jensen 1976) should contribute to our understanding of antigenic variation.

ANTIGENIC VARIATION AND RED CELL PENETRATION

Merozoites from erythrocytic parasites only penetrate other red cells. Thus, there must be an erythrocyte-specific target site recognized by merozoites. This site is species-specific and apparently is important in determining the host distribution of the parasite species (McGhee 1953; Butcher et al. 1973). Very limited experiments involving pretreatment of erythrocytes with enzymes of the parasite species (Miller et al. 1973) and concanavalin A (Trigg & Shakespeare 1975) suggest that the receptor site for *P. knowlesi* may be tentatively identified as a minor membrane glycoprotein with less than 8% carbohydrate and very little sialic acid.

The merozoite surface coat, visible by electron microscopy, is the first point of contact with the erythrocyte. It seems inevitable that this protein or glycoprotein coat initiates erythrocyte recognition and penetration (Miller et al. 1975). Serum from infected monkeys, which agglutinates merozoites by their surface coats, inhibits invasion of red cells (Miller et al. 1975).

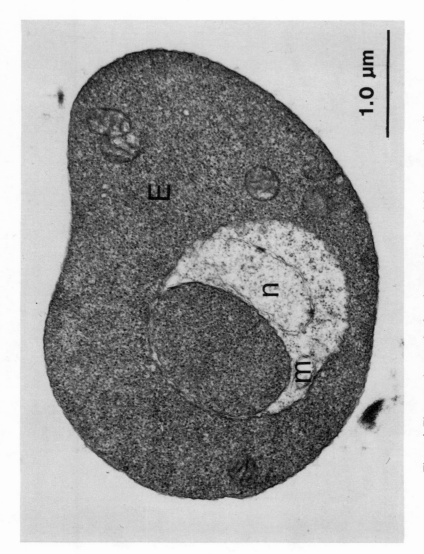

Figure 4. Electronmicrograph of erythrocyte infected with immature "ring" stage of *P. knowlesi*. These cells are not agglutinated in the SICA test. E = erythrocyte, n = nucleus, m = mitochondrion.

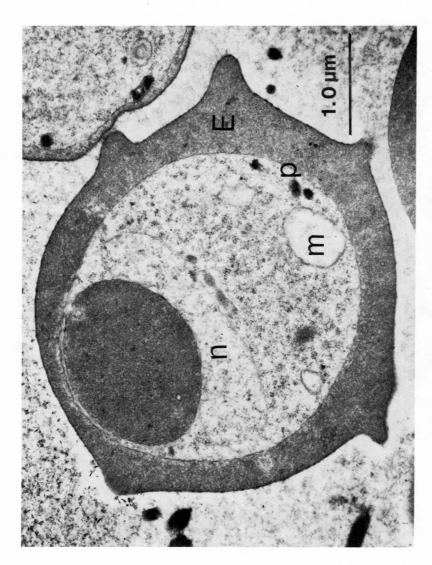

Figure 5. Electronmicrograph of erythrocyte infected with trophozoite of *P. knowlesi.* These cells are not usually agglutinated in the SICA test. E = erythrocyte, n = nucleus, m = mitochondrion, p = pigment.

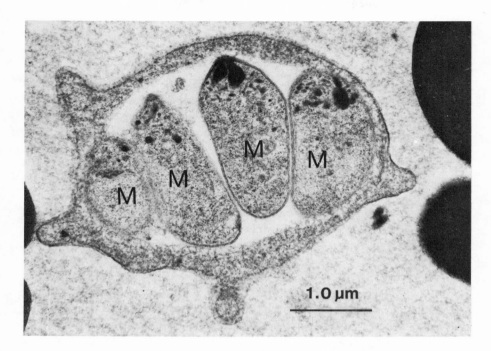

Figure 6. Electronmicrograph of erythrocyte infected with schizont of *P. knowlesi*. These cells are agglutinated in the SICA test. M = merozoite.

There is an apparent paradox in the phenomenon of red cell invasion. Erythrocytic infections are nearly always chronic, with erythrocyte invasion continuing over many months in the presence of antiplasmodial antibody. Furthermore, rhesus monkeys subjected to prolonged immunization with preparations of schizont-infected cells or merozoites of one variant type of *P. knowlesi* in Freund's complete adjuvant (FCA) still develop a parasitemia on challenge with another antigenic variant of the same strain. These observations strongly imply that the merozoite surface coat is a variable antigen, since, if antigenicity were constant, the antimerozoite antibodies could be expected to block red cell invasion and thus preclude chronic infection. *In vitro*, at least, antibodies that do combine with the surface coat inhibit red cell penetration (Miller et al. 1975), but the variant-specificity of this response has yet to be studied.

On the other hand, if the surface coat is a variable antigen, it presumably has some exposed region that is common to all variants and that serves as a recognition site for the red cell receptor. One can only suppose that this putative recognition site does not stimulate an antibody response specific for itself or, if it does, the antibodies produced are of such low avidity that, although possibly detectable *in vitro* (Butcher & Cohen 1972), *in vivo* they can be readily displaced by red cell receptor molecules.

VARIANT-SPECIFIC ANTIBODY SYNTHESIS AND
PROTECTIVE IMMUNITY

From the work outlined above, it is evident that there are at least two types of variant-specific antibody responses: agglutinating and opsonizing. Agglutination, detected by the SICA test, correlates with induction of antigenic variation; the opsonizing test (OT), also involving schizont-infected cells, correlates with parasite destruction (Brown et al. 1970b; Brown 1971; Brown & Hills 1974).

These responses appear qualitatively different, although the difference has not been analyzed in detail. Whether the difference is due to antibody class, affinity, or some other characteristic is not known. Clearly, the relative rate at which these two types of antibody are synthesized in response to the presence in the blood of a particular antigenic variant will determine the number of parasites in that variant population which will survive and give rise to alternative antigenic variants.

In most malaria infections, if the host survives the initial phase of high parasitemias, the infection is normally reduced to a relatively low, although fluctuating, level. In *P. knowlesi* in rhesus monkeys, induction of protective immunity is a particularly prolonged process, which makes this a very useful model for studying changes in the rate of synthesis of variant-specific SICA and opsonizing antibodies in relation to control of the parasitemia. It has been shown (Brown & Hills 1974) that in the initial phase, when parasitemias are high and must be controlled by antimalarial drugs, the synthesis of SICA antibodies (which correlates with the variation-inducing element in the total antibody response) precedes the synthesis of opsonizing antibodies. Later, when the infection is maintained at a relatively low level, both types of antibody respond to new variants more quickly, and variant-specific opsonizing and SICA antibodies are synthesized simultaneously (Figure 7). Presumably, when this stage is reached fewer parasites of each antigenic type survive, and subsequent variants stimulate rapid and effective specific antibody response.

LYMPHOCYTE SUBPOPULATIONS AND IMMUNITY
TRANSCENDING ANTIGENIC VARIATION

If a host survives the initial phase of high parasitemia, then despite continuous antigenic variation by the parasite, the infection is mostly restricted to subclinical levels. From the evidence outlined above, this change reflects an increased rate of protective antibody response to new variants. Presumably, each variant population initiates expansion of B-cell clones specific for itself.

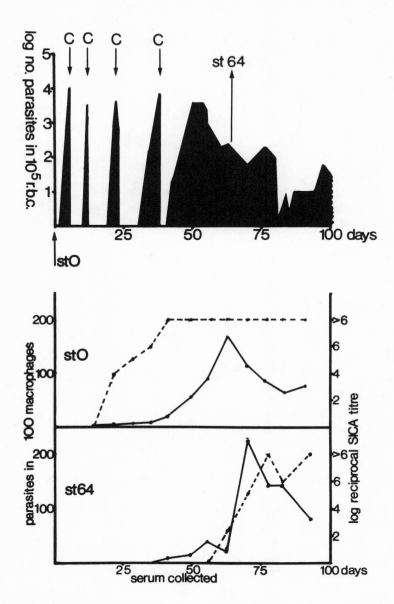

Figure 7. Schizont-infected red cell agglutination test (SICA) and opsonizing test (OT) response in rhesus monkey to stabilate st0, used to infect on day 0, and stabilate st64, isolated on day 64. C = parasitemia controlled with subcurative chloroquine therapy, (-------) = SICA response, (————) = OT response. (From Brown & Hills 1974.)

T cells play a key role in the development of protective immunity to malaria. Animals depleted of T cells (either before infection or during the chronic phase) are unable to control parasite numbers satisfactorily (Brown et al. 1968; Stechschulte 1969; Brown 1971). Analysis of the evidence indicates that the role of T cells is that of "helper" in variant-specific antibody synthesis (Brown 1971, 1974).

It is possible that T cells respond to antigenic determinants common to all variable antigens, and that once sensitized by the initial parasitemias, splenic T cells are helpers in the synthesis by B cells of antibodies specific to later antigenic variants. These responses to antigenic variants not previously experienced by the host would thus have the features of a secondary antibody response. That is, they would be rapid, predominantly IgG rather than IgM, and mostly high-affinity antibody. An underlying assumption of this interpretation is that the features recognized by T cells, while common to all variants, are not normally available as antibody binding sites, perhaps only becoming exposed after the death of the parasite. If they were available for antibody binding, then non-variant-specific antibodies would presumably neutralize the parasites and eliminate the infection.

The role of T cells in protective immunity has been explored using rodent malarias. Protective immunity that restricts the parasite to low-level chronic infections can be transferred from chronically infected rats to nonimmune recipients using spleen cells (Stechschulte 1969; Phillips 1970) (Figure 8), or by a subpopulation of lymphocytes which are presumably T cells, since they lack surface immunoglobulins (Brown et al. 1976) (Figures 9 and 10). A satisfactory positive marker for rat spleen T cells was not available for these experiments. These cells are detectable quite early in the infection but the transferred immunity is more effective after prolonged infection (Figure 9). This is presumably due to an increase in the number of sensitized T cells in the total spleen cell population and/or an increase in T-cell affinity.

One difficulty in these experiments is that no simple serologic tests have been developed to detect antigenic variation in rodent malarias. Thus, the role of transferred T cells in these systems has not yet been related to the rate of antibody response to particular antigenic variants.

Although the presence of T cells is crucial for control of the parasitemia, B-cell memory is undoubtedly important in the longer term. When the donors are rats that have suffered and finally cleared a chronic *P. berghei* infection, comparisons of transferred T cells with equivalent numbers of unfractionated spleen cells have shown that the T-plus-B cells are even more effective than T cells alone.

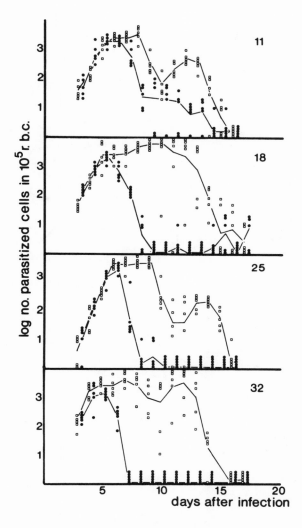

Figure 8. Transfer to nonimmune recipients of unfractionated spleen cells from rats infected
with *P. berghei* for varying periods. Spleens were transferred at a ratio of 1:1, donor:recipient.
Recipients were challenged with 10^6 *P. berghei*-infected erythrocytes. ● = spleen
cell recipients, □ = controls. Solid line indicates geometric mean of
parasitemia in each group. Numbers (11,18,25,32) indicate length
of time, in days, of infection in spleen donors. Infective inoculum
of donors and recipients was 10^6 parasitized cells.

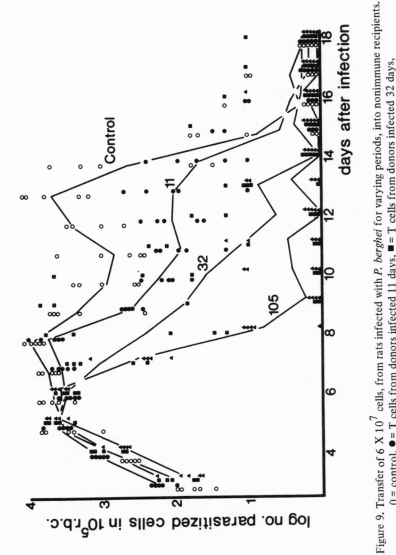

Figure 9. Transfer of 6×10^7 cells, from rats infected with *P. berghei* for varying periods, into nonimmune recipients. 0 = control, ● = T cells from donors infected 11 days, ■ = T cells from donors infected 32 days, ▲ = T cells from donors infected 105 days. Donors and recipients were infected with 10^6 parasitized cells. Solid lines indicate geometric mean of parasitemia in each group. Numbers indicate length of infection in cell donor in days.

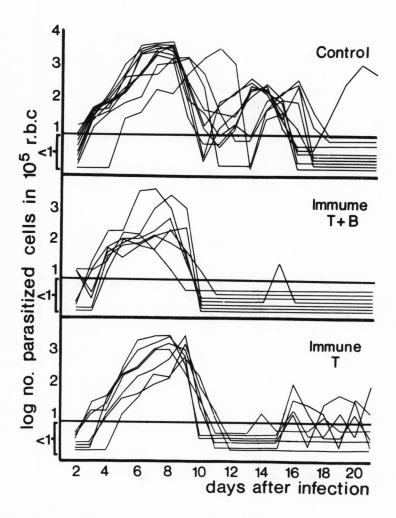

Figure 10. Parasitemia in rats receiving 4 X 10[6] immune T cells, 5 X 10[6] unfractionated immune spleen cells (T and B), or normal spleen cells (donor:recipient ratio 1:1 [control]), as neonates and challenged with 10[6] *P. berghei*-infected erythrocytes 56 days later. Donor rats have cleared their original chronic infections by day 213 and a subsequent reinfection by day 225. Cells collected on day 242.

Under the conditions of these experiments, in which 4 X 10^6 cells were transferred to neonatal rats which were then challenged 8 weeks later, T-cell recipients controlled the parasitemia very effectively compared to controls. However, their subsequent parasitemias tended to be higher than in recipients of T and B cells (Figure 10). All recipients developed a chronic infection. These experiments suggest that B-cell memory of the variants experienced by the donors may affect the multiplication of the antigenic variants that appear in the recipients.

Using another rodent malaria (*P. chabaudi*) in mice, McDonald & Phillips (1975) have confirmed the effect of transferred T cells and obtained evidence, by transfer into irradiated recipients (an experiment which cannot be carried out in the *P. berghei* system), that T cells function as helpers in antibody synthesis. Nevertheless, the problem remains of relating these findings to the rates of synthesis and biological properties of variant-specific antibodies.

GAMETOCYTES, ANTIGENIC VARIATION, AND PROTECTION

Although Hawking et al. (1966) produced circumstantial evidence that antigenic variation may occur in gametocytes as well as in asexual blood stages, this possibility has not been explored. Thus, how far the considerations discussed above apply to the gametocyte production and transmission of the infection has simply not been studied. The strains used are poor producers of gametocytes, and although gametogenesis is related to number of asexual parasites, the relationship is not necessarily direct.

ANTIGENIC VARIATION AND IMMUNIZATION
AGAINST MALARIA

Artificial immunization against particular strains of malaria parasites is relatively easy to achieve under laboratory conditions with certain parasite-host combinations. Infection and cure, and immunization with irradiated erythrocytic parasites or dead antigen (Corradetti 1974) can be used. Challenge infection usually produces a subclinical chronic infection with presumed continuance of antigenic variation, although immunization with attenuated strains can produce a sterile immunity (Weiss 1968).

With *P. knowlesi* in the rhesus monkey (an unnatural host that is very slow to develop appreciable immunity even when infected) artificial immunization has been reported only when the parasite material used was incorporated in

FCA or FIA along with Bacillus Calmette-Guerin (BCG) or high doses of poly A: poly U (Freund et al. 1945; Targett & Fulton 1965; Brown et al. 1970a; Mitchell et al. 1974; Brown & Tanaka 1975). The antigen used has been either schizont-infected erythrocytes or a merozoite preparation. Even after prolonged immunization, these animals are more susceptible to infection with an antigenic variant different from that used to immunize than with homologous variants, indicating that non-variant-specific immunity is difficult to obtain even by these draconian methods of immunization. But to add further confusion to the situation, after the initial challenge infection (which is often cleared completely from the circulation) these animals become refractory not only to other variants of the same strain, but also to other strains of *P. knowlesi* (Brown et al. 1970a; Mitchell et al. 1974). This is in marked contrast to immunity following chronic infection, which is almost entirely strain-specific.

The nature of this response is obscure but it is apparently only effective against *P. knowlesi* and not against other species of *Plasmodium*. Obviously, these observations require urgent investigation. There appear to be three levels of protective response. The first, variant-specific, either totally destroys or appreciably reduces in number parasites of a homologous variant. The second effect is an enhanced response to any heterologous intrastrain variants that might multiply in the blood. These two responses are also characteristic of animals immunized by infection. The third response to immunization with FCA produces complete clearance of the parasite and protection against other strains of the same species. The mechanism of this reaction is obscure, but the possibility that it has an autoimmune component must be considered. The requirement for FCA, and its somewhat labile nature, with later challenge sometimes giving rise to chronic subpatent infections rather than sterile immunity, suggests an autoimmune response. The argument that this protection is species-specific, and therefore cannot be autoimmune, is not necessarily valid. Antibodies produced against an unusual configuration resulting from parasite antigen on the membrane of schizont-infected cells, or from binding of merozoite surface-coat protein with erythrocyte membrane contaminants in the preparation (perhaps equivalent to the interaction between the merozoite recognition site and the red cell receptor), might have the effect of lysing schizont-infected cells or red cells that are in the process of being penetrated by a merozoite. Such antibodies, because they recognize, in part, red-cell membrane determinants, could have autoimmune characteristics, and may occur in noticeable amounts only when the parasite-erythrocyte antigenic complexes are present in the circulation.

CONCLUSION

Antigenic variation is of paramount importance in any consideration of protective immunity to protozoan parasites. Clearly, many hosts can produce a protective response that transcends variation to some extent, thus controlling parasite numbers, but the infection is rarely eliminated in the first few weeks. Studies on *P. knowlesi* indicate that changes in the rate of protective variant-specific antibody responses are responsible for this wider, although incomplete, immunity, which is usually specific for a given strain and its variants.

Studies on rodent malarias have demonstrated that T cells play a crucial role in this response. These cells are presumed to respond to a feature common to all variant-specific antigen molecules of a given strain, features possibly not exposed as antibody-combining sites on the live parasite but perhaps made available to the host immune system after release from the parasite. Thus, resistance to malaria parasites, and possibly other protozoan parasites capable of antigenic variation, will depend in large measure on effective recognition by T cells of common determinants on variant-specific molecules. Since immune recognition by T cells and histocompatibility type seem to be linked, the relationship of tissue type to susceptibility to infection with various strains and species of protozoa should be explored. Immunization with parasite antigen in FCA and subsequent infection leads to development of a protective immunity effective against strains of *P. knowlesi* and their variants. This is an encouraging sign that very effective protection, cutting across variant and strain differences, may be possible even in very susceptible hosts. Characterization of the antigens, both variable and constant, involved in protective immunity is urgently required.

BIBLIOGRAPHY

Briggs, N.T. & Wellde, B.T. 1969. Some characteristics of *Plasmodium berghei* "relapsing" in immunized mice. *Mil. Med.* 134: 1243-1248.

Brown, I.N., Brown, K.N. & Hills, L.A. 1968. Immunity to malaria: the antibody response to antigenic variation by *Plasmodium knowlesi. Immunology* 14: 127-138.

Brown, K.N. 1971. Protective immunity to malaria parasites: a model for the survival of cells in an immunological hostile environment. *Nature* (Lond.) 230: 163-167.

Brown, K.N. 1973. Antibody induced variation in malaria parasites. *Nature* (Lond.) 242: 49-50.

Brown, K.N. 1974. Antigenic variation and immunity to malaria. *In* Parasites in the Immunized Host: Mechanisms of Survival. Ciba Foundation Symposium 25 (new series. Porter, R. & Knight, J., Eds.: 35-51. Associated Scientific Publishers. Amsterdam, The Netherlands.

Brown, K.N. & Brown, I.N. 1965. Immunity to malaria: antigenic variation in chronic infections of *Plasmodium knowlesi. Nature* (Lond.) 208: 1286-1288.

Brown, K.N., Brown, I.N. & Hills, L.A. 1970a. Immunity to malaria. I. Protection against *Plasmodium knowlesi* shown by monkeys sensitized with drug-suppressed infections or by dead parasites in Freund's adjuvant. *Exp. Parasitol.* 28: 304-317.

Brown, K.N., Brown, I.N., Trigg, P.I., Phillips, R.S. & Hills, L.A. 1970b. Immunity to malaria. II. Serological response of monkeys sensitized by drug-suppressed infections or by dead parasitized cells in Freund's complete adjuvant. *Exp. Parasitol.* 28: 318-338.

Brown, K.N. & Hills, L.A. 1974. Antigenic variation and immunity to *Plasmodium knowlesi:* antibodies which induce antigenic variation and antibodies which destroy parasites. *Trans. R. Soc. Trop. Med. Hyg.* 68: 139-142.

Brown, K.N., Jarra, W. & Hills, L.A. 1976. T cells and protective immunity to *Plasmodium berghei* in rats. *Infec. Immun.* 14: 858-871.

Brown, K.N. & Tanaka, A. 1975. Vaccination against *Plasmodium knowlesi* malaria. *Trans. R. Soc. Trop. Med. Hyg.* 69: 350-353.

Butcher, G.A. & Cohen, S. 1972. Antigenic variation and protective immunity in *Plasmodium knowlesi* malaria. *Immunology* 23: 503-521.

Butcher, G.A., Mitchell, G.H. & Cohen, S. 1973. Letter: Mechanism of host specificity in malaria infection. *Nature* (Lond.) 244: 40-41.

Corradetti, A. 1974. Prospect of vaccination in human malaria. *In* Proceedings of the Symposium on Malaria Research. Rabat, Morocco, 287. World Health Organization, Geneva, Switzerland.

Cox, H.W. 1959. A study of relapse *Plasmodium berghei* infections isolated from white mice. *J. Immunol.* 82: 209-214.

Cross, G.A.M. 1975. Identification, purification and properties of clone-specific glycoprotein antigens constituting the surface coat of *Trypanosoma brucei. Parasitology* 71: 393-417.

Dennis, E.D., Mitchell, G.H., Butcher, G.A. & Cohen, S. 1975. *In vitro* isolation of *Plasmodium knowlesi* merozoites using polycarbonate sieves. *Parasitology* 71: 475-481.

Eaton, M.D. 1938. The agglutination of *Plasmodium knowlesi* by immune serum. *J. Exp. Med.* 67: 857-870.

Freund, J., Thomson, K.J., Sommer, H.E., Walter, A.W. & Pisani, T.M. 1945. Immunization of monkeys against malaria by means of killed parasites with adjuvants. *Am. J. Trop. Med.* 28: 1-22.

Hawking, F., Worms, M.J., Gammage, K. & Goddard, P.A. 1966. The biological purpose of the blood-cycle of the malaria parasite *Plasmodium cynomolgi. Lancet* 2: 422-424.

McDonald, V. & Phillips, R.S. 1975. Immunity to *Plasmodium vinckei chabaudi* in mice: attempts to understand the role of different lymphoid cell types. *J. Protozool.* 22: 54A.

McGhee, R.B. 1953. The infection by *Plasmodium lophurae* of duck erythrocytes in the chicken embryo. *J. Exp. Med.* 97: 773-782.

Miller, L.H., Dvorak, J.A., Shiroishi, T. & Durocher, J.R. 1973. Influence of erythrocyte membrane components on malaria merozoite invasion. *J. Exp. Med.* 138: 1597-1601.

Miller, L.H., Aikawa, M. & Dvorak, J.A. 1975. Malaria (*Plasmodium knowlesi*) merozoites: immunity and the surface coat. *J. Immunol.* 114: 1237-1242.

Mitchell, G.H., Butcher, G.A. & Cohen, S. 1973. Isolation of blood-stage merozoites from *Plasmodium knowlesi* malaria. *Int. J. Parasitol.* 3: 443-445.

Mitchell, G.H., Butcher, G.A. & Cohen, S. 1974. A merozoite vaccine effective against *Plasmodium knowlesi* malaria. *Nature* (Lond.) 252: 311-313.

Phillips, R.S. 1970. *Plasmodium berghei:* passive transfer of immunity by antisera and cells. *Exp. Parasitol.* 27: 479-495.

Stechschulte, D.J. 1969. *Plasmodium berghei* infection in thymectomized rats. *Proc. Soc. Exp. Biol. Med.* 131: 748-752.

Taliaferro, W.H. & Cannon, P.R. 1936. The cellular reactions during primary infections and superinfections of *Plasmodium brasilianuum* in Panamanian monkeys. *J. Infect. Dis.* 59: 72-125.

Taliaferro, W.H. & Mulligan, A.W. 1937. The histopathology of malaria with special reference to the function and origin of the macrophages in defence. *Indian Med. Res. Mem.* 29: 138.

Targett, G.A., & Fulton, J.D. 1965. Immunization of rhesus monkeys against *Plasmodium knowlesi* malaria. *Exp. Parasitol.* 17: 180-193.

Trager, W. & Jensen, J.B. 1976. Human malaria parasites in continuous culture. *Science* 193: 673-675.

Trigg, P.I. & Shapespeare, P.G. 1975. Factors affecting the invasion of erythrocytes by *Plasmodium knowlesi in vitro. J. Protozool.* 22: 57A.

Voller, A. & Rossan, R.N. 1969a. Immunological studies on simian malaria. III. Immunity to challenge and antigenic variation in *P. knowlesi. Trans. R. Soc. Trop. Med. Hyg.* 63: 507-523.

Voller, A. & Rossan, R.N. 1969b. Immunological studies with simian malarias. I. Antigenic variants of *Plasmodium cynomolgi bastianelli. Trans. R. Soc. Trop. Med. Hyg.* 63: 46-56.

Weiss, M.L. 1968. Active immunization of mice against *Plasmodium berghei.* Cross-resistance to a recently isolated strain. *Am. J. Trop. Med. Hyg.* 17: 516-521.

2

ANTIGENIC VARIATION IN *BABESIA*

John J. Doyle*

*World Health Organization Immunology
Research and Training Center
CH-1011 Lausanne, Switzerland*

As babesiosis has been the subject of several recent reviews (Mahoney 1972; Riek 1968; Ristic 1970) and is the subject of another chapter in this volume (Callow, Chapter 8), I will only briefly present the evidence now available to show that antigenic variation also occurs in this disease. Parasites of the genus *Babesia,* intraerythrocytic parasites in the mammalian host, are transmitted by ixodid ticks. They represent a widespread problem in domestic animal husbandry, causing a disease characterized by erythrocyte destruction with anemia, jaundice, and hemoglobinemia. The patterns of morbidity and mortality depend on the conditions under which the animals are maintained.

Cattle infested with *Babesia* spp. commonly have a long period of subclinical infection either after recovery from the clinical disease or following their infection as passively protected calves. Cyclical variations in the level of detectable parasitemia can be observed during these chronic infections.

Curnow (1973) used a parasitized erythrocyte agglutination test in a series of experiments with chronic *Babesia argentina* infections in calves to study both the possibility of the occurrence of antigenic variation and the effect of tick transmission on the antigenic type of the parasite. It was found that parasites isolated from the relapsing peaks of parasitemia were in fact antigenically distinct, six different relapse populations being isolated over 180 days of infection of a calf originally infected with a single strain. When these relapse populations were transmitted by ticks there was a reversion to a common antigenic type.

*Present address: International Laboratory for Research on Animal Diseases, P.O. Box 30709, Nairobi, Kenya.

There was, however, little antigenic similarity between the common antigenic types obtained by tick transmission of relapse populations of different strains. Phillips (1971) also demonstrated the occurrence of antigenic variation in chronic rodent infections with *B. rhodaini*. Antigenic differences between relapse populations were demonstrated by cross-protection tests following vaccination with irradiated parasites.

The relevance of antigenic variation in *Babesia* spp. to the acquisition of a protective immunity in infected animals is at present uncertain, and little is known about the antigens involved in this phenomenon apart from the fact that they are displayed on the surface of the parasitized erythrocytes. It is interesting to note, however, that on transmission through the insect vector there is reversion of the antigenically distinct relapse populations of a strain to a common antigenic type in a manner similar to that described for salivarian trypanosomes. This reversion to what is recognized by the host's immune response as a common antigen occurs at the time when the parasite changes from multiplication in the insect environment, i.e., salivary gland cells, to multiplication in the mammalian environment, i.e., erythrocytes. Again, as in the case of the trypanosomes, one wonders about a possible relationship between function and antigenicity.

The phenomenon of antigenic variation, originally described in African trypanosomiasis, has now been described in malaria and babesiosis, and further investigations may detect its occurrence in other chronic protozoal diseases such as anaplasmosis and Chagas' disease. It would appear that the ability to undergo what is recognized by the host as antigenic variation has evolved in these parasites through the need to establish the chronic infections necessary for the parasite's ultimate survival.

We have now gone some little way in trying to elucidate the mechanisms by which this process occurs at the level of the individual parasite but unfortunately, with the exception of malaria, we have very little idea of the means by which some hosts eventually develop a protective immunity to these parasites. It will be important in the future, therefore, to try to discover the parasite antigens which in each disease eventually induce a protective immunity, and to delineate the relationship of these antigens to the antigens responsible for antigenic variation. It is not inevitable that they should be the same antigens.

The relevance of the phenomenon of antigenic variation to the pathogenesis, epidemiology, and immunity of these diseases should preferably, therefore, be clearly defined when considering possible approaches to their immunologic control. In some cases it may be of fundamental importance, in others it may be possible to circumvent it.

BIBLIOGRAPHY

Curnow, J.A. 1973. Studies on antigenic changes and strain differences in *Babesia argentina* infections. *Aust. Vet. J.* 49: 279-283.

Mahoney, D.F. 1972. Immune response to hemoprotozoa. II. *Babesia* spp. *In* Immunity to Animal Parasites. Soulby, E.J.L., Ed.: 301-341. Academic Press, Inc. New York, N.Y.

Phillips, R.S. 1971. Antigenic variation in *Babesia rodhani* demonstrated by immunization with irradiated parasites. *Parasitol.* 63: 315-322.

Riek, R.F. 1968, Babesiosis. *In* Infectious Blood Diseases of Man and Animals, Vol. 2. Weinman, D. & Ristic, M., Eds.: 219-268. Academic Press, Inc. New York, N.Y.

Ristic, M. 1970. Babesiosis and Theileriosis. *In* Immunity to Parasitic Animals, Vol. 2. Jackson, G.J., Herman, R., & Singer, I., Eds.: 831-780. Appleton-Century-Crofts, New York, N.Y.

3

ANTIGENIC VARIATION IN THE SALIVARIAN TRYPANOSOMES

John J. Doyle*

*World Health Organization Immunology
Research and Training Center
CH-1011 Lausanne, Switzerland*

ANTIGENIC VARIATION IN THE HEMOPROTOZOA

The term "antigenic variation" has been widely used to describe a phenomenon in which, during infection of the final host by what is taxonomically considered a single species of pathogenic protozoa, there arises a succession of parasite populations, each recognized as antigenically different by the host's immune response. This results in the formation of antibodies, specific for each population, which are demonstrable by tests recognizing surface antigens of the parasite or parasitized cell such as agglutination and lysis.

The ability to undergo antigenic variation during the course of infection is best recognized in members of the genus *Trypanosoma,* especially the salivarian trypanosomes, etiological agents of sleeping sickness in man and animals. Certain mechanically transmitted species of trypanosomes such as *Trypanosoma equiperdum,* responsible for the disease dourine in horses and donkeys, also show antigenic variation. The evidence, however, for a similar phenomenon in the stercorarian trypanosomes as exemplified by *Trypanosoma cruzi,* causative agent of Chagas' disease, is still equivocal. Antigenic variation has also been described as occurring during infection with members of at least two other genera, *Plasmodium* and *Babesia.* In the genus *Plasmodium,* antigenic variation has been detected during infection with *Plasmodium berghei, Plasmodium knowlesi,* and *Plasmodium cynomologi.* In the genus *Babesia,* the phenomenon occurs during infection with *Babesia rhodhaini* and *Babesia argentina.*

The life cycles of the hemoprotozoa are highly complex, often including both a final and intermediate host, where in both hosts the parasite undergoes a series of complex morphological and physiological changes to ensure its successful further transmission. As of yet it is not clear whether the process of antigenic

*Present address: International Laboratory for Research on Animal Diseases, P.O. Box 30709, Nairobi, Kenya.

variation represents solely the loss and acquisition of antigenically different molecules on the surface of the parasite or parasitized cell or whether parasite populations recognized as antigenically different by the host also differ in other physiological and biochemical parameters that ensure their survival and eventual transmission from host to host.

The fact remains that the ability to undergo antigenic variation apparently confers on these parasites a remarkable advantage in ensuring their survival in and transmission from an immunocompetent host. The establishment of chronic infections in the final host favors the efficient onward transmission of the parasite to the intermediate host, so completing the parasite cycle. Indeed it is noticeable that both *Trypanosoma rhodesiense* and *Trypanosoma simiae,* which cause an acute and peracute disease in man and the domestic pig, respectively, both infect wild animals where the disease runs a chronic course and thereby facilitates parasite transmission and hence parasite survival.

This paper will briefly review the current knowledge of the phenomenon of antigenic variation in the genera *Trypanosoma* and *Babesia* with special reference to the possible mechanisms involved, the role of insect vectors, and the relevance of antigenic variation to the possible control of disease by immunologic means.

The greater part of this review will be concerned with antigenic variation in the salivarian trypanosomes, as they represent major pathogens of man and animals and a great deal of literature has accumulated on this subject. Antigenic variation in *Plasmodium* and *Babesia* will be reviewed in two other papers in this volume.

ANTIGENIC VARIATION IN THE SALIVARIAN TRYPANOSOMES

Introduction

Antigenic variation in salivarian trypanosomes has been the subject of several recent reviews (de Raadt 1974; Desowitz 1970; Lumsden 1972a; Seed 1974; Vickerman 1971, 1974). It is not intended in this contribution to repeat the ground covered in previous reviews but rather to present their overall findings and discuss where appropriate the major papers cited in these reviews with respect to new information which has since appeared. The effect of cyclical transmission (where a large amount of new information has recently appeared) will be the subject of a more detailed review.

The species of salivarian trypanosome to be considered are those causing sleeping sickness in man and animals (n'gana). These are *Trypanosoma (Trypanozoon) brucei, Trypanosoma (Trypanozoon) gambiense, Trypanosoma (Trypanozoon) rhodesiense, Trypanosoma (Nannomonas) congolense,* and *Trypanosoma*

(Duttonella) vivax. Trypanosoma gambiense and *Trypanosoma rhodesiense* are human pathogens, the remainder are solely animal pathogens.

Life Cycle

The life cycle of these trypanosomes is indirect, with a member of the genus *Glossina* as the intermediate host. *Trypanosoma brucei, Trypanosoma gambiense,* and *Trypanosoma rhodesiense* ingested by the tsetse in a blood meal taken from an infected mammal develop initially in the fly midgut and then in the salivary glands where the cycle of development is completed by the appearance of meta-cyclic forms again infective for the mammalian host. After ingestion *Trypanosoma congolense* develops in the midgut and then in the mouth parts where metacyclic forms appear. *Trypanosoma vivax,* however, undergoes all of its developmental stages in the mouth parts of an infected fly. The period of development in the fly varies according to the external temperature and varies between 17 and 53 days for *Trypanosoma congolense* and the subgenus *Trypanozoon,* but is considerably shorter (5 to 13 days) in the case of *Trypanosoma vivax* (Hoare 1970). The parasite returns to the mammalian host with the injection of metacyclic forms during the feeding of an infected fly.

In the mammalian host, infection with *Trypanosoma brucei, Trypanosoma gambiense,* and *Trypanosoma rhodesiense* occurs predominately in the blood-stream and tissue spaces, whereas with *Trypanosoma congolense* and *Trypanosoma vivax* the infection appears to be confined solely to the vascular system (Losos & Ikede 1972). In the final host, the infection is characterized by a relapsing parasitemia which continues to the death or recovery of the host. The interval between parasitemic peaks varies both with the species of parasite and the host but is, in general, only several days. Each new wave of parasites is recognized by the immune system of the host as being antigenically different, hence the phenomenon of "antigenic variation."

In the case of infection with members of the subgenus *Trypanozoon,* the parasites also undergo complex morphological and physiological changes during the course of each wave of parasitemia. In the initial rising phase of the parasi-temia, the trypanosomes have a long slender appearance, whereas in the descend-ing phase they have a shorter, more stumpy appearance. This morphological change is accompanied by an increase in size of the trypanosome mitochondrium and changes in respiratory metabolism which appear to facilitate the establish-ment of an infection in the fly by this form of the parasite (Boehringer & Hecker 1974a; Boehringer & Hecker 1974b; Bowman 1974; Brown et al. 1973; Vickerman 1965, 1970, 1971, 1974a). These stumpy forms appear, however, to be capable of only limited further development in the mammalian host, since parasites taken from a descending parasitemia have a greatly reduced infectivity for a new mammalian host (Ashcroft 1960; Balber 1972; Luckins 1972; Wijers 1959). The parasite appears, therefore, to have developed a mechanism which both ensures its further transmission to the intermediate host and establishes a chronic infection in the mammalian host by limiting the numbers in each parasitemia (Ormerod et al. 1974). In the case of *Trypanosoma congolense* and *Trypanosoma vivax,* little is known about their morphological and biochemical changes except that bloodstream forms of both species appear to resemble the stumpy forms of *Trypanosoma brucei* in their respiratory physiology (Vickerman 1971).

Antibodies to each population can be detected in the serum shortly after the disappearance of the variant population. In view of the fact that the levels of peak parasitemia are higher in immunosuppressed animals (Balber 1974; Otieno 1973; Ormerod et al 1974; Doyle, unpublished results), it is probable that antibodies are present during the latter part of a parasitemic wave and contribute to the elimination of the parasite. In the period of antigen excess, however, antibodies would not be detectable by the commonly used tests such as agglutination, which demonstrate only the presence of unbound antibodies.

An ultrastructural feature of salivarian trypanosomes relevant to the phenomenon of antigenic variation is the existence of an electron-dense layer or "coat" immediately external to the limiting trilaminar membrane. This surface coat is dense in the bloodstream forms of *Trypanosoma brucei, Trypanosoma rhodesiense,* and *Trypanosoma congolense* but less dense in the case of *Trypanosoma vivax* (Vickerman 1971, 1974a, 1974b; Wright & Hales 1970). Following ingestion by the fly, this surface coat is lost, only to reappear with the development of metacyclic forms (Steiger 1971; Vickerman 1969, 1971, 1974a, 1974b). In the case of *Trypanosoma vivax,* however, metacyclic forms do not appear to possess a surface coat (Vickerman 1974a; Vickerman & Evans 1974).

Several terms commonly used to describe certain types of trypanosome populations may be conveniently introduced at this point. A "strain" is a population derived from a wild population of organisms which has been maintained in the laboratory by passage, cyclical or noncyclical, in culture or laboratory animals (Lumsden 1972b). A "clone" is a population derived from a single organism which has been allowed to multiply in a series of laboratory animals. Cloned populations are usually obtained by injection of a single trypanosome into a laboratory animal with subsequent passage at 2- to 3-day intervals.

THE ANTIGENS OF SALIVARIAN TRYPANOSOMES

Variant Antigens

The fact that tests such as agglutination can distinguish between successive populations of bloodstream trypanosomes is presumptive evidence that the antigens responsible for these antigenic differences are located on the surface of the living parasite. This was confirmed when immunoelectron microscopy showed that labeled antivariant antibodies reacted with the surface coat of bloodstream trypanosomes (Fruit et al. 1974; Vickerman & Luckins 1969).

A considerable amount of work has been carried out to elucidate both the biochemical nature of these antigens and their relationship to the surface coat (Desowitz 1970; Seed 1974). It was shown initially that the variable antigens of *Trypanosoma brucei* were glycoprotein in nature with D-mannose, D-galactose and glucosamine as the major sugar components (Allsopp 1973; Allsopp & Njogu 1971, 1973, 1974; Allsopp et al. 1971; Njogu 1972, 1974; Njogu et al. 1974) and later that these glycoproteins were located on the external surface of the parasite (Njogu et al. 1974). More detailed information has now become available on the nature of these glycoproteins in cloned populations derived at weekly intervals from a rabbit infected with *Trypanosoma brucei*. It was shown that a characteristic predominant glycoprotein could be isolated from each clone and that this molecule was the major constituent of the parasite surface coat (Cross 1973, 1975). Each glycoprotein had a molecular weight of approximately 65,000 and consisted of about 600 amino acid residues and 20 monosaccharide residues. The sugars were again galactose, mannose, and glucosamine. Although these clone-specific glycoproteins had a similar molecular weight, they differed considerably in their isoelectric point (pI 8.19-6.46) and preliminary structural studies indicated that there were large differences in the amino acid sequences dispersed over more than one half of the polypeptide chain (Cross 1975; Cross & Johnson 1976). It has been proposed that the variant-specific surface antigen of *Trypanosoma brucei* may have a major and minor protein component (Allsopp 1973). This apparent discrepancy may be due, however, to enzymatic breakdown of the glycoprotein during preparation (Cross 1975; Cross & Johnson 1976). Immunization with purified clone-specific glycoproteins gave complete protection against challenge with the homologous but not heterologous clones and resulted in the formation of both precipitating and agglutinating antibodies.

A number of investigators have also tested the ability of parasite fractions obtained by various biochemical and physical means from bloodstream trypanosomes to induce protective immune responses in animals vaccinated with these fractions. It has been shown, for example, that a soluble fraction obtained by column chromatography from the supernatant of disrupted bloodstream forms of *Trypanosoma brucei* was strongly immunogenic and protected mice against challenge with the homologous variant but not against challenge with a heterologous variant or strain. Immunization gave rise to both agglutinating and precipitating antibodies. Immunodiffusion and electrophoresis showed the fraction to consist of at least four separate components (Lanham & Taylor 1972; Taylor & Lanham 1972). Seed, however, (see review 1972, 1974) has proposed that variant antigens are located on the surface of African trypanosomes but that separate antigens are responsible for the formation of protective and agglutinating antibodies. The species studied were *Trypanosoma gambiense, Trypanosoma rhodesiense,* and *Trypanosoma equiperdum.*

Van Meirvenne et al. (1973) have recently shown by immunoelectrophoresis that, of the 22 antigenic components found when the serum from rabbits hyperimmunized with lyophilized variant populations of *Trypanosoma brucei* was reacted with the soluble fraction of these preparations, only one component (V) was unique to each variant population. These antisera would, however, in the presence of complement lyse only their homologous population. The ability to precipitate the specific component V and cause immune lysis of the homologous population could not be removed by absorption with a heterologous variant population but was readily removed by absorption with the homologous population (Le Ray et al. 1973).

Antigens Other Than Variant-Specified

As would be expected these parasites contain many antigenic components apart from those responsible for the antigenic specificity of the variant bloodstream populations. Common antigens exist between different variant populations of the same strain, between different strains of the same species, and between different species (see reviews de Raadt 1974; Desowitz 1970; Seed 1974). Antibodies to these various common antigenic components have been detected by tests such as complement fixation and immunofluorescence using fixed trypanosomes as the antigen (see review de Raadt 1974). It has been postulated that the common antigens are internal constituents of the parasite, such as enzymes and nucleic acids, which are released following the death of the parasite (de Raadt 1974; Desowitz 1970; Seed 1974). There is as of yet no evidence for the existence in living bloodstream trypanosomes of common surface antigens between either variants of the same strain or species of parasite.

Antisera raised against lyophilized variant populations and culture forms of *Trypanosoma brucei* demonstrated the existence by immunoelectrophoresis of 21 common antigenic components in the soluble fractions of different variant populations of the same strain. Twenty of these antigens were also present in the soluble fraction of the culture form of this trypanosome (Van Meirvenne et al. 1973).

There is evidence that bloodstream forms of a rodent-adapted strain of *Trypanosoma vivax* and a laboratory strain of *Trypanosoma gambiense* have serum components of their laboratory animal host closely associated with the parasite surface coat. These host components are not antibodies as judged by their size, electrophoretic mobility, and occurrence in immunosuppressed animals (Ketteridge 1971, 1972; Seed 1974; Vickerman 1974b). The precise nature of these components, their relation to the parasite surface structures, and their relevance to parasite survival is not yet clear. Whether or not host components can be similarly demonstrated in bloodstream trypanosomes recovered from infections of their natural host by recently isolated strains of either of these species is also at present unknown.

Antigens and Protection

Antibodies to common antigens have not, as of yet, been clearly shown to play a part in protection of the host against either reinfection or continuation of an existing infection. The subject of vaccination against salivarian trypanosomes will be considered in Chapter 11 of this book. But with regard to the possible protective roles of variant-specific and common antigen-specific antibodies, one consistent fact has emerged from the experiments described in the literature. It appears that the protection induced by immunizing a host with bloodstream trypanosomes (living or attenuated), their metabolic products, or biochemical fractions is limited solely to challenge with the homologous population of trypanosomes whether it be a clone or a strain. No significant degree of protection has been demonstrated either against heterologous variants of the same strain or against heterologous strains of the same species (see reviews Desowitz 1970; Gray 1967; Lumsden 1970, 1972a; Seed 1974 and recent publications Cross 1975; Duxbury et al. 1972, 1973, 1974; Uilenberg & Giret 1973; Wellde et al. 1973, 1975).

Spectrum of Variant Types

The total number of variant types which can arise during the course of infection by a clone or strain of the pathogenic salivarian trypanosomes is at present unknown. The highest number so far recorded is 22 variants obtained by passage of a strain of *Trypanosoma gambiense* in mice (Osaki 1959). Variation was induced by treatment of infected mice with a suitable dose of human serum or a chemotherapeutic agent. The greatest number of variants which appeared before the death of a single infected mouse was seven and each was antigenically distinct. Indeed there is only one description in the literature of the occurrence of the same variant twice during the course of an experimental infection of a single animal (Wilson & Cunningham 1972). The appearance of an antigenic type which resembled that initiating the infection immediately preceded the disappearance of detectable trypanosomes from this animal and its recovery from the disease.

In a more general sense, however, if protection against infection in the field is mediated by antivariant-specific antibodies in a similar manner to the immunity induced in experimental animals, there may be a limit to the number of variants produced by a species in a given area (Wilson & Grainge 1967). In the case of cattle, animals can recover from infection and thereafter trypanosomes cannot be detected in their blood even though the animals are still exposed to challenge by infected flies. The ability to acquire a resistance to natural infections appears to require that cattle be born and maintained in an infected area (Desowitz 1959, 1970). It appears that cattle of N'dama bred together with the West African shorthorns are more resistant to the disease than are the humped Zebu cattle or imported European species (Desowitz 1959, 1970; Fiennes 1970). The importance of genetic background with regard to the ability to resist various pathogens has also been noted in other diseases of man and animals (Behin et al. 1975; Bradley 1974; McDevitt & Bodmer 1974).

Another possible indication of the existence of a finite number of antigenic variants was the demonstration of the occurrence of apparently the same antigenic type in two series of variant populations derived in laboratory animals from two strains of *Trypanosoma brucei* isolated 6 years apart in the same district of Uganda (Van Meirvenne et al. 1975b). The topic of the interrelationships of trypanosome populations isolated in a given locality will be discussed after consideration of the effect of cyclical transmission on the antigenic type of the metacyclic population.

CYCLICAL TRANSMISSION AND ANTIGENIC VARIATION

The information available with regard to the effect of cyclical transmission on antigenic variation and its relevance to the epidemiology of the disease will be considered separately for each of the subgenera.

Subgenus *Trypanozoon*

It was observed initially that there were extensive cross-reactions between the first trypanosome populations which arose in rats each infected with salivary gland material from tsetses infected originally with different variants of a strain of *Trypanosoma brucei*. While cross-reactions occurred in "cyclical substrains" derived from antigenically different variants of a given strain, there were no cross-reactions between "cyclical substrains" derived from different strains of *Trypanosoma brucei* (Broom & Brown 1940). The serologic test used to identify and differentiate variant populations was the red cell adhesion test where antisera to the variant and transmitted populations were tested for their ability to cause trypanosome adhesion to erythrocytes in infected blood (Fairbairn & Culwick 1946).

Gray (1965a) then studied the effect of cyclical transmission on the antigenic variant of a strain of *Trypanosoma brucei* and observed that the trypanosome populations transmitted by different tsetse flies possessed a common or "basic" antigen and that this antigen type was relatively stable during cyclical transmission, whereas other variant antigens tended to revert to the basic type during transmission. The basic antigen also appeared early in the course of a syringe-passaged infection of the other variant antigen types; hence, he termed the basic antigen the "predominant" antigenic type of the strain. These experiments were based on agglutination testing of trypanosome populations, derived from subpassage of the blood of infected animals into laboratory animals, against either serum derived from the infected animals or antisera raised against the passaged populations by infection of rabbits.

Cunningham (1966) isolated metacyclic forms from individual tsetse flies infected with *Trypanosoma rhodesiense* by allowing the flies to feed on blood through a membrane. The metacyclic forms were then preserved at low temperatures. Antisera to ten of these metacyclic stabilates was raised by infecting individual sheep with a different stabilate and bleeding 14 days later. These sera were then tested for their ability to prevent infection with the stored metacyclic stabilates. The results showed that metacyclic stabilates from all flies contained a similar antigenic type although some contained at least two types. Several stabilates from the same fly were all of the same type. Cross-reactions were not obtained with metacyclic stabilates of different strains of *Trypanosoma rhodesiense.*

The question of the range of antigenic diversity of a given species in a confined locality or in a country, and the relevance of the possible appearance of a basic antigen after cyclical transmission in limiting the antigenic heterogenicity has been approached in several ways. Some workers have studied the antigenic relationships of trypanosome populations isolated from infected mammals, while others have studied the antigenic character of the parasite populations isolated from infected flies.

Gray (1966a) used the agglutination test to study the effect of cyclical transmission of six clones of trypanosomes derived from six rodent-adapted strains of *Trypanosoma brucei* originally isolated from the same area in Nigeria. Using antisera taken from cyclically infected rabbits up to a month after their infection, he found that two clones possessed apparently similar basic antigens, and two other clones possessed different basic antigens but were taken to be related to the first two cloned populations, as antisera obtained from all four rabbits after 4 weeks of infection agglutinated the homologous and heterologous clones. The two remaining clones were unrelated to each other and to any of the other four clones ingested by the flies. Six strains of *Trypanosoma brucei* from different areas were compared by infecting rabbits with each strain and testing serum taken at intervals of up to one month after infection for its ability to agglutinate heterologous strains. This method was based on the premise that the predominant antigens of any strain occur early in a syringe-passaged infection (Gray 1965a). On this basis only two of the six strains tested had antigens in common.

In a further study using the same technique for isolation and maintenance of original isolates and the production of antiserum to basic and predominant antigens of strains of *Trypanosoma brucei,* Gray studied the antigenic relationships in 37 isolates of *Trypanosoma brucei* collected over an interval of 5 years from a herd of cattle kept in the same locality in Nigeria (Gray 1970). Four isolates collected in one year apparently belonged to the same strain, while a further 27 isolates collected 3 years later appeared to belong to three different strains. An isolate obtained in the first year of the experiment was closely related to four of the isolates obtained 2 years later but, in general, there was little demonstrable antigenic relationship between the trypanosomes isolated from year to year and at least seven distinct strains were identified in this 5-year period. It is interesting to note that in order to provide sufficient material for agglutination testing, adaptation to laboratory animals was required which took a mean time of 88 days and 15 passages.

Gray (1972) then studied the variant antigens of *Trypanosoma gambiense* isolates collected at different places in Nigeria. Again the isolates were rodent-adapted over 6 to 46 passages in nursling rats and then maintained in adult rats. Sufficient numbers of trypanosomes for agglutination testing were raised again in nursling rats. Of 122 samples obtained from sleeping sickness patients, 97 patent infections were established; prepatent periods varied from 6 to 79 days but 94% of infected animals became patent in less than 22 days. Antisera to predominant antigens were obtained from several bleedings over a period of 5 weeks from rabbits infected with the rodent-adapted strains. From 48 isolates Gray identified 19 serologically different populations which produced antibodies to at least seven common variant antigens. A further nine antigens were also widely distributed among the isolates from different areas. The remaining three antigens occurred only in isolates obtained from one limited area. Gray considered that all the isolates were representatives of a single strain of *Trypanosoma gambiense* on the basis of their ability to produce similar variant antigens but that the strain comprised two substrains, only one of which had the ability to produce the three variant types isolated from the same locality. On this occasion it was shown that sera from eight sleeping sickness patients in two areas of Nigeria and antisera raised in rabbits infected directly with lymph node biopsy material from infected patients would agglutinate some of the rodent-adapted variants of *Trypanosoma gambiense*. When three isolates of this strain of *Trypanosoma gambiense* (P.10 substrain A; M8; M10 substrain B) were cyclically transmitted to rabbits and monkeys, the first agglutinating antibodies detected in the sera of these animals all agglutinated one of the 19 original isolates (C2) of the strain (Gray 1975). Gray suggested that this isolate then represented the basic antigen of the strain. There was also a tendency for agglutinating antibodies to five of the original isolates to appear in a similar sequence during the course of infection of these six cyclically infected animals. Gray (1974) also found that antisera raised against rodent-adapted isolates from sleeping sickness patients in Senegal, Zaire, and Uganda cross-reacted with 8 to 12 of these 15 rodent-adapted isolates from Nigeria.

In another type of survey, Dar and his coworkers in East Africa compared the antigenic types of *Trypanosoma brucei* subgroup originally isolated from infected wild tsetse flies in four separate areas (Dar & Wilson 1973; Goedbloed et al. 1973). It would perhaps be useful at this point to give the definitions used by these workers to describe their various types of trypanosome populations and their antisera. "Metacyclic" trypanosomes were cryopreserved from macerated salivary gland material, "primary parasitemic" trypanosomes were harvested from animals after infection with "metacyclic" trypanosomes, and the "final parasitemic" trypanosomes were harvested at peak parasitemia after 3 to 14 three-day passages of metacyclic trypanosomes. Antiserum to each population was obtained by treating infected rats after an interval of 3 days and collecting serum 6 days later. The serologic test used with each population was primarily agglutination, supplemented on occasion by neutralization and immune lysis.

The investigators first established the relationship between the three populations—metacyclic, primary, and final—derived from a single isolate of *Trypanosoma brucei*. Each antiserum could neutralize the infectivity of each of the three parasite populations. When, however, antisera to the three populations derived from each of 13 isolates were tested by agglutination against the final antigen of these isolates, 5 of either the metacyclic or primary antisera failed to agglutinate their final population. The final populations of isolates collected in each area were then compared by testing by agglutination against all the final antisera of isolates in the area. In the first area five of ten final antigens and antisera exhibited some degree of cross-reactivity. In the second area, 4 of 13 final antigens and antisera cross-reacted, and while the 2 final antigens collected from the third area were unrelated, all 13 final antigens in the fourth area reacted with at least 2 of the final antisera.

The cross-reactivity between isolates obtained from the different areas were then studied by testing the final antigens of each area against the final antisera obtained from the other areas. In the first area, five of the final antigens cross-reacted with 6 of 13 antisera from the second area, two final antigens cross-reacted with sera from the third area, and in the fourth area only 1 of the 13 antisera cross-reacted with two antigens of the first area. In the second area, eight final antigens cross-reacted with six antisera from the first area and one antisera from the fourth area. The two final isolates from the third area did not cross-react with antisera from any other area, while two final antigens from the fourth area cross-reacted with two antisera from the first area and one apiece from the second and third areas.

It is perhaps rather surprising that the majority of cross-reactions obtained in all of these tests were, as the authors termed, "unilateral" in that an antiserum raised against a final antigen would agglutinate one or more other final antigens but that antisera raised against these cross-reacting antigens did not recognize the former antigen. The number of cross-reactions obtained would have been significantly increased if, as would have been expected, reciprocal agglutination took place.

The difficulties in carrying out this type of survey should be noted in that of 102 isolates obtained from infected flies only 38 could be eventually prepared in a form suitable for test, the remaining 64 being either not infective for laboratory rodents or lost in the process of antigen preparation. Of the 38 isolates, nine proved difficult to maintain in normal laboratory rodents and a regime of immunosuppression had to be carried out to try to obtain sufficient parasite numbers for test.

Subgenus *Nannomonas*

Wilson (1967) cyclically passaged two variant populations of a strain of *Trypanosoma congolense* through separate groups of *Glossina morsitans,* identified an infected fly in each group, and allowed each fly to feed artificially through a membrane into defibrinated bovine blood. Each pool of blood was then used to infect a group of four mice. Trypanosomes were first detected in the blood of infected mice 17 to 20 days after infection and these populations were stored as the first cyclical populations of the eight mice. Antiserum to each of the original populations and the cyclical populations was obtained by infection and treatment of rats. These sera were then tested for their ability to inhibit the infectivity of the various populations. It was found that all the cyclical populations were antigenically different from each of the original variants. The cyclical populations could be differentiated into three different antigenic types, but three populations were identical even though derived originally from different variant populations.

This possibility of reversion to a basic type on cyclical passage of variant populations of *Trypanosoma congolense* was further investigated by Uilenberg et al. (Uilenberg 1973, 1974; Uilenberg & Giret 1972). In their initial experiments they used a strain of *Trypanosoma congolense* (EATRO 325-I) which had been passaged 40 times through laboratory animals and 7 times cyclically in the 9 years since its original isolation. Six sheep were each cyclically infected by a population of *Glossina morsitans* which had ingested a variant of this strain. Six different variants were tested, one per sheep. Populations of trypanosomes were obtained from each sheep by subinoculation of blood into laboratory animals. The first positive infection in laboratory animals occurred with blood taken from the sheep 7 to 10 days after cyclical infection and these took 10 to 14 days to become patent, whereas trypanosome populations were readily obtained in 2 to 3 days in laboratory animals inoculated with blood taken after patency of the infection in the sheep, which occurred 13 to 17 days after their infection.

Serum was obtained from each sheep at intervals after infection and the sheep were treated 3 to 6 weeks after infection. When sera taken early in the infection were tested for their ability to inhibit the infectivity of the various trypanosome populations, it was found that the first populations—that is those obtained before patency—were antigenically similar and different from the variant populations ingested by the flies. The populations obtained at patency of the sheep infections were antigenically different, but sera taken later in the infection from each sheep recognized the variant types which subsequently appeared in the other sheep. In an attempt to repeat the findings of Wilson, metacyclic trypanosomes were obtained from the flies used to infect the sheep, by allowing feeding through a membrane and the infected blood then inoculated into mice. The first patent parasitemic populations in these mice were then tested against the sera obtained from the sheep, but no antigenic similarity could be demonstrated to the basic antigen which appeared in the sheep. The mice populations, however, were recognized by sera taken later in the sheep infections.

These experiments were then repeated using the same strain of *Trypanosoma congolense,* but on this occasion a sample which had remained cryopreserved since its original isolation (EATRO 325-II) and had not undergone extensive passage in the laboratory was used. On this occasion, however, cyclically transmitted variant populations did not appear to return to the same basic antigen as previously. The first populations of trypanosomes isolated from the second group of sheep by subinoculation into mice were not recognized by early antisera taken from the first group of sheep. They appeared to consist of four different types as recognized by sera taken from the first sheep later in the course of infection. An experiment of inoculation of mice with metacyclic types was also carried out with the modification that blood from these mice was subinoculated before patency. Trypanosome populations could be isolated 2 days before patency. These again did not carry the basic antigen recognized by early sera from the first group of sheep but appeared to resemble the types which succeeded the basic population in the original sheep.

It is interesting to note that these investigators isolated populations of trypanosomes from the lesion at the site of the fly bite which were antigenically different from the population isolated from the blood only 3 days previously.

Little information is available on the effect of cyclical transmission on the epidemiology of *Trypanosoma congolense* in the wild. One survey has been carried out to investigate the antigenic types of *Trypanosoma congolense* obtained from wild tsetse flies in four areas of East Africa (Wilson et al. 1973). Metacyclic forms isolated from wild flies were titrated for their infectivity in mice and bovines. The trypanosomes of the first patent parasitemia were termed primary populations and stored; the animals were then treated and serum obtained 7 days later. These sera were tested against seven primary populations; cross-reactions occurred with 11 of the antisera but these were limited to five of the seven primary populations. Two antisera recognized trypanosomes collected from different areas. Two similar primary populations were also isolated in different areas with an interval of 15 months between the isolations.

Again there were difficulties in obtaining sufficient material for test, since of 140 isolates obtained only 7 provided enough material for all tests. Only 24 isolates provided enough material for antiserum production and homologous tests, while the infectivity of the remainder (75%) was too low for any useful experimental work.

Subgenus *Duttonella*

Jones & Clarkson (1972a, 1972b) obtained variant populations at weekly intervals from a calf experimentally infected with a West African strain of *Trypanosoma vivax*. Five of these variant populations were then cyclically transmitted to sheep by *Glossina morsitans,* one variant population per sheep. The sheep were treated with dexamethosone until the appearance of trypanosomes in the blood, 10 to 14 days after transmission, when the infected blood was cryopreserved. An immune lysis technique was used to test the sera, taken from the sheep at weekly intervals after infection, directly against the preserved trypanosome populations in the presence of complement. The first populations isolated from two sheep were similar to the variants used to infect the flies, the four remaining first populations were similar to each other and different from any of the variant types isolated initially from the calf. The same workers later showed that, in a calf cyclically infected with the same strain of

Trypanosoma vivax, parasites could first be detected in the bloodstream 10 days after infection, but thereafter new variant populations succeeded each other at 2- to 3-day intervals (Jones & Clarkson 1974). They did not, however, describe the antigenic relationship of the variant population detected 10 days after transmission with the original strain used to infect the fly, but made the point that in *Trypanosoma vivax* infections in cattle, populations isolated more than 10 days after infection may be already different from those present at the time of infection.

This may be of relevance to the results of the only survey carried out to investigate the antigenic types of *Trypanosoma vivax* isolated from infected wild flies in two areas of East Africa (Dar et al. 1973). In this survey metacyclic trypanosomes from infected proboscides were used to infect cattle which were then treated 1 to 3 days after the first appearance of trypanosomes in the blood (6 to 33 days) and serum collected 7 days later. The first trypanosome populations to appear were stored as the primary parasitemic antigen and some of these were tested against the various antisera by immune lysis. Of the 107 primary populations obtained, only 23 provided sufficient trypanosomes for homologous and heterologous testing. When the 23 primary populations were tested against the 23 homologous antisera, some degree of cross-reactivity was obtained with each population reacting both with its homologous and one or more heterologous sera. The 23 populations were then tested against 50 other sera for which there were insufficient numbers in the primary population to allow testing. Twenty-one of these antisera showed some cross-reactivity with one or more of the 23 primary populations and 13 of the 23 primary populations cross-reacted with one or more of the antisera. Cross-reactions occurred both with isolates obtained from within each of the two areas and with isolates obtained from different areas. The investigators point out that the cross-reactions were mostly of a partial nature, where the test antigen evidently contained a mixture of antigenic types, some of which were not recognized by the cross-reacting serum.

Discussion

The effect of cyclical transmission on the antigenic character and epidemiology of the pathogenic salivarian trypanosomes has therefore been investigated in a variety of ways, with significant differences in experimental design, techniques, and results. The information currently available only allows very broad statements to be made about the effect of the tsetse transmission on the phenomenon of antigenic variation and its relevance to the epidemiology of the disease. It would appear, in general, that perhaps the majority of trypanosomes transmitted by the fly have an antigenic type different from that of the population ingested by the fly. The "basic" antigenic character of this new population may be relatively constant in a given strain of trypanosomes even though different variant populations of the strain are ingested by the fly. The relevance of this finding to the epidemiology of the natural disease is as of yet unclear, since what little is known of the epidemiology would seem to indicate only that there is some degree of antigenic relationship between variable numbers of individual populations of any one species isolated in a given area and that this relationship can also be extended to include populations isolated in different geographic areas. There is also evidence that trypanosome populations of a given antigenic type may remain in an area for some years. In general, most investigators have concluded that the number of antigenically different populations of a given species which exist in an area is too numerous to envisage the development of a successful vaccine and that cyclical transmission does not appear to reduce the spectrum of variants to more manageable proportions.

The major point which comes out of this review, however, is the fact that in only one instance (Cunningham 1966) were the metacyclic forms obtained directly from the vector tested for their antigenic character. In the other experiments populations derived by cyclical transmission or infection with metacyclic forms in laboratory or domestic animals were the source of the antigens. The relationship between these populations and the metacyclic forms derived from the fly is with one exception (Goedbloed et al. 1973) unknown. The sensitivity and specificity of the serologic tests used to investigate the antigenic composition of these trypanosome populations will be discussed in more detail in the next section but it should be noted that all the tests used are severely restricted in their ability to demonstrate the existence of minor variant populations in the test populations.

Conclusive evidence on the role of cyclical transmission in the phenomenon of antigenic variation would seem to require information based on the precise identification of the antigenic character(s) of the metacyclic trypanosomes obtained directly from the infected fly rather than on the antigenic character(s) of populations derived from those metacyclic populations in experimental animals.

MECHANISMS OF ANTIGENIC VARIATION

Divergent opinions as to the possible inductive or selective role of host antibodies in the phenomenon of antigenic variation were published as early as 1909 by Ehrlich et al. (1909) and Levaditi & McIntosh (1909). This controversy has persisted to the present day despite the considerable amount of literature which has since accumulated on this subject.

The basic question still to be answered is the genetic basis of the phenomenon in the individual parasite. Here two broad choices exist. Either each parasite has in its genome the information required to synthesize a series of variant antigens, thereby making antigenic variation phenotypic in nature, or the parasite genome codes only for a single variant antigen and the appearance of new variants is the result of random spontaneous mutations in this gene.

As the literature concerning antigenic variation has been the subject of recent reviews, each of which proposes a different mechanism as underlying this phenomenon (de Raadt 1974; Vickerman 1974b), I wish initially simply to summarize the experimental results generally cited to support either a phenotypic or random basis for antigenic variation and later discuss some of these results in more detail.

Support for the latter hypothesis is generally based on the work of several investigators (Cantrell 1958; Inoki et al. 1956; Seed & Gam 1966; Watkins 1964) who showed that only a small number (less than 1×10^{-4}) of a given population of trypanosomes appeared to be capable of producing new variant types and the rate of appearance of these trypanosomes was similar to that of appearance of mutants in bacterial populations (Cantrell 1958; Watkins 1964).

Support for a phenotypic basis to antigenic variation is based on the results of a number of workers who showed that in early stages of the disease there tended to be some order in the sequence of variant populations which appeared in experimental animals initially infected with the same parasite populations (Gray 1962, 1965b; Inoki 1960; Inoki et al. 1952, 1956, 1957; Osaki 1959).

It is somewhat surprising, however, to realize that in only four of the experiments cited above were the trypanosome populations studied derived at some point from a single trypanosome. The remainder were carried out using strains of parasites which are likely to consist of a mixture of different variant populations. This has recently been confirmed with the important additional finding that the various variant populations making up a strain have different multiplication rates, some types being much more virulent than others (McNeillage & Herbert 1968; McNeillage et al. 1969). Indeed the similar sequential appearance early in the infection of variant types in animals infected with a strain could, as proposed by de Raadt, be the result of the differential growth of the various initial constituents of the strain (de Raadt 1974).

It is proposed therefore to review only the results of experiments carried out with populations derived at the same point from a single trypanosome.

Osaki (1959) observed that the first relapse populations induced in mice infected by a single trypanosome of *Trypanosoma gambiense* by treatment with drugs or human serum consisted of a mixture of three to four antigenic types with a high incidence of certain types in all the relapse populations studied. The antigenic types were recognized by agglutination testing using sera obtained 4 to 7 days after treatment of infected mice.

Cantrell (1958) obtained relapse populations of *Trypanosoma equiperdum* by challenging rats previously immunized with drug-treated parasites of the strain with approximately 10^8 trypanosomes from populations derived in rats originally infected with a single parasite of this strain. It was concluded that since the new populations arising in the challenged rats were antigenically different from the immunizing population they could be composed of mutant types which had occurred with an incidence of 2 X 10^{-6} during the course of infection of the donor rats. The new relapse populations were shown by cross-immunization experiments to consist of several different antigenic types, some antigenic types being common to the populations recovered from differently challenged rats.

Gray (1965b) derived two antigenically different clones of *Trypanosoma brucei* by inoculation of single organisms into mice with subsequent mouse passage. These cloned populations were then used to infect individual rabbits. These rabbits were bled one week later, the blood passaged into another rabbit and also into mice where subpassage occurred until sufficient trypanosomes were obtained for use in the agglutination test. This process was repeated with each newly infected rabbit so the clone was passaged at weekly intervals in five separate rabbits. Serum was collected from each of the infected rabbits at weekly intervals. It was found that when the sera obtained from the 10 rabbits one week after infection were tested against the trypanosome populations isolated in mice, each of these populations cross-reacted with more than one serum. Gray proposed that these common cross-reacting antigenic types from each clone be termed the predominant antigens.

More recently Van Meirvenne et al. (1975a) described a series of experiments in which antigenically different clones were derived from single organisms of *Trypanosoma brucei,* the isolation of these clones taking 12 to 24 three-day passages in mice. Antisera to clones were raised by infecting rabbits with 10^6 trypanosomes and bleeding 6 days later. It was found that when 10^4 to 10^7 trypanosomes from these clones were incubated *in vitro* with their homologous antisera and the mixture then inoculated into mice, antigenically different relapse populations developed in the recipient mice. Up to 10 antigenically different variant populations were identified in the relapse populations by immune lysis tests and indirect immunofluorescence of air-fixed trypanosomes in blood smears. Again several predominant types were common to the populations derived from mice inoculated with antibody-treated clones which were antigenically distinct. These different relapse types also appeared to have different multiplication rates in infected mice. Five mice were then each infected with 10^3 trypanosomes of a single clone and the infections allowed to relapse naturally. In the first natural-relapse populations obtained 8 days after infection, the same major antigenic type was present in three mice. The two remaining mice had different major antigenic types, but six minor types were common to all five first relapse populations and three further minor types were present in some of these populations.

Perhaps it is pertinent at this point to consider some results of current work at Lausanne. It would seem fundamental to work on antigenic variation that the population used in each experiment be shown to be entirely homogenous for the variant antigen under study, in view of the suggestion that the antigenic character of a trypanosome population could vary during passage in normal mice (Gray 1965a). As tests such as agglutination (Cunningham & Vickerman 1962) and immune lysis give no indication of antigenic character at the level of individual parasites, an immunofluorescent technique originally developed for the study of surface antigens of *Leishmania* parasites (Doyle et al. 1974) was modified to allow identification of the variant antigen carried by individual living bloodstream trypanosomes *in vitro*.

The parasite populations used in this study were originally obtained by harvesting the first (B) and second (C) relapse populations which occurred in a rabbit originally infected with a clone (A) of *Trypanosoma brucei*. Clones were derived from these populations in both normal mice and mice whose immune response was ablated by prior exposure to 900 rads of total body gamma-irradiation. Antisera to each clone were obtained by infecting a rabbit with 10^7 organisms of the clone and bleeding 6 days later. These sera showed little cross-reactivity for the heterologous clones but each was extensively cross-absorbed so that at the time of use no heterologous cross-reactions could be detected by agglutination, immunofluorescence (I/F), or neutralization tests at dilutions as low as 1:4.

In the first series of experiments, the sensitivities of agglutination and I/F tests were defined by testing their ability to detect the presence of the minor population in a mixture of two antigenically different clones. The I/F test consistently detected a minor variant population which represented only 0.1% of the test population. The agglutination test detected the presence of the minor population only when it represented more than 5% of the test population (10^5 parasites), but a new variant population could compose as much as 90% of the test population before there was a significant reduction in the agglutination titer of the antiserum to the original variant.

The second series of experiments was designed to investigate the stability of cloned populations derived and passaged in normal mice at 2- to 3-day intervals as compared to the stability of similar clones derived and passaged in lethally irradiated mice. It was found that trypanosomes carrying new variant antigen, not recognized by the homologous clone-specific antiserum, could be detected after 10 passages (four of 3 days, six of 2 days) from injection of the original trypanosome. Parallel experiments using lethally irradiated mice did not at the limit of sensitivity of the immunofluorescence test reveal the appearance of a new variant population even after 38 days of passage. In a further series of experiments where normal mice were initially infected with 10^3 trypanosomes of the same clone, a new variant population not recognized by the homologous antiserum again occurred after as few as five passages (two of 3 days, three of 2 days). That these new parasites were not present in the original inoculum was clearly shown by the fact that preexposure of similar numbers of parasites of the clone to low dilutions of the clone-specific antisera completely neutralized their infectivity when inoculated into new mice.

A clone (D) was derived in lethally irradiated mice from the new population which appeared on passage of clone C in a normal mouse. An antiserum raised to this new clone recognized trypanosomes in the new populations which appeared on the six occasions clone C was passaged in normal mice.

In the third series of experiments, the homogeneity of populations cloned and passaged in lethally irradiated mice was studied using a neutralization test. Donor mice were infected with 10^2 trypanosomes of clone C and the homogeneity of this number of organisms with respect to the antigen(s) recognized by anti-C was shown by the fact that prior exposure to anti-C completely abolished their infectivity when inoculated into control mice. When the donor mice became parasitemic, their trypanosomes were recovered and aliquots of 10^6 to 10 trypanosomes were incubated with the same dilution of anti-C prior to reinoculation into new mice. All the mice used in these experiments received 900 to 1,200 rads of whole body inoculation 24 hours prior to use.

The results of three experiments of this type using a total of 18 donor mice have been remarkably consistent in that the recipient mice which were inoculated with 10^4 to 10 antibody-treated trypanosomes did not become infected. On occasions mice (3/19) infected with 10^5 treated parasites became parasitemic but on every occasion mice receiving 10^6 treated parasites subsequently developed a parasitemia. A 25-fold increase in the amount of antibody used to treat the parasites failed to protect these mice even though the time of patency of these infections was consistent with the survival of only 1 to 100 parasites. When the antigenic composition of these new populations was studied by I/F, no trypanosomes were found which were recognized by the original antiserum (anti-C), but the populations comprising a mixture of antigenic types, some recognized by anti-D, occurred in 21/27 of the new populations examined. Surprisingly, trypanosomes recognized by anti-B, that is, antiserum to the clone of the population which appeared prior to population C in the original rabbit, were detected in at least three of these new populations. There were also variable numbers of trypanosomes in these populations which were not recognized by any of the available antisera.

In an attempt to obviate the possibility that these new populations (D and B) originated from trypanosomes which had appeared during the infection of the lethally irradiated donor mice, the experiments were repeated with the modification that the aliquots of trypanosomes from the donor mice were incubated in lethal concentrations of anti-D and anti-B prior to incubation with anti-C and injection into the lethally irradiated recipient mice. On four occasions populations containing trypanosomes of antigenic types D or B developed on these recipient mice. This would suggest that these trypanosomes were not originally present in the inoculum derived from the donor mice.

Discussion

The present state of knowledge of the mechanisms underlying the phenomenon of antigenic variation can be summarized by stating that when populations of trypanosomes, derived originally from a single organism, have been exposed *in vitro* to a sufficient quantity of their homologous antivariant antibodies prior to reinoculation into new animals, the populations of trypanosomes which developed in these recipient animals contained a number of variant types antigenically different from the original populations. It would appear that these new variant populations were derived from a small number, possibly no greater than 1×10^{-5} of the antibody-treated populations.

The proviso must be made that since there are severe intrinsic limitations in the techniques which have been used to investigate this phenomenon, the conclusions which will be drawn may only be relevant in a general way to the mechanisms of antigenic variation as they occur in the infected host.

As regards the genetic basis for this phenomenon in the individual parasite, several facts would appear to militate against its being the result of truly random mutations in a gene coding for only a single variant antigen.

It is difficult to reconcile the following findings with a mechanism based on random errors in the translation of the DNA content of a single gene: the ability of trypanosomes derived from a single organism to display an antigen carried by a population which appeared earlier in the course of infection than the population from which the original organism was derived, i.e., the parasites do not lose their ability to display a previously expressed antigen; the apparent order in the appearance of new types in the case when a variant population is exposed to its homologous antivariant antibodies; the ability of different populations to express a similar antigen following cyclical transmission; and finally the marked structural heterogeneity of the variant-specific glycoproteins. This, however, is essentially a simplistic approach to a problem which appears similar to that of the mechanism underlying the generation of antibody diversity in mammals where even though the genetic basis has been studied in detail there is still no general agreement on the mechanisms involved (Osher & Neal 1975).

As we can only draw general conclusions about the genetic basis of this phenomenon on the basis of the evidence at present available, so we can only speculate about any role for host antibodies in antigenic variation other than that of selection against the predominant variant(s) at any given time. There is yet no absolutely conclusive evidence to support the proposed inductive role for antibodies in this phenomenon (Vickerman 1974b). The experiments generally cited to support this view are those of Gray (1962) and Takayangi & Enriquez (1973). Gray was able to suppress the sequential appearance of a variant population in a rabbit infected with a strain of *Trypanosoma brucei* by the passive administration of antiserum to this variant population prior to infection. This could most simply be explained by proposing the selective removal of parasites carrying that variant antigen from the strain population when it is initially injected into the rabbit. The probability that the sequential appearance of variant types early in infections with a strain is due to different virulences of the different variant populations making up the strain has been discussed earlier. The most convincing evidence so far for the possible inductive role of antibodies in the phenomenon of antigenic variation is the work of Takayangi & Enriquez who exposed 10^4 parasites of a strain of *Trypanosoma gambiense in vitro* to increasing amounts of IgG or IgM fractions of an antiserum raised by mouse infection prior to reinoculation of these parasites into new mice. It was found that exposure to high levels of antibody completely inhibited the subsequent infectivity of the treated parasites. Exposure to low levels of antibodies allowed the development of the original strain in the recipient mice. Exposure to intermediate levels of antibodies resulted with the development of a new variant population in the recipient mice. Since, however, antiserum was raised to a strain rather than a clone of parasites, it is probable that it would consist of varying amounts of antibodies to the various components of the strain. It is difficult, therefore, to exclude the possibility that subsequent dilution of these antibodies could reduce an originally low but efficient concentration of antibodies to a minor variant population of the strain, to a point compatible with survival of at least some of the organisms in the test population.

The lack of detectable variation in trypanosome populations maintained in lethally irradiated, hence immunosuppressed, mice as compared with the variation which occurs in parasites maintained in normal mice indicates only that the immune response may play a part in this phenomenon but does not indicate whether it is inductive, selective, or both.

It has been proposed that antibodies could not be inductive on the basis of the fact that only small numbers of trypanosomes in large populations exposed to the same concentration of homologous antivariant antibodies apparently give rise to new variant populations (Seed & Gam 1966). It could equally as well be stated that these results show that only small numbers of trypanosomes exist under these experimental conditions which are capable both of resisting the cytotoxic effect of the antibodies and being induced to change their variant antigens. In future experiments it may be relevant to note that in mammalian cells susceptibility to complement-mediated lysis depends on such factors as the stage of the cell in the cell cycle, cells being most susceptible in G_1 and most resistant in mitosis, the class of antibodies used, and the concentration of antigenic determinants on the cell surface (Citkes & Friberg 1971; Kerbel et al. 1975; Lerner et al. 1971; Rubio 1974). It is also intriguing to note that in the mammalian model system where hepatoma cells are exposed to corticosteroids to induce the formation of a specific enzyme (tyrosine aminotransferase) induction is only possible during a certain part of the cell cycle (S-G_1) (Tompkins et al. 1969). It is conceivable therefore that if antibody does induce antigenic variation in the individual parasite it may be possible only at a very limited stage of the cell cycle where the parasites will be both resistant to the cytotoxic effect of the antibody and be capable of being induced to change their antigen. Antibody type or class may also be important in this respect as will be discussed in relation to antigenic variation in *Plasmodium*.

Parallels have been drawn between the phenomenon of antigenic variation in trypanosomes and the ability of free-living protozoa of the genus *Paramecium* to change a surface antigen following exposure to various stimuli such as temperature, salt concentration, and antibodies. This process is under genetic control and appears to be associated with the processes by which the protozoan adapts to a hostile environment (see reviews, Beale 1954; Beale 1974; Sommerville 1970). Many aspects of the work done on this protozoan may eventually prove relevant to our understanding of the phenomenon of antigenic variation in the salivarian trypanosomes, but it should be noted that in the case of *Plasmodium aurelia* exposure to antibody does not always induce a change in its surface antigens. It generally requires that some other parameter be modified at the same time, such as feeding or temperature, and there are occasions when antibodies appear to stabilize the expression of a particular antigen on the surface of the parasite.

In conclusion it can be said that at the present time our knowledge of the mechanisms underlying the phenomenon of antigenic variation at the level of the individual is very limited. This situation has arisen because of the limitations imposed by the techniques used to investigate this phenomenon both as regards maintenance of the parasite and identification of its antigens. The first requirement for a valid investigation of this phenomenon is the development of a defined *in vitro* culture system for the bloodstream forms of the salivarian trypanosomes which would allow analysis of the phenomenon without the undefined variables introduced by the present necessity to maintain the trypanosomes in living animals either normal or immunosuppressed. A major advance in this respect has been the development at the International

Laboratory for Research on Animal Diseases of a culture system which allows the long-term cultivation of infective bloodstream forms of *Trypanosoma brucei in vitro* (Hirumi et al. 1976). The second requirement is that the immunologic techniques used to investigate the mechanisms underlying antigenic variation be related to the antigen(s) carried by an individual parasite rather than parasite populations and that their limits of sensitivity be clearly defined. It would be preferable that antisera used in such investigations be derived from isolated, purified, and biochemically characterized antigens. The results of neutralization tests, especially those using large numbers of parasites, should be considered equivocal until it is clearly shown whether antibody does or does not induce antigenic variation. In short what is required of this study of parasite surface antigens is that it develop the degree of precision necessary for the immunological and biochemical investigation of surface antigens of mammalian cells.

CONCLUDING REMARKS

The phenomenon of "antigenic variation" in salivarian trypanosomes is a complex process which we are now only beginning to understand at the molecular level. The antigens responsible for the differences between successive bloodstream populations during the course of infection have been shown, at least in the case of *Trypanosoma brucei,* to be surface glycoproteins of similar size but different amino acid composition. The genome of an individual trypanosome codes apparently for a number (as of yet unknown) of the antigenically different surface glycoproteins.

The factor(s) which induce an individual bloodstream trypanosome to undergo antigenic variation are at present unknown. Host antibodies have been implicated but their possible inductive role has not been clearly established. As the parasites undergo a complex series of physiological, biochemical, and morphological changes in their cycle of infection through intermediate and final hosts, it may be as well not to lose sight of the possibility that what the host's immune system recognizes as "antigenic variation" may be only a part of a series of physiological changes by which the parasites adapt to a hostile environment. Variant populations have in fact been shown to differ not only immunologically but also physiologically with respect to multiplication rates, drug sensitivities, etc. (Gray 1966b; McNeillage & Herbert 1968; Soltys 1959).

A more detailed understanding at the molecular level of the processes underlying the phenomenon of antigenic variation would appear to be required before possible protective measures, either immunologic or chemotherapeutic, can be successfully devised. A wide variety of new techniques in molecular biology have been developed in such fields as immunology, virology, bacterial genetics, and eukaryote cell function and it is very likely that application and modification of these techniques to investigate the molecular biology of parasites would result in the elucidation of some of the major problems involved in the control of host-parasite relationships.

BIBLIOGRAPHY

Allsopp, B.A. 1973. Separation of the components of *Trypanosoma brucei* subgroups 4S (surface) antigen. *Trans. R. Soc. Trop. Med. Hyg.* 67: 270-271.

Allsopp, B.A. & Njogu, A.R. 1971. Studies on the surface sugar composition of the antigens of *Trypanosoma brucei* subgroup. *E. Afr. Trypanosomiasis Res. Organ. Annu. Rep.* 1971: 21-33.

Allsopp, B.A. & Njogu, A.R. 1973. Sugar composition of *Trypanosoma brucei* subgroup 4S (surface) antigens. *Trans. R. Soc. Trop. Med. Hyg.* 66: 347.

Allsopp, B.A. & Njogu, A.R. 1974. Monosaccharide composition of the surface glycoprotein antigens of *Trypanosoma brucei*. *Parasitology* 69: 271-281.

Allsopp, B.A., Njogu, A.R. & Humphryes, K.C. 1971. Nature and location of *Trypanosoma brucei* subgroup exoantigen and its relationship to 4S antigen. *Exp. Parasitol.* 29: 271-284.

Aschroft, M.T. 1960. A comparison between a syringe-passaged and a tse-tse fly-transmitted line of a strain of *Trypanosoma rhodesiense*. *Ann. Trop. Med. Parasitol.* 54: 44-53.

Balber, A.E. 1972. *Trypanosoma brucei:* fluxes of the morphological variants in intact and X-irradiated mice. *Exp. Parasitol.* 31: 307-319.

Balber, A.E. 1974. *Trypanosoma brucei:* attenuation by corticosteroids of the anaemia of infected mice. *Exp. Parasitol.* 35: 209-218.

Beale, G.H. 1954. *The Genetics of Paramecium Aurelia.* Cambridge University Press. Cambridge, England.

Beale, G.H. 1974. Genetics of antigenic variation in *Paramecium:* a model system. *In* Parasites in the Immunized Host: Mechanisms of Survival, Porter, R. & Knight, J., Eds.: 21-27. Ciba Foundation Symposium 25 (new series). Associated Scientific Publishers. Amsterdam, The Netherlands.

Behin, R., Mauel, J., Biroum-Noerjasin & Rowe, D.S. 1975. Studies on cell-mediated immunity to cutaneous leishmaniasis of guinea-pigs and mice by *Leishmania enriettii*. *Ann. Parasitol. Hum. Comp.* In press.

Boehringer, S. & Hecker, H. 1974a. Quantitative ultrastructural differences between blood and midgut forms of *Trypanosoma bruce brucei*. *In* Proceedings of the 3rd International Congress on Parasitol. 1: 21-22.

Boehringer, S. & Hecker, H. 1974b. Quantitative ultrastructural differences between strains of *Trypanosoma brucei* subgroup during transformation in the blood. *J. Protozool.* 21: 694-698.

Bowman, I.B.R. 1974. Intermediary metabolism of pathogenic flagellates. *In* Trypanosomiasis and Leishmaniasis: 255-271. Ciba Foundation Symposium 20 (new series). Associated Scientific Publishers. Amsterdam, The Netherlands.

Bradley, D.J. 1974. Letter: Genetic control of natural resistance to *Leishmania donovani. Nature* (Lond.) 250: 353-354.

Broom, J.C. & Brown, H.C. 1940. Studies in trypanosomiasis. IV. Notes on the serological characters of *Trypanosoma brucei* after cyclical development in *Glossina morsitans. Trans. R. Soc. Trop. Med. Hyg.* 34: 53-64.

Brown, R.C., Evans, D.A. & Vickerman, K. 1973. Changes in oxidative metabolism and ultrastructure accompanying differentiation of the mitochondrion in *Trypanosoma brucei. Int. J. Parasitol.* 3: 691-704.

Cantrell, W. 1958. Mutation rate and antigenic variation in *Trypanosoma equiperdum. J. Infect. Dis.* 103: 263-271.

Citkes, M. & Friberg, S., Jr. 1971. Expression of H-2 and Moloney Leukemia virus determined cell-surface antigens in synchronized cultures of a mouse cell line. *Proc. Nat. Acad. Sci. U.S.A.* 68: 566-569.

Cross, G.A.M. 1973. Identification and purification of a class of soluble surface proteins from *Trypanosoma brucei. Trans. R. Soc. Trop. Med. Hyg.* 67: 261.

Cross, G.A.M. 1975. Identification, purification and properties of clone-specific glycoprotein antigens constituting the surface coat of *Trypanosoma brucei. Parasitology* 71: 393-417.

Cross, G.A.M. & Johnson, J.G. 1976. Structure and organization of the variant specific surface antigens of *Trypanosoma brucei. In* Proceedings of the 2nd International Symposium on the Biochemistry of Host Parasite Relationships. Van den Bossche, H., Ed.: 413-420. Elsevier Publishing Company. Amsterdam, The Netherlands.

Cunningham, M.P. 1966. The preservation of viable metacyclic forms of *Trypanosoma rhodesiense* and some studies of the antigenicity of the organisms. *Trans. R. Soc. Trop. Med. Hyg.* 60: 126.

Cunningham, M.P. & Vickerman, K. 1962. Antigenic analysis in the *Trypanosoma brucei* group, using the agglutination reaction. *Trans. R. Soc. Trop. Med. Hyg.* 56: 48-59.

Dar, F.K., Paris, J. & Wilson, A.J. 1973. Serological studies on trypanosomiasis in East Africa. IV. Comparison of antigenic types of *Trypanosoma vivax* group organisms. *Ann. Trop. Med. Parasitol.* 67: 319-329.

Dar, F.K., & Wilson, A.J. 1973. Serological studies on trypanosomiasis in East Africa. I. Introduction and techniques. *Ann. Trop. Med. Parasitol.* 67: 21-29.

De Raadt, P. 1974. Immunity and antigenic variation: clinical observations suggestive of immune phenomena in African trypanosomiasis. *In* Trypanosomiasis and Leishmaniasis: 199-216. Ciba Foundation Symposium 20 (new series). Associated Scientific Publishers. Amsterdam, The Netherlands.

Desowitz, R.S. 1959. Studies on immunity and host-parasite relationships. I. The immunological response of resistant and susceptible breeds of cattle to trypanosomal challenge. *Ann. Trop. Med. Parasitol.* 53: 293-313.

Desowitz, R.S. 1970. African trypanosomes. *In* Immunity to Parasitic Animals, Jackson, G.J., Herman, R. & Singer, I. Eds. Vol. 2: 551-596. Appleton-Century-Crofts, New York, N.Y.

Doyle, J.J., Behin, R., Mauel, J. & Rowe, D.S. 1974. Antibody-induced movement of membrane components of *Leishmania enriettii. J. Exp. Med.* 139: 1061-1069.

Duxbury, R.E., Sadun, E.H. & Anderson, J.S. 1972. Experimental infections with African trypanosomes. II. Immunization of mice and monkeys with a gamma-irradiated, recently isolated human strain of *Trypanosoma rhodesiense. Am. J. Trop. Med. Hyg.* 21: 885-888.

Duxbury, R.E., Anderson, J.S., Wellde, B.T., Sadun, E.H. & Muriithi, I.E. 1972. *Trypanosoma congalense* — Immunisation of mice, dogs and cattle with gamma-irradiated parasites. *Exp. Parasitol.* 32: 527-533.

Duxbury, R.E., Sadun, E.H., Schoenbechler, M.J. & Stroupe, D.A. 1974. *Trypanosoma rhodesiense:* protection in mice by inoculations of homologous parasite products. *Exp. Parasitol.* 36: 70-76.

Ehrlich, P., Roehl, W. & Gulblausen, R. 1909. Ueber serumfeste Trypanosomenstaemme. *Z. Immunitaetsforsch.* 3: 296-299.

Fairbairn, H. & Culwick, A.T. 1946. A new approach to trypanosomiasis. *Ann. Trop. Med. Parasitol.* 40: 421-452.

Fiennes, R.N. 1970. Pathogenesis and pathology of animal trypanosomiasis. *In* The African Trypanosomiasis, Mulligan, H.W., Ed.: 729-750. Allen & Unwin. London, England.

Fruit, J.N., Van Meirvenne, N., Petitprez, A., Afchain, D., Le Ray, D. & Bout, D. 1974. Antigenic studies on the surface coat of *T.(T).b.brucei. In* Proceedings of the 3rd International Congress on Parasitology. 2: 1095.

Goedbloed, E., Ligthart, G.S., Minter, D.M., Wilson, A.J., Dar, F.K. & Paris, J. 1973. Serological studies of trypanosomiasis in East Africa. II. Comparisons of antigenic types of *Trypanosoma brucei* subgroup organisms isolated from wild tsetse flies. *Ann. Trop. Med. Parasitol.* 67: 31-43.

Gray, A.R. 1962. The influence of antibody on serological variation in *Trypanosoma brucei. Ann. Trop. Med. Parasitol.* 56: 4-13.

Gray, A.R. 1965a. Antigenic variation in a strain of *Trypanosoma brucei* transmitted by *Glossina morsitans* and *G. palpalis. J. Gen. Microbiol.* 41: 195-214.

Gray, A.R. 1965b. Antigenic variation in clones of *Trypanosoma brucei. Ann. Trop. Med. Parasitol.* 59: 27-36.

Gray, A.R. 1966a. The antigenic relationships of strains of *Trypanosoma brucei* isolated in Nigeria. *J. Gen. Microbiol.* 44: 263-271.

Gray, A.R. 1966b. Antigenic variation in clones of *Trypanosoma brucei.* II. The drug sensitivities of variants of a clone and the antigenic relationships of trypanosomes before and after drug treatment. *Ann. Trop. Med. Parasitol.* 60: 265-275.

Gray, A.R. 1967. Some principles of the immunology of trypanosomiasis. *Bull. WHO* 37: 177-193.

Gray, A.R. 1970. A study of the antigenic relationships of isolates of *Trypanosoma brucei* collected from a herd of cattle kept in one locality for five years. *J. Gen. Microbiol.* 62: 301-313.

Gray, A.R. 1972. Variable agglutinogenic antigens of *Trypanosoma gambiense* and their distribution among isolates of the trypanosome collected in different places in Nigeria. *Trans. R. Soc. Trop. Med. Hyg.* 66: 263-284.

Gray, A.R. 1974. Antigenic similarities among isolates of *Trypanosoma gambiense* from different countries in Africa. *Trans. R. Soc. Trop. Med. Hyg.* 68: 150-151.

Gray, A.R. 1975. A pattern in the development of agglutogenic antigens of cyclically transmitted isolates of *Trypanosoma gambiense. Trans. R. Soc. Trop. Med. Hyg.* 69: 131-138.

Hirumi, H. et al. 1977 Salivarian trypanosoma: *in vitro* cultivation of bloodstream forms using bovine fibroblast monolayers. *Science.* In press.

Hoare, C.A. 1970. The mammalian trypanosomes of Africa. *In* The African Trypanosomiases. Mulligan,H.W.,Ed.: 3-59. Allen & Unwin. London, England.

Inoki, S. 1960. Studies on antigenic variation in the Welcome strain of *Trypanosoma gambiense.* II. On the first relapse appearing in mice treated with human plasma. *Biken J.* 3: 223-228.

Inoki, S., Kitaura, T., Nakabayashi, T. & Kurogochi, H. 1952. Studies on the immunological variations in *Trypanosoma gambiense.* I. A new variation system and a new experimental method. *Med. J. Osaka Univ.* 3: 357-371.

Inoki, S., Nakabayashi, T., Osaki, H. & Fukukita, S. 1957. Studies on the immunological variation in *Trypanosoma gambiense. Med. J. Osaka Univ.* 7: 731-743.

Inoki, S., Osaki, H. & Nakabayashi, T. 1956. Studies on the immunological variation in *Trypanosoma gambiense* II. Verifications of the new variation system by Ehrlich's and *in vitro* methods. *Med. J. Osaka Univ.* 7: 165-173.

Jones, T.W. & Clarkson, M.J. 1972a. The effect of tsetse passage on variants of *Trypanosoma vivax*. *Trans. R. Soc. Trop. Med. Hyg.* 66: 336.

Jones, T.W. & Clarkson, M.J. 1972b. The effect of syringe and cyclical passage on antigenic variants of *Trypanosoma vivax*. *Ann. Trop. Med. Parasitol.* 66: 303-312.

Jones, T.W. & Clarkson, M.J. 1974. The timing of antigenic variation in *Trypanosoma vivax*. *Ann. Trop. Med. Parasitol.* 68: 485-486.

Kerbel, R.S., Birbeck, M.S.C., Robertson, D. & Cartwright, P. 1975. Ultra-structural and serological studies on the resistance of activated B cells to the cytotoxic effects of antiimmunoglobulin serum. Patch and cap formation of surface immunoglobulin on mitotic B lymphocytes. *Clin. Exp. Immunol.* 20: 161-177.

Ketteridge, D.S. 1971. Studies on rodent-adapted *Trypanosoma vivax*. Ph.D. thesis. University of Glasgow. Glasgow, Scotland.

Ketteridge, D.S. 1972. *Trypanosoma vivax:* surface interrelationships between host and parasite. *Trans. R. Soc. Trop. Med. Hyg.* 66: 324.

Lanham, S.M. & Taylor, A.E.R. 1972. Some properties of the immunogens (protective antigens) of a single variant of *Trypanosoma brucei brucei*. *J. Gen. Microbiol.* 72: 101-116.

Le Ray, D., Van Meirvenne, N. & Jadin, J.B. 1973. Immunoelectrophoretic characterization of common and variable antigens of *Trypanosoma brucei*. *Trans. R. Soc. Trop. Med. Hyg.* 67: 273-274.

Lerner, R.A., Oldstone, M.B. & Cooper, N.R. 1971. Cell cycle-dependent immune lysis of Moloney virus-transformed lymphocytes: presence of viral antigen, accessibility to antibody and complement activation. *Proc. Nat. Acad. Sci. U.S.A.* 68: 2584-88.

Levaditi, C. & McIntosh, J. 1909. Le mécanisme de la création des varietés de trypanosomes resistants aux anticorps. *Compt. R. Soc. Biol.* 66: 49-51.

Losos, G.J. & Ikede, B.O. 1972. Review of pathology of diseases in domestic and laboratory animals, caused by *Trypanosoma congolense, T. vivax, T. brucei, T. rhodiense,* and *T. gambiense. Vet. Pathol.* Suppl. 9: 71.

Luckins, A.G. 1972. Effects of x-irradiation and cortisone treatment of albino rats on infections with *brucei*-complex trypanosomes. *Trans. R. Soc. Trop. Med. Hyg.* 66: 130-139.

Lumsden, W.H.R. 1970. Biological aspects of trypanosomiasis research, 1965: a retrospect, 1969. *Adv. Parasitol.* 8: 227-249.

Lumsden, W.H.R. 1972a. Immune response to hemoprotozoa. *In* Immunity to Animal Parasites. Soulsby, E.J.L., Ed.: 287-289. Academic Press, Inc. New York, N.Y.

Lumsden, W.H.R. 1972b. Trypanosomiasis. *Brit. Med. Bull.* 28: 34-48.

McDevitt, H.O. & Bodmer, W.F. 1974. HL-A, immune-response genes, and disease. *Lancet* 1: 1269-1275.

McNeillage, G.J.C. & Herbert, W.J. 1968. Infectivity and virulence of *Trypanosoma (trypanozoon) brucei* for mice. II. Comparison of closely related trypanosome antigenic types. *J. Comp. Pathol.* 78: 345-349.

McNeillage, G.J.C., Herbert, W.H. & Lumsden, W.H.R. 1969. Antigenic type of first relapse variants arising from a strain of *Trypanosoma (trypanozoon) brucei. Exp. Parasitol.* 25: 1-7.

Njogu, A.R. 1972. Purification of the 4S antigens of *brucei* subgroup trypanosomes. *Trans. R. Soc. Trop. Med. Hyg.* 66: 347-348.

Njogu, A.R. 1974. The immunochemistry of the variable antigens of *Trypanosoma brucei. In* Proceedings of the 3rd International Congress on Parasitology. 2: 1094.

Njogu, A.R., Itazi, O.K., Enyaru, J.C. & Abonga, L. 1974. Direct evidence that the 4S (surface) antigens are located on the outer surface of the *Trypanosoma brucei* subgroup cell membrane. *Trans. R. Soc. Trop. Med. Hyg.* 68: 147-148.

Ormerod, W.E., Venkatesan, S. & Carpenter, R.G. 1974. The effect of immune inhibition on pleomorphism in *Trypanosoma brucei rhodesiense. Parasitology* 68: 355-367.

Osaki, H. 1959. Studies on the immunological variation in *Trypanosoma gambiense* (serotypes and the mode of relapse). *Biken J.* 2: 113-127.

Osher, F.C. & Neal, W.C. 1975. Theories of antibody diversity: the great debate. *Cell. Immunol.* 17: 552-559.

Otieno, L.H. 1973. Effects of immunosuppressive agents on the course of *Trypanosoma (trypanozoon) brucei* infections in heat-stressed mice. *Trans. R. Soc. Trop. Med. Hyg.* 67: 856-869.

Rubio, N. 1974. Surface H-2 antigenic concentration requirement of somatic hybrid cells for IgM-mediated cytotoxicity. *Nature* (Lond.) 249: 461-463.

Seed, J.R. 1972. *Trypanosoma gambiense* and *T. equiperdum:* characterization of variant specific antigens. *Exp. Parasitol.* 31: 98-108.

Seed, J.R. 1974. Antigens and antigenic variability of the African trypanosomes. *J. Protozool.* 21: 639-646.

Seed, J.R. and Gam, A.A. 1966. Passive immunity to experimental trypanosomiasis. *J. Parasitol.* 52: 1134-1140.

Soltys, M.A. 1959. Immunity in trypanosomiasis. III. Sensitivity of antibody resistant strains to chemotherapeutic drugs. *Parasitology* 49: 143-152.

Sommerville, J. 1970. Serotype expression in *Paramecium. Adv. Microb. Physiol.* 4: 131-178.

Steiger, R. 1971. Some aspects of the surface coat formation in *Trypanosoma brucei. Acta Trop.* 28: 341-346.

Takayanagi, T. & Enriquez, G.L. 1973. Effects of the IgG and IgM immunoglobu-lins in *Trypanosoma gambiense* infections in mice. *J. Parasitol.* 59: 644-647.

Taylor, A.E.R. & Lanham, S.M. 1972. Partial purification of immunogenic (protective) antigens of *Trypanosoma brucei brucei. Trans. R. Soc. Trop. Med. Hyg.* 66: 345-346.

Tomkins, G.M., Gelehrter, T.D., Granner, D., Martin, D., Jr., Samuels, H.H. & Thompson, E.B. 1969. Control of specific gene expression in higher organisms. *Science* 166: 1474-1480.

Uilenberg, G. 1974. Summary of studies on the immunology of *Trypanosoma congolense* infection carried out at Maisons-Alfort (I.E.M.V.T.) France, 1970-1972. *In* Control Programmes for Trypanosomes and Their Vectors. *Rev. Élevage Méd. Vét. Pays. Trop.* Suppl.: 207-208.

Uilenberg, G. & Giret, M. 1972. Etudes immunologiques sur les trypano-somes. 1. Existence d'un type antigenique de base chez une souche de *Trypanosoma congolense* Broden, 1904. Variation après transmission cyclique. *Rev. Élevage Méd. Vét. Pays. Trop.* 25: 37-52.

Uilenberg, G. & Giret, M. 1973. Etudes immunologiques sur les trypanosomes. 3. Essais d'immunisation de moutons contre l'infection cyclique par *Trypanosoma congolense. Rev. Élevage Méd. Vét. Pays. Trop.* 26: 37-42.

Uilenberg, G., Maillot, L. & Giret, M. 1973. Etudes immunologiques sur les trypanosomes. 2. Observations nouvelles sur le type antigenique de base d'une souche de *Trypanosoma congolense. Rev. Élevage Méd. Vét. Pays Trop.* 26: 27-36.

Van Meirvenne, N., Janssens, P.G. & Magnus, E. 1975a. Antigenic variation in syringe-passaged populations of *Trypanosoma (Trypanozoon) brucei.* I. Rationalization of the experimental approach. *Ann. Soc. Belge Med. Trop.* 55: 1-23.

Van Meirvenne, N., Janssens, P.G., Magnus, E., Lumsden, W.H.R. & Herbert, W.J. 1975b. Antigenic variation in syringe-passaged populations of *Trypanosoma (Trypanozoon) brucei.* II. Comparative studies on two antigenic type collections. *Ann. Soc. Belge Med. Trop.* 55: 25-30.

Van Meirvenne, N., LeRay, D., Janssens, P.G. & Magnus, E. 1973. Immunogenic properties of common and variable antigens of *T. brucei, Trans. R. Soc. Trop. Med. Hyg.* 67: 274-275.

Vickerman, K. 1965. Polymorphism and mitochondrial activity in sleeping sickness trypanosomes. *Nature* (Lond.) 208: 762-766.

Vickerman, K. 1969. On the surface coat and flagellar adhesion in trypano-somes. *J. Cell Sci.* 5: 163-193.

Vickerman, K. 1970. Ultrastructure of *Trypanosoma* and relation to function. *In* The African Trypanosomiases. Mulligan, H.W., Ed.: 60-66. Allen & Unwin. London, England.

Vickerman, K. 1971. Morphological and physiological considerations of extra-cellular blood protozoans. *In* Ecology and Physiology of Protozoal Parasites. Fallis, A.M., Ed.: 58-89. University of Toronto Press. Toronto, Canada.

Vickerman, K. 1974a. The ultrastructure of pathogenic flagellates. *In* Trypanosomiasis and Leishmaniasis: 171-190. Ciba Foundation Symposium 20 (new series), Associated Scientific Publishers. Amsterdam, The Netherlands.

Vickerman, K. 1974b. Antigenic variation in African trypanosomes. *In* Parasites in the Immunized Host: Mechanisms of Survival. Porter, R. & Knight, J., Eds.: 53-80. Ciba Foundation Symposium 25 (new series). Associated Scientific Publishers. Amsterdam, The Netherlands.

Vickerman, K. & Evans, D.A. 1974. Studies on the ultrastructure and respiratory physiology of *Trypanosoma vivax* trypomastigote stages. *Trans. R. Soc. Trop. Med. Hyg.* 68: 145.

Vickerman, K. & Luckins, A.G. 1969. Localization of variable antigens in the surface coat of *Trypanosoma brucei* using ferritin conjugated antibody. *Nature* (Lond.) 224: 1125-1126.

Watkins, J.F. 1964. Observations on antigenic variation in a strain of *Trypanosoma brucei* growing in mice. *J. Hyg.* 62: 69-80.

Wellde, B.T., Duxbury, R.E., Sadun, E.H., Langbehn, H.R., Lötzsch, R., Deindl, G. & Warui, G. 1973. Experimental infections with African trypanosomes. IV. Immunization of cattle with gamma-irradiated *Trypanosoma rhodesiense. Exp. Parasitol.* 34: 62-68.

Wellde, B.T., Schoenbechler, M.J., Diggs, C.L., Langbehn, H.R. & Sadun, E.H. 1975. Trypanosoma rhodesiense: variant specificity of immunity induced by irradiated parasites. *Exp. Parasitol.* 37: 125-129.

Wijers, D.J.B. 1959. Polymorphism in *Trypanosoma gambiense* and *Trypanosoma rhodesiense,* and the significance of the intermediate forms. *Ann. Trop. Med. Parasitol.* 53: 59-68.

Wilson, A.J. 1967. An immunological study of *T. congolense* group organisms on cyclical passage through *G. morsitans. E. Afr. Trypanosomiasis Res. Organ. Annu. Rep.* 1967: 21-22.

Wilson, A.J. & Cunningham, M.P. 1972. Immunological aspects of bovine trypanosomiasis. I. Immune response of cattle to infection with *Trypanosoma congolense* and the antigenic variation of the infecting organisms. *Exp. Parasitol.* 32: 165-173.

Wilson, A.J., Dar, F.K. & Paris, J. 1973. Serological studies on trypanosomiasis in East Africa. 3. Comparison of antigenic types of *Trypanosoma congolense* organisms isolated from wild flies. *Ann. Trop. Med. Parasitol.* 67: 313-317.

Wilson, A.J. & Grainge, E.B. 1967. Immunological relationship of *Trypanosoma brucei* subgroup isolates obtained from different areas of East Africa as judged by the agglutination test. *East Africa Trypanosomiasis Res. Organ. Annu. Rep.* 1967: 20-21.

Wright, K.A. & Hales, H. 1970. Cytochemistry of the pellicle of bloodstream forms of *Trypanosoma (Trypanozoon) brucei. J. Parasitol.* 56: 671-683.

4

CELLULAR IMMUNITY AND THE PARASITE

G. B. Mackaness

Trudeau Institute, Inc.
Saranac Lake, New York 12983

INTRODUCTION

When acquired resistance cannot be demonstrated to depend on antibody, it is legitimate to ask whether specifically reactive lymphyocytes are at work as the mediators of immunity, hence to consider the possibility that we are dealing with an example of cell-mediated immunity (CMI). This, however, is not the only sense in which the term "cellular immunity" is applied. It is also used to describe a defense mechanism in which the phagocytic cells of the immune host display abnormally high levels of antimicrobial activity. In this circumstance the ultimate effector cell is an altered macrophage. These two concepts of cellular immunity are related but they are not identical. Although CMI often works through its capacity to potentiate the antimicrobial capacity of host macrophages, other effector mechanisms may also operate in CMI.

THE NATURE OF CMI

It is essential to separate the two distinct functions that are implied when we speak of the mediation and expression of cellular immunity. This distinction is dictated by the widely different origins and functions of the cell types that must cooperate with each other in the implementation of this type of acquired resistance. As a rule, the *mediators* of cellular immunity are activated T cells. The cells through which antiparasitic resistance is expressed are phagocytic cells.

If CMI is suspected of being a factor in the host's acquired defenses, it is first necessary to ask how it might operate against the parasite. There are obvious limitations to a defense mechanism that depends upon the functional attributes of two interacting cell populations. One or the other must presumably intervene directly between host and parasite. So far as we know, specifically reactive lymphocytes (activated T cells) cannot neutralize, opsonize, or detoxify a parasite as antibodies can. They seem, in fact, to be singularly ill-equipped for disposing of intruding parasites. It is, however, both plausible and truthful to suggest that activated T cells can destroy host cells in which an obligate intracellular parasite is living. It has often been demonstrated *in vitro* that immunologically reactive lymphocytes can lyse infected host cells. Destroying the host cell would obviously deny the parasite a means of sustaining itself; but as a means of self-defense such a mechanism would have limited value if unaccompanied by the production of a neutralizing antibody that could interfere with the subsequent parasitization of adjacent cells. Without this protection the latter would obviously be doomed to destruction, either by the virus or by the host's own immunological attack. Cutting off one's nose to spite one's face is not a practical way to deal with an infectious agent.

Even in circumstances in which an activated T cell is demonstrably capable of destroying a parasitized host cell *in vitro,* it is more than likely that this function is normally performed by mononuclear phagocytes. Unlike the activated T cell, which gives the phagocyte its immunological directives, the "professional" phagocyte is capable of ingesting and disposing entirely of an ailing host cell and its whole content of parasitic forms.

These ideas do not preclude the possibility that immunologically reactive cells could interact with antigenic constituents in the plasma membrane of protozoan parasites, thereby destroying them in a manner analogous to the lympholytic destruction of allogeneic cells or of syngeneic cells which have been antigenically changed by infection or neoplastic transformation. There is no convincing evidence, however, that cell-mediated immunity ever operates in this way against hemoparasites. It is nonetheless possible that hemoparasites could be dealt with if infected erythrocytes were sequestered and destroyed before they could replicate. Such a mechanism presupposes that the infected host cell display an antigenic difference very soon after becoming parasitized.

Since there is little to indicate that activated T cells (or any other class of reactive lymphocytes) act directly to interfere with the life cycle of protozoan parasites, it is necessary to postulate that resistance caused by CMI results from the host's capacity to stage a concerted attack upon entrenched parasites in the tissues. The cellular and vascular responses involved in this process are the familiar ones we recognize as inflammation. It is appropriate and mechanistically correct to speak of "immunological inflammation" when it results from allergic hypersensitivity. In the case of CMI, it is delayed-type hypersensitivity (DTH) that provides the immunological basis for the inflammatory reaction. Delayed-type hypersensitivity is simply a manifestation of increased irritability purposefully directed against the source of the antigens to which the host has responded immunologically.

When considering the *modus operandi* of a defense mechanism that is based on CMI and is directed against hemoparasites, we must think of a moving target which does not lend itself to the focalized type of inflammatory reaction that can be successfully deployed against a fixed target in the tissue. Tuberculosis is the classic instance of this form of acquired immunity. No doubt its counterpart exists in many parasitic diseases; for example, *Trypanosoma cruzi* in the heart. It seems also likely that successful immunization with sporozoites depends upon CMI directed against preerythrocytic stages of malaria parasites in the liver. The granulomas which develop in the livers of immunized animals may be indicative of a defensive response involving CMI.

As Dr. Bloom has stressed, the assembly of mononuclear phagocytes at the site of a DTH reaction is a predictable consequence of the local release of pharmacologically active molecules when specifically sensitive lymphocytes are stimulated by antigen. The fact that activated T cells, regardless of specificity, can enter any area of inflammation would obviously facilitate the staging of a defensive response at an infective focus. It would also allow the host to give expression to its specific capacity to defend itself, for the entry of specifically reactive lymphocytes would further enhance the inflammatory reaction. Dr. Bloom has also pointed out, however, that the staging of a local inflammatory response by virtue of cell-mediated hypersensitivity may not be the only protective effect that stems from CMI. During the interaction between antigen and specifically sensitized T cells, the same spectrum of pharmacologically active molecules is probably released to the systemic circulation. Macrophage inhibitory factor and an interferon-like molecule are readily detected in the circulation 24 hours after tuberculin has been injected into tuberculin-sensitive animals. It seems certain that one consequence of disseminating substances that stimulate mononuclear phagocytes is the intense hyperplasia and hyperactivity of the reticuloendothelial system (RES) seen in chronically infected animals. Since the Taliaferros made their enlightening observations on the tissue reaction to malaria, we have known that reticuloendothelial hyperplasia is a conspicuous feature of this disease. But it is not known whether these tissue changes have an immunological origin or are merely an adaptation to the greatly increased numbers of red blood cells that must be scavenged. In short, we do not know if the changes in the reticuloendothelial system that accompany many hemoparasitic infections result from the host's immunological response to its infection or themselves contribute significantly to the host's acquired defenses. Activation of the RES might improve its phagocytic and parasitocidal powers, but antibodies may be indispensable in promoting an effective interaction between circulating parasites and the stimulated RES.

IDENTIFYING THE IMPORTANT ANTIGENS

Merely to have demonstrated that acquired resistance to a particular parasite is T-cell-dependent does not prove that CMI is involved. The production of antibodies usually requires helper-cell activity. Some antibody classes require much stronger helper-cell activity. It may transpire, therefore, that a protective immune response is contingent upon the induction of an abnormally vigorous T-cell response because of this need for helper cells. We do not yet know for certain whether or not the cells which serve as helper cells and the mediators of cellular immunity are one and the same. Most indications suggest that they are. From a practical viewpoint it may not matter which of the two functional states of the activated T-cell population is involved so long as we have managed to create an effector mechanism that interacts definitively with one or more parasitic antigens.

Most parasites are antigenically complex, but very few of the antigens in a trypanosome, for example, have much influence on the host-parasite relationship. An antigen exposed at the surface might provoke production of an antibody that fixes complement and results in lysis of the parasite, whereas an antigenic nucleoprotein that is not exposed to the immunological apparatus unless the parasite dies is most unlikely to provoke a protective response from the host. This does not mean that all manner of concealed antigens do not act collectively to aid in the building of a defensive response by the host. Imagine, for example, that delayed-type hypersensitivity develops against 10 antigenic components of an organism and that all of them are eventually released at infective foci. Each would contribute something to the intensity of the hypersensitivity reaction developed in the vicinity of the parasite, thereby increasing the effectiveness of the local defenses. In general, however, we must reason that the most important antigens are probably those that are revealed to the immunological apparatus by living parasites. Obviously immunity could not be allowed to depend on the response to antigens that are not released until the parasite dies. This is illustrated in the case of mice infected with tubercle bacilli. The fact that virtually every infecting organism is alive and can be accounted for in the tissues until DTH develops is evidence enough that CMI develops in response to antigens that are shed by living organisms.

The question of selecting the most important antigen for provoking a prophylactic immune response is thus both crucial and difficult. The only obvious approach at present is to identify the antigens to which the actively infected animal actually responds during the early phases of infection. It is during this period that decisive events are shaping the outcome of the host-parasite relation. It is clearly less important to know what happens after the host has learned to kill parasites, hence releasing a multitude of secondary antigens which the immunological apparatus can sense and to which it will no doubt respond. Delayed-type hypersensitivity, or a correlate that can be measured *in vitro*, must be used to test antigenic fractions of the parasite for their capacity to react with specifically sensitized lymphocytes formed in response to infection. We have used DTH as an approach to the problem of determining which antigens are important to the initiation of a protective response to *Listeria monocytogenes*. Actively growing *Listeria* release at least four antigens to their environment; the host responds to each of them. This means that the defense mechanism consists of a composite response to several antigens, each tending to strengthen the host's defensive posture.

HOW TO INDUCE CELL-MEDIATED IMMUNITY

If we have reason to suppose that cell-mediated immunity has an important part to play in acquired resistance to a particular parasite, and the antigens which are important in this respect have been identified, the next and equally difficult problem is to use them for inducing CMI. Herein lies a special problem because antigenic stimulation usually produces little overt evidence of a T-cell response. As a rule, the production of humoral antibody greatly overshadows all other manifestations of immunity. There are exceptions, of course. Natural infections, for example, are commonly associated with DTH, the most conspicuous manifestation of CMI. It is perhaps for this reason that vaccination with living attenuated organisms often provides better protection than do other artificial immunizing procedures.

The reasons for the difficulties encountered in attempting to induce CMI are gradually coming to light as we learn more about the mechanisms involved in the induction and regulation of the immune response. This subject has been difficult to investigate because DTH does not commonly occur except under the distorting influence of adjuvants and is not easily quantified *in vivo* and *in vitro*.

REGULATION OF T-CELL ACTIVITY

Fortunately, the unmodulated immune response of mice to heterologous red cells is attended by strong peripheral manifestations of T-cell activity in the form of DTH. If the dose and route of immunization are suitably chosen, DTH to sheep red blood cells (SRBC) develops consistently without the use of an adjuvant. Whereas small doses of SRBC produce strong DTH in tests performed

4 or 5 days after intravenous immunization, high doses do not. The absence of DTH in animals receiving a large intravenous dose of SRBC is due to the formation of factors that block the cellular mediators of DTH (activated T cells). Blocking is caused by complexes formed between antigen and antibody. Those formed with IgM are the most active in this regard. This inhibitory influence of immune complexes gains emphasis from the fact that splenectomy or differential suppression of B cells by drugs such as cyclophosphamide (CY) results in the development of very high levels of DTH in response to doses of antigen that cause complete suppression of DTH in normal animals.

The conventional way of enhancing the T-cell response is by the use of adjuvants. Freund's complete adjuvant is the time-honored agent for inducing CMI. The idea of using mycobacteria or mycobacterial products to modulate the immune response in favor of T cells had its origins in the discovery that tuberculous animals respond to antigenic stimulation with the development of what was then known as bacterial allergy (i.e., DTH). It transpires that living Bacillus Calmette-Guerin (BCG) is even more effective than Freund's complete adjuvant as a modulator of the immune response, at least to some antigens. To be effective, BCG must be given in advance of the antigenic stimulus because its modulating influence depends, in part at least, upon changes induced in responding lymphoid tissues. Thus, a prior infection of BCG into the footpad causes maximum effect on the subsequent response to an injection of SRBC or soluble microbial antigens given 2 weeks later.

The effects of BCG are probably complex but they certainly include an alteration in susceptibility to T-cell blocking by immune complexes. Mice systemically infected with BCG are almost completely resistant to the blocking effects of specific immune complexes. Although this is almost certainly not the only mode of action of BCG as a modulating agent, it certainly seems to be an important factor, which explains why DTH develops so consistently in this and other infections that impinge directly on the RES. It also explains why high levels of DTH develop when antigens are injected into BCG-infected animals despite the fact that even higher levels of antibody are produced. It is apparent, therefore, that DTH can develop in the presence of a vigorous antibody response, presumably because any complexes that are formed cannot block the formation of activated T cells. It is apparent that since increased levels of T-cell activity can be achieved either by blocking antibody production with CY or by infecting with BCG (a procedure which actually enhances antibody production), it follows that these two agents must act in different ways to potentiate the T-cell response. It is not suprising, therefore, that extraodinary levels of DTH develop when BCG and CY are used jointly to modulate the immune response to SRBC, *Listeria* antigens, and *Plasmodium berghei*.

BCG is a practical agent that could conceivably be used to induce a vigorous T-cell response to antigens which have been properly chosen for their importance in host resistance to a particular parasitic disease. BCG, however, is not the only agent having this effect. Components of the cell walls of mycobacteria, Formalin-killed *Corynebacterium parvum,* carrageenan, dextran sulphates, and *Bordetella pertussis* also are strong modulating agents. Most of them, however, have objectionable side effects that make them less acceptable as modulators of the immune response. It is far from certain, however, that BCG offers the best approach to the solution of this important problem. It is to be hoped that when the constituents which are responsible for the remarkable modulating effects of BCG have been identified, we may be able to modulate immune responses at will for the purpose of achieving virtually any desired effect.

THE IMPORTANCE OF A VIGOROUS T-CELL RESPONSE

Although it is difficult to perceive ways in which CMI can protect against parasites which do not become associated with fixed tissue elements, there are indications that a vigorous T-cell response may be important for an entirely different reason. We know that antibodies which react with viruses do not necessarily provide protection. Nonneutralizing antibodies are found in a number of slow virus infections and in virus carriers of the type seen in congenitally infected subjects. Yet in other circumstances neutralizing antibodies are produced which provide excellent protection against the same virus. Lymphocytic choriomeningitis virus (LCMV) infection of mice provides a good example. Congenitally infected mice become carriers. They form antibodies which react with the virus to form circulating complexes that remain infectious. By analogy with what we know of the effect of immune complex on CMI, the virus-antibody complex would suppress all evidence of DTH and leave the host bereft of any defenses that depend on activated T-cells. An animal in the carrier state, if transfused with T cells from a recently infected adult, is cured of its viremia to the accompaniment of a very vigorous antibody response. The new antibody, however, has virus-neutralizing properties. There is a distinct possibility that the disappearance of virus is due to the formation of a new class of antibodies made possible by the helper function supplied by the transferred cells. This seems to be a more likely explanation of the therapeutic effect of adoptive immunization than to argue, as most do, that CMI is responsible for immunity to LCMV.

Much of what we know about immunity in malaria has a similar ring to it. Immunization has been clearly shown to give rise in both simian and rodent malaria to protective antibodies. Others will have much to say about this subject. It is important to point out, however, that the conditions needed for the induction of a protective antibody response are those that make use of modulating agents which encourage the development of CMI. It is a mistake to conclude on evidence such as this that CMI forms the basis of acquired resistance in this disease. It seems no less likely that the requirement for modulating agents that enhance the T-cell response relates more to formation of antibodies that can protect against malaria than to any direct role of T cells in the mechanism of acquired resistance. This view is based, of course, on a preconception of the ways in which CMI operates. Our present concept holds that specifically reactive T cells increase the supply of mononuclear phagocytes, marshal them at sites of infection, and stimulate them to increase metabolic activity. A mechanism of this sort is ideally suited to combat hemoparasites which exist in an extraerythrocytic phase and are located in extravascular tissues.

CRITERIA BY WHICH TO JUDGE THE IMPORTANCE OF CMI IN HOST RESISTANCE TO INFECTION

I should like to end by proposing a new set of criteria for judging the importance of CMI in any particular infection: (1) There should be no evidence that protection can be conferred by passive transfer of antibody alone. (2) Resistance should be immediately operative in animals immunized adoptively with thymus-derived lymphocytes from immune donors. For this purpose purified T cells should be used with an assay procedure that enables the observer to determine the fate of the parasite before any antibody can be formed in the recipient. (3) The absence of discernible (by immunofluorescence) antibody-forming cells at reactive foci of infection in adoptively immunized subjects. This criterion seems necessary because of the theoretical capacity of activated T cells to promote the local formation of antibody in small but significant amounts. (4) A tissue reaction at sites of infection that is consistent with a T-cell-mediated hypersensitivity reaction. This implies the predominance of monocytes. Radioactive labeling of monocyte precursors helps greatly in evaluating this aspect of the defense mechanism. (5) An inability of the parasite to survive in normal or activated macrophages. This criterion may be difficult to satisfy, but a role for CMI in the defense mechanism is not automatically negated by finding that antibody is also required for an effective defense. There are several examples of parasites that can survive in activated macrophages if they have not been exposed to specific antibody. Their ability to do so appears to result from a paralyzing influence the parasite has on endocytic processes. (6) The most certain indication of CMI, not yet achieved in any known instance, would be to demonstrate that specific immune complexes can abolish DTH and with it the host's resistance to infection. This criterion might be tested in one of two possible ways: (a) The serum of chronically infected subjects may contain the blocking complexes that would prevent adoptive immunization by cell transfer. Only in a very few experimental situations could this test be made. (b) If a purified antigen that gives a DTH reaction in recently infected or convalescent subjects and which provides protection when used to immunize under appropriate modulating conditions is available, immune complexes made with it would interfere with the induction of a protective immune response. The strength of this argument for CMI lies in the fact that immune complexes are strongly immunogenic in their own right. They can provoke a vigorous antibody response.

5

IMMUNOPROPHYLAXIS OF MALARIA: SPOROZOITE-INDUCED IMMUNITY

Ruth S. Nussenzweig

Department of Preventive Medicine
New York University School of Medicine
New York, New York 10010

This chapter reviews the state of knowledge of immunization against malaria using sporozoites as immunizing agents and summarizes recent progress in this field. The demonstration of the immunogenicity of the sporozoite stage and of the occurrence of sporozoite-induced protection was first provided by the classical experiments of Mulligan et al. (1941) on avian malaria. Since then, a considerable amount of information on sporozoite-induced immunity has been obtained through experimental work using the rodent and, more recently, the simian malaria system. We intend to critically review these findings and to correlate them with the information obtained in preliminary vaccination attempts in humans, performed by immunization through the bite of infected irradiated mosquitoes (Clyde et al. 1973a, 1973b, 1975; Rieckmann et al. 1974). Furthermore, we will delineate what we consider to be some of the basic deficiencies in our knowledge of sporozoite-induced immunity and indicate some potentially productive future experimental approaches directed primarily at clarifying protective mechanisms and potentiating the sporozoite-induced immune response.

Progress in two particular research areas will be of considerable importance in determining future advances in sporozoite immunization: (1) Cultivation of the sporogonic cycle of *Plasmodium*, which would result in an adequate parasite supply, and (2) clarification of the initial stages of parasite-host interaction which succeed sporozoite inoculation and determine parasite development in liver cells. To date, few research groups have devoted their efforts to attempt the *in vitro* cultivation of the sporogonic cycle of *Plasmodium* and success has been limited. As for the investigation of sporozoite-host cell interaction, this has recently become feasible due to advances in the *in vitro* maintenance and growth of differentiated hepatocytes and other cell types, and the development of methods of sporozoite purification and concentration.

SPOROZOITE-INDUCED PROTECTIVE IMMUNITY IN RODENT
MALARIA: SOME OF ITS CHARACTERISTICS
AND POSSIBLE MECHANISMS

One of the outstanding characteristics of the protection obtained in sporozoite-immunized mice is that it affords complete resistance against infection. In fact, this immunization does not result in a milder and/or shorter course of parasitemia, but rather the absence of any detectable parasite development upon sporozoite challenge. This has been confirmed by subinoculation of large blood volumes as well as by splenectomy, both of which have failed to reveal the occurrence of subpatent blood infections in the immunized challenged animals (Nussenzweig et al. 1967, 1969a).

Another rather important characteristic of this immune response is that in rodents it provides cross-protection against sporozoites of various other rodent malarial species and subspecies. Thus, it has been observed that immunization of mice with sporozoites of *P. berghei berghei* also protects them against challenge with sporozoites of *P. vinckei vinckei* (Nussenzweig et al. 1969b) and *P. vinckei chabaudi* (Nussenzweig et al. 1972). The latter study also showed the reverse to be true, namely, that immunization with irradiated sporozoites of *P. vinckei chabaudi* produces considerable protection of the mice against challenge with sporozoites of *P. berghei berghei*.

This protection was found to be strictly stage-specific, active only when sporozoites were used as the challenging inoculum. When sporozoite-immunized and protected animals were challenged with erythrocytic stages of the same parasite strain, these animals were fully susceptible, and invariably succumbed after a course of infection which was in every way similar to that of control mice (Nussenzweig et al. 1969b).

It was further determined that sporozoites only acquire the protective antigen(s) at a late stage of their morphogenesis; namely, at the time of their migration to the mosquito's salivary glands, being absent in oocyst sporozoites. Timewise, this coincides with the development of sporozoite invasiveness, since oocyst sporozoites of *P. berghei* almost always fail to induce patent infections. This "maturation" can also be evidenced by serologic means, since antisera produced by immunization with oocyst sporozoites react mainly with the homologous stage and little, if at all, with salivary gland sporozoites (Vanderberg et al. 1972).

Most of these results were obtained through immunization with sporozoites which had been exposed to x-rays or a gamma source of irradiation, so that the parasites had lost their capacity to develop into recognizable liver forms and cause patent blood infections (Vanderberg et al. 1968). It was also observed that the route of immunization was of primary importance, and that in the absence of adjuvants, a reproducible high degree of protection could only be obtained upon repeated intravenous immunization (Spitalny & Nussenzweig 1972), or through the repeated bite of infected irradiated mosquitoes (Vanderberg et al. 1970).

Recently Verhave and Meuwissen (1974) have shown that the injection of viable sporozoites of *P. berghei* into rats or mice, or the exposure of these animals to the bite of infected mosquitoes, followed by suppressive drug treatment, also produced a significant antisporozoite immune response. The effects of this immunity were detectable by a considerable reduction of the number of tissue stages which developed upon sporozoite challenge. The extent of this protection was dose-dependent and increased considerably with the number of immunizing doses, to the point of completely preventing the development of the erythrocytic cycle. These animals also produced detectable antisporozoite antibody levels, but the antibody response to irradiated parasites appeared to be of longer duration than the one induced by infective sporozoites (Spitalny & Nussenzweig 1973a).

The mechanism of sporozoite-induced protection still remains to be fully understood, but it is known to be, at least in part, antibody-mediated. This contention is based on (1) the effects which passive transfer of immune sera have on sporozoite-induced infection, and (2) the *in vitro* effects of immune sera on sporozoite morphology and infectivity.

The transfer of large amounts of immune sera to normal mice just prior to their intravenous inoculation with viable sporozoites resulted in rapid clearance and/or neutralization of the circulating parasites, which after a few minutes were undetectable by blood subinoculation (Nussenzweig et al. 1972). In addition, we found a marked reduction in the number of exoerythrocytic forms in the liver of these animals as compared to normal serum recipients. However, all the immune serum recipients eventually developed fatal patent infections, whereas most of the actively immunized animals remained negative in spite of the large challenging dose. This seems to indicate that in the actively immunized animals an additional and as yet undefined mechanism of protection is operating (besides the humoral immunity) which can be passively transferred by serum.

The *in vitro* effects of immune serum on sporozoite morphology have been examined with the help of phase contrast optics and most recently also by electron microscopy. Sporozoites incubated with immune serum rapidly form a long threadlike precipitate, clearly recognizable under phase microscopy. This has been designated as the circumsporozoite (CSP) reaction (Vanderberg et al. 1969). The precipitate is usually detected at one end of the parasite.

The antibody responsible for this CSP reactivity of immune sera is precipitable by addition of 40% ammonium sulfate. Its activity is increased upon addition of the "CSP cofactor," present in both immune and normal serum, in a fraction nonprecipitable by 40% ammonium sulfate (Spitalny & Nussenzweig 1975a).

The CSP antibodies possess the same species and stage specificity characteristic of protective immunity (Vanderberg et al. 1969). However, there are instances in which animals form CSP antibodies in the absence of any detectable degree of protection, as for example upon immunization with sonicated or otherwise disrupted sporozoites. The reverse has also been observed to occur, that is, the presence of protection in the absence of detectable CSP antibodies, although in most instances these two manifestations of the immune response do coincide.

An example of dissociation of these two phenomena occurs during the early stage of immunization after the administration of a single dose of irradiated sporozoites. Under these conditions, a variable percentage of mice develop protection against challenge at a time (7 days after immunization) when no CSP antibodies can be detected in their sera (Spitalny & Nussenzweig 1973b). Sporozoite immunization of splenectomized mice constitutes another example of this dissociation, since a considerable proportion of these animals becomes protected in the absence of detectable CSP activity (Spitalny & Nussenzweig 1975b).

The *in vitro* incubation of sporozoites with immune sera also results in loss of sporozoite infectivity, detectable by the inoculation of the parasites into normal recipients. This has been designated as sporozoite-neutralizing activity (SNA), found to reside in the immunoglobulin fraction of the sera of sporozoite-immunized animals. Both the sporozoite-neutralizing activity and the CSP reaction are complement-independent, i.e., occur in the absence of participation of components of the complement system (Spitalny & Nussenzweig 1975a).

Protection, as well as the humoral antisporozoite immune response, is thymus-dependent. Thymectomized sporozoite-immunized mice fail to become protected against challenge. Their sera fail to develop SNA, and only a minimal CSP reactivity can be detected in the sera of some of these animals. The immunization of nude mice with viable sporozoites corroborated these results (Spitalny et al. 1975).

Ultrastructural observations of sporozoites incubated in immune, as compared to normal, serum have shown the outer surface membrane of the parasite to be the site of interaction with antibody. Upon immune serum incubation, there is deposition of a very prominent surface coat, which can be revealed both by transmission and scanning electron microscopy. Negative staining and scanning electron microscopy have further shown that this deposition occurs along most of the sporozoite's surface except for the anterior end which frequently appears to be relatively free of precipitate (Cochrane et al. 1975). The threadlike formation that corresponds to the CSP reaction seen under phase microscopy consists of a prolongation of this coat originating from the posterior end of the parasite.

Coat formation was also observed on the surface of metabolically inactive, nonsecreting parasites, such as formalin-treated sporozoites and parasites kept on ice during their incubation with immune serum. This observation indicates that the antibody responsible for coat formation is directed against antigen(s) present on the parasite's surface membrane, and that this reaction does not depend on the secretion of antigen(s) initiated by antibody-parasite interaction. A positive CSP reaction failed, however, to occur under both of these experimental conditions. This reaction was observed to be highly temperature-dependent, and occurred when the temperature of the sporozoite-immune serum mixture was changed from 4 C to 37 C.

The role of the surface properties of sporozoites, and the effect of the surface coat on the tropism of these parasites and their potential for subsequent development within hepatocytes or interaction with other cell types, are entirely open to investigation.

SIMIAN MALARIA IMMUNIZATION: RESULTS IN THE
P. CYNOMOLGI - RHESUS MONKEY SYSTEM

The main purpose of this approach has been to verify if, and to what extent, the findings on sporozoite-induced protective immunity in rodent malaria reflect a more general phenomenon, and are also applicable to a plasmodial-primate system. The use of one or more simian malaria systems in these investigations would permit the establishment of optimal conditions for sporozoite immunization, the investigation of possible potentiators of this immune response, and serve, it is to be hoped, as a model which might produce findings applicable to vaccination attempts in humans.

In addition, it has become important to determine if sporozoites of some simian malarial species would prove to be closely related among themselves, or antigenically related to sporozoites of the human malarial species. If so, then these simian malarias would constitute a potential source for mosquito infections for vaccination purposes and also the *in vitro* cultivation of the sporogonic stages.

The question of the species and strain specificity of the immune response to sporozoites of simian and human malaria was approached by determining the extent of their humoral cross-reactivity using the formation of the circumsporozoite precipitate (CSP reaction) as a parameter of the immune response. This was greatly facilitated by the finding that rats produced CSP antibodies very rapidly and consistently in response to the intravenous injection of sporozoites of various simian and human malarial species (Nussenzweig et al. 1973; Nussenzweig & Chen 1974).

No cross-reactivity was detected among sporozoites of six different species of simian malaria. Even between *P. fieldi* and *P. simiovale,* two malarial species believed to be closely related, no cross-reactivity was observed. Neither did any of these antisera react with sporozoites of two different geographic isolates of the human malarias *P. falciparum* and *P. vivax.* However, antisera produced by immunization with sporozoites of the B strain of *P. cynomolgi* cross-reacted strongly with sporozoites of both the Cambodian and Ceylonensis strains of the same malarial species (Chen 1974).

In addition, antisera produced by immunization of rats with the Thau strain of *P. falciparum* reacted intensively also with sporozoites of the Mark strain of this parasite. No cross-reaction occurred with sporozoites of *P. vivax* nor with any of the various simian malarial species (Nussenzweig & Chen 1974). Based on all these results, the humoral response to sporozoites of simian and human malaria appears to be strictly species-specific and is further characterized by an extensive cross-reactivity among the different geographic isolates (strains) of the same malarial species.

Within the context of the development of a malarial vaccine, it also became important to determine when and where during their sporogonic development sporozoites of simian malaria become infective and immunogenic. The establishment of these parameters is also of importance for studies on the *in vitro* cultivation of *Plasmodium*, providing the possibility of determining functionally the degree of sporozoite maturation reached under certain conditions of *in vitro* cultivation. For the purpose of this investigation, sporozoites of *P. cynomolgi* collected at various periods after an infective blood meal were recovered from mosquito midguts, abdominal hemocele, thoracic hemocele, and salivary glands. Studies on the development of sporozoite antigens during the sporogonic cycle and sporozoite migration in the mosquitoes were conducted using stage-specific antisera obtained in CFN rats injected intravenously with sporozoites of *P. cynomolgi.*

Basically, it was found that salivary gland sporozoites were most immunogenic, i.e., able to induce antisporozoite (CSP) antibody formation, and most reactive when incubated with known antisera. Sporozoites obtained from the hemocele of the thoracic region were less reactive than those obtained from the abdominal hemocele. Midgut sporozoites failed completely to induce CSP antibodies and were totally nonreactive when incubated with antibody-containing antisera.

The capacity of the sporozoites to induce antibody formation tended to increase with length of stay within the salivary glands, reaching maximal levels between the 21st and 25th day after mosquito infection. A further confirmation that sporozoite maturation continued after salivary gland penetration was provided by the finding that salivary gland sporozoites obtained on the 10th day of infection were poorly reactive when tested with known antisera.

In view of these findings, as well as our prior work on the sporogonic stages of *P. berghei* (Vanderberg et al. 1972), sporozoite maturation appears to be gradual, possibly involving various steps. This still leaves unsolved the basic question concerning the nature and identification of the factors that lead to the formation, expression, and/or release of certain sporozoite antigens. Studies of surface antigens of sporozoites and further investigations of the nature of the interaction of these parasites with antibodies might provide some of these answers.

Development of sporozoite infectivity was determined by inoculating sporozoite populations recovered at various times, from different mosquito regions, into rhesus monkeys. In each experiment a monkey injected with salivary gland sporozoites served as a control of infectivity for the sporozoites obtained on the same occasion from the remaining mosquito regions. Besides patency, the length of the prepatent period was used as an additional parameter to evaluate sporozoite infectivity.

We found a certain delay of patency in the monkeys injected with hemocele sporozoites, suggesting that the parasites had a lower degree of infectivity prior to their localization in the salivary glands. Monkeys injected with midgut sporozoites repeatedly failed to become patent.

Vaccination against simian malaria by immunization with sporozoites has been attempted by several groups of investigators in recent years. All of these studies have made use of the same host-parasite system, namely, immunization of the rhesus (*Macaca mulatta*) with irradiated sporozoites of *P. cynomolgi*.

The preliminary reports of two of these attempts indicate that in both instances the authors failed to observe total protection against sporozoite challenge. Collins and Contacos (1972) observed a certain delay in patency in the two rhesus which had been immunized by the intravenous injection of five doses totaling approximately 1×10^5 salivary gland sporozoites. This delay in patency was interpreted by the authors to be suggestive of a reduction in the number of sporozoites able to develop into tissue stages in the immunized animals.

The other report (Ward & Hayes 1972) is based on the immunization of three rhesus by the bite of *P. cynomolgi*-infected irradiated *Anopheles stephensi*. Each rhesus was submitted on three occasions to the bite of 25 to 30 infected irradiated mosquitoes, and challenged also by mosquito bite less than 2 months after the first immunizing dose. The total number of irradiated parasites introduced in the immunized animals consisted, according to the author's estimate, of a maximum of 9×10^4 sporozoites. This is a very small immunizing dose if we consider that indeed it is considerably less than the dosage we determined to be necessary to protect a mouse against sporozoite challenge.

Our own investigation involving the vaccination of rhesus with sporozoites of *P. cynomolgi* was mainly directed at (1) determining optimal conditions of immunization with regard to schedule and route of antigen administration and (2) establishing various parameters of the sporozoite-induced immune response and their possible correlation with protection. The results of these vaccination attempts were evaluated by determining the rate of development of antisporozoite antibodies and the degree of protection of these animals against challenge.

Two distinct types of antisporozoite antibody activities were detected and quantitated in the immunized animals: (1) the presence of CSP antibodies; and (2) sporozoite-neutralizing activity (SNA), which resulted in loss of infectivity upon incubation of the sporozoites with immune serum. The criterion for protection of these animals was either complete resistance to an intravenous challenge with viable sporozoites, or partial resistance resulting in delayed patency and possibly also in an altered course of infection.

The length of the period of immunization of any given group of animals was based on titers of CSP antibodies and, whenever possible, also on the degree of sporozoite-neutralizing activity. The experiments were also planned so that we could obtain data on the efficiency of various time and dose schedules of immunization in an attempt to define optimal conditions to obtain protection. The challenge doses, either 1×10^3 or 2×10^4 sporozoites, varied in the course of our vaccination attempts due to changes in sporozoite infectivity.

Our results, based on the immunization of 18 animals, demonstrate that extensive or total protection of rhesus monkeys against sporozoite challenge was obtained only after a period of immunization of several months and the administration of multiple immunizing doses (Chen 1974).

The use of relatively large individual and total immunizing doses certainly favors the development of protective immunity. The two animals which were totally protected against challenge had received a total of 4.0×10^7 and 1.7×10^8 sporozoites over a period of 9.5 and 13.5 months, respectively.

On the basis of preliminary results, three conditions of immunization appeared to be quite promising with regard to the possibility of inducing a more efficient immune response: (1) multiple immunization, at short intervals, by the bite of irradiated infected mosquitoes; (2) pretreatment of the monkeys with *Corynebacterium parvum*, a potent reticuloendothelial system stimulant; and (3) incubation of the irradiated sporozoites with normal serum prior to their inoculation into rhesus monkeys. These experimental conditions induce an unusually rapid CSP antibody response in the immunized rhesus and are known to enhance resistance to sporozoite-induced rodent malaria (unpublished results).

We have also tested the neutralizing activity of serum samples obtained at various stages of the immunization of five rhesus monkeys. In each experiment, we included sporozoites incubated with normal monkey serum as a control. By injecting these preincubated sporozoites into normal recipients, it was noticed that the animals which received sporozoites incubated in normal serum consistently developed early patency (mean, 9.5 days). In all but one instance, the prepatent period of the animals injected with sporozoites pretreated with immune serum was considerably longer (mean, 12.6 days). Incubation of sporozoites with two serum samples obtained on different dates from a totally protected rhesus resulted in complete neutralization, i.e., loss of parasite infectivity (Chen 1974).

These data on sporozoite neutralization in immunized rhesus are still limited, but the results appear to be similar to those obtained in rodent malaria and seem to indicate that SNA correlates well with protective immunity. The mechanism of this serum-mediated loss of sporozoite infectivity, and its possible role in sporozoite induced protection *in vivo* still remains to be clarified. Present investigations of the effects of serum pretreatment on sporozoite-cell interaction will hopefully provide some insight into the nature of SNA.

The animals' immune response to sporozoite vaccination was also monitored by titrating the CSP activity of their sera. Considerable individual variations in their antibody responses became evident when we compared serum samples of rhesus submitted to similar schedules of immunization. The time-span after which we first found detectable CSP antibodies varied considerably in our series of animals, i.e., from the 10th up to the 200th day after the first injection of irradiated sporozoites of *P. cynomolgi*. In most animals, however, this time-span ranged between 1.5 and 3 months after their initial immunizing dose.

This differs quite markedly from the rather constant pattern of CSP antibody response which we have observed in mice and rats immunized with irradiated sporozoites of *P. berghei* (Spitalny & Nussenzweig 1973). Furthermore, these rodents frequently had detectable CSP antibodies 2 to 3 weeks after a first immunizing dose and never failed to become CSP-positive 3 to 4 days after the second sporozoite injection.

The observed pattern of CSP antibody response in rhesus is certainly not due to lack of antigenicity of the sporozoites of *P. cynomolgi*, since rats as well as mice produce, within 2 weeks, a detectable CSP antibody response to these parasites (Nussenzweig et al. 1973). The variability of the CSP antibody response of rhesus monkeys to immunization with sporozoites of *P. cynomolgi* might therefore be a peculiarity of this particular host-parasite association. Alternatively, it is also quite possible that our initial immunizing dose (sporozoite number) was, in many instances, close to a minimal threshold below which the individual differences of responsiveness of the animals became considerably amplified.

In this regard, it might be noteworthy to recall that this variability of the CSP antibody response of the sporozoite-immunized rhesus monkeys resembles the results obtained in a very limited series of humans, where only two out of four volunteers on the same schedule of immunization produced detectable CSP antibody levels (Clyde et al. 1973a, 1975).

We find it conceivable, however, that the immunization of rhesus with sporozoites of another simian malarial species might produce quite different results, not only with regard to the development of antisporozoite antibodies, but also protection. In fact, a more acute and severe simian malarial infection would present greater similarities with the rodent system in which sporozoite immunization is highly effective. Since an acute severe simian malaria would also present greater analogies with the course of *P. falciparum* infections in man, such a simian malaria might well constitute a better model for sporozoite immunization than the presently used *P. cynomolgi*-rhesus system.

IMMUNIZATION OF MAN AGAINST SPOROZOITE-INDUCED MALARIA

Two groups of investigators have reported results on the immunization of man against malaria through the bite of infected irradiated mosquitoes. Clyde et al. (1973a, 1975) immunized four volunteers against *P. falciparum*, two of whom developed CSP antibodies and became protected against sporozoite challenge for a period of several months. Antisporozoite antibodies as well as protective immunity were both species-specific, since these volunteers were not protected against challenge with *P. vivax*, nor did their sera cross-react with sporozoites of this malarial species. The protection was, however, fully effective against a number of isolates (strains) of *P. falciparum*, from widely different geographic areas, including a strain not used for the immunization (Clyde et al. 1973b, 1975). The sera of these volunteers also reacted strongly with the sporozoites of all these various geographic isolates of *P. falciparum*. This is analogous to what we had observed with regard to the cross-reactivity of different strains of *P. cynomolgi*, and the interstrain reactivity of antibodies to human malaria sporozoites produced in rats (Chen 1974, Nussenzweig & Chen 1974).

One of the volunteers was subsequently also immunized against sporozoites of *P. vivax*. He became protected for a period between 3 and 6 months and developed the same type of geographically broad interstrain protection and serum reactivity (Clyde et al. 1975). An additional case of successful immunization with sporozoites of *P. falciparum* was recently reported by Rieckmann et al. (1974), who used irradiated mosquitoes infected with an Ethiopian strain of this malarial species.

CONCLUSION

Considering all the presently available information on sporozoite-induced immunity, the following conclusions regarding the present state of the art as well as future research goals seem to be justified:

1. That the preliminary results of the immunization of volunteers with sporozoites of *P. falciparum* and *P. vivax* have corroborated much of the earlier evidence on sporozoite-induced protection in experimental animals and demonstrated the occurrence of this protection in man.

2. That this protection is relatively short-lived and occurs only in a certain percentage of individuals and thus needs to be enhanced or potentiated. This might possibly be achieved through the use of sporozoite preparations of greater immunogenicity, and/or through the concomitant use of an appropriate adjuvant.

3. That the mechanism of this protection still fails to be fully understood although the experimental models have permitted the obtaining of some information regarding its mode of action. The identification of the type of immune response responsible for protection might permit a more rational approach toward the goal of increasing its effectiveness, and thus be of considerable value for the development of a malarial vaccine.

4. That virtually nothing is known with regard to the nonspecific mechanisms of resistance, including the mode of sporozoite-host cell interaction in a nonimmune host. Such knowledge might provide clues enabling us to interfere with the development of sporozoites into tissue stages.

5. That further progress in sporozoite immunization and any perspective of practical application of a malarial vaccine is contingent upon advances in the *in vitro* cultivation of these parasite stages.

BIBLIOGRAPHY

Chen, D. 1974. Aspects of host-parasite interactions in the rhesus *P. cynomolgi-A. stephensi* system. Ph.D. Thesis. New York University School of Medicine.

Clyde, D.F., Most, H., McCarthy, V.C. & Vanderberg, J.P. 1973. Immunization of man against sporozoite-induced falciparum malaria. *Am. J. Med. Sci.* 266: 169-177.

Clyde, D.F., McCarthy, V.C., Miller, R.M. & Hornick, R.B. 1973b. Specificity of protection of man immunized against sporozoite-induced falciparum malaria. *Am. J. Med. Sci.* 266: 398-403.

Clyde, D.F., McCarthy, V.C., Miller, R.M. & Woodward, W.E. 1975. Immunization of man against falciparum and vivax malaria by use of attenuated sporozoites. *Am. J. Trop. Med. Hyg.* 24: 397-401.

Cochrane, A.H., Aikawa, M. & Nussenzweig, R.S. 1976. Ultrastructural observations on sporozoite-antibody interaction in rodent and simian malaria. *J. Immunol.* 116: 859-867.

Collins, E.W. & Contacos, P.G. 1972. Immunization of monkeys against *Plasmodium cynomolgi* by x-irradiated sporozoites. *Nat. New Biol.* 236: 176-177.

Mulligan, H.W., Russell, P.F. & Mohan, B.N. 1941. Active immunization of fowls against *Plasmodium gallinaceum* by injections of killed homologous sporozoites. *J. Malar. Inst. India.* 4: 25-34.

Nussenzweig, R.S., Vanderberg, J., Most, H. & Orton, C. 1967. Protective immunity produced by injection of x-irradiated sporozoites of *Plasmodium berghei. Nature* (Lond.). 216: 160-162.

Nussenzweig, R., Vanderberg, J. & Most, H. 1969a. Protective immunity produced by the injection of x-irradiated sporozoites of *Plasmodium berghei.* IV. Dose response, specificity and humoral immunity. *Mil. Med.* 134: 1176-82.

Nussenzweig, R.S., Vanderberg, J.P., Most, H. & Orton, C. 1969b. Specificity of protective immunity produced by x-irradiated *Plasmodium berghei* sporozoites. *Nature* (Lond.). 222: 488-489.

Nussenzweig, R., Vanderberg, J., Spitalny, G.L., Rivera, C.I.O., Orton, C. & Most, H. 1972a. Sporozoite-induced immunity in mammalian malaria. A review. *Am. J. Trop. Med. Hyg.* 21: 722-728.

Nussenzweig, R.S., Vanderberg, J.P., Sanabria, Y. & Most H. 1972b. *Plasmodium berghei:* accelerated clearance of sporozoites from blood as part of immune-mechanism in mice. *Exp. Parasitol.* 31: 88-97.

Nussenzweig, R., Montuori, W., Spitalny, G.L. & Chen, D. 1973. Antibodies against sporozoites of human and simian malaria produced in rats. *J. Immunol.* 110: 600-601.

Nussenzweig, R.S. & Chen, D. 1974. The antibody response to sporozoites of simian and human malaria parasites: Its stage and species specificity and strain cross-reactivity. *Bull. WHO* 50: 293-297.

Rieckmann, K., Carson, P., Beaudoin, R., Cassels, J. & Sell, K. 1974. Sporozoite-induced immunity in man against an Ethiopian strain of *Plasmodium falciparum* (Letter). *Trans. R. Soc. Trop. Med. Hyg.* 68: 258-259.

Spitalny, G. & Nussenzweig, R. 1972. Effect of various routes of immunization and methods of parasite attenuation on the development of protection against sporozoite-induced rodent malaria. *Proc. Helminthol. Soc. Wash.* 39: 506-514.

Spitalny, G. & Nussenzweig, R.S. 1973. *Plasmodium berghei:* relationship between protective immunity and antisporozoite (CSP) antibody in mice. *Exp. Parasitol.* 33: 168-178.

Spitalny, G.L. & Nussenzweig, R.S. 1975a. Properties of antisporozoite antibodies against *Plasmodium berghei.* Submitted for publication.

Spitalny, G.L. & Nussenzweig, R.S. 1976. *Plasmodium berghei:* Role of the spleen in the development and expression of sporozoite-induced immunity. *Exp. Parasit.* 40: 179-188.

Spitalny, G.L., Verhave, J.P., Meuwissen, J.H.E. Th. & Nussenzweig, R.S. 1977 T-cell dependence of sporozoite-induced immunity in rodent malaria. *Exp. Parasitol.*

Vanderberg, J., Nussenzweig, R., Most, H. & Orton, C. 1968. Protective immunity produced by the injection of x-irradiated sporozoites of *Plasmodium berghei.* II. Effects of radiation on sporozoites. *J. Parasitol.* 54: 1175-1180.

Vanderberg, J., Nussenzweig, R. & Most, H. 1969. Protective immunity produced by the injection of x-irradiated sporozoites of *Plasmodium berghei.* V. *In vitro* effects of immune serum on sporozoites. *Mil. Med.* 134: 1183-1190.

Vanderberg, J., Nussenzweig, R. & Most, H. 1970. Protective immunity produced by the bite of x-irradiated mosquitoes infected with *Plasmodium berghei.* *J. Parasitol.* 56: 350-351.

Vanderberg, J., Nussenzweig, R., Sanabria, Y., Nawrot, D. & Most, H. 1972. Stage specificity of antisporozoite antibodies in rodent malaria and its relationship to protective immunity. *Proc. Helminthol. Soc. Wash.* 39: 514-525.

Verhave, J.P. & Meuwissen, J.H.E. Th. 1974. Inhibition of exo-erythrocytic form development following reinoculation with sporozoites of *P. berghei.* *In* The Proceedings of the International Congress on Parasitology: 1243-1244.

Ward, R.A. & Hayes, D.E. 1972. Attempted immunization of rhesus monkeys against cynomolgi malaria with irradiated sporozoites. *Proc. Helminthol. Soc. Wash.* 39: 525-529.

6

IMMUNIZATION AGAINST ERYTHROCYTIC FORMS OF MALARIA PARASITES

S. Cohen, G. A. Butcher, and G. H. Mitchell

Department of Chemical Pathology
Guy's Hospital Medical School
London, SE1 9RT

INTRODUCTION

It is almost 20 years since a worldwide program of malaria eradication was formally adopted by the 8th World Health Assembly and its implementation coordinated by the World Health Organization (WHO). The strategy of eradication involved widespread indoor spraying with residual insecticides and elimination of remaining foci using antimalarial drugs and further spraying. The success of this international endeavor can be judged from a recent WHO report showing that malaria has been eradicated or controlled in almost 80% of originally malarious zones.* However, the remaining areas where eradication could not be implemented include 66 countries covering vast tracts of the developing world, notably in Africa, inhabited by about 500 million people. Reliable data are not available from these areas, but it seems likely that malaria at present produces a morbidity rate of 100 million and mortality of about 1 million per annum, mainly among young children. Moreover, the resurgence of malaria in Pakistan, Bangladesh, Sri Lanka, and several Indian provinces that all had advanced eradication programs is a source of much alarm. It is clear that tropical areas still harbor a vast reservoir of malarial infection and that its eradication or even containment is no longer feasible with available health facilities.

Under these circumstances, attempts to find alternative ways of attacking the malaria parasite are obviously of interest and importance. Clinical observations on acquired resistance to human malaria and experimental studies had long indicated that vaccination against malaria may be feasible, but no practical method could be envisaged for developing a human vaccine.

---

*WHO Technical report series Number 549, 1974.

MALARIA LIFE CYCLE

Four species of malaria infect man, *Plasmodium falciparum, P. vivax, P. ovale,* and *P. malariae* (Table 1), the first being by far the most lethal. Certain simian malarias may infect man, but these are not of epidemiologic importance. The parasite has a complex life cycle involving man and the mosquito (Figure 1). Sporozoites inoculated by female *Anopheles* mosquitoes disappear within 1 hour from the circulation and develop within hepatic parenchymal cells into schizonts (preerythrocytic forms). One sporozoite of *P. falciparum* may produce 40,000 merozoites, whereas those of *P. vivax, P. ovale,* and *P. malariae* yield approximately 10,000, 15,000, and 2,000, respectively (Miller 1975). The preerythrocytic merozoites liberated from parenchymal cells enter the bloodstream and invade erythrocytes. Within red cells the parasite develops into an asexual, multinuclear schizont that contains 6 to 24 merozoites, depending on the species.

Table 1

Summary of the Biologic and Clinical Characteristics
of the Four Human Malarias[a]

	P. falciparum	*P. vivax*	*P. ovale*	*P. malariae*
Worldwide incidence	common	common	uncommon	uncommon
Incubation period	7-27 days	10-40 days	12-26 days	18-76 days
Persistence of infection	$<$3 years	$<$3 years	$<$3 years	many years
Cycle in red cell	48 hours	48 hours	48 hours	72 hours
Red cell age preference	all ages	young	young	old
Parasitemia	high (up to 60%)	low ($<$1%)	low ($<$1%)	low ($\ll$1%)
Mortality	high	low	low	low
Chloroquine resistance	present	absent	absent	absent

(a) From Miller et al. (1975).

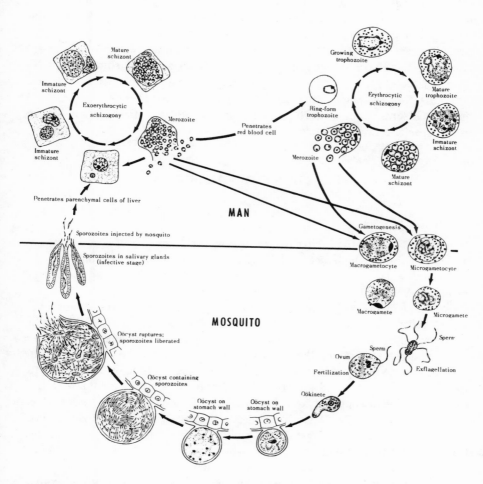

Figure 1. The sexual and asexual cycles of the malaria parasite. (From Sadun 1976.)

Each merozoite released from the ruptured erythrocyte rapidly invades another red cell. The asexual cycle continues at 48-hour (*P. falciparum, P. vivax,* and *P. ovale*) or 72-hour (*P. malariae*) intervals. Clinical disease and naturally acquired immunity in malaria are associated with the cycle in the erythrocyte. Exoerythrocytic development within the liver causes no clinical symptoms and apparently induces no immunity. For reasons that are undefined, some merozoites differentiate into male and female gametocytes that complete the life cycle within the *Anopheles* mosquito (Figure 1). Whether or not relapse infections from hepatic schizonts occur after the primary process of development in any human malaria species is now uncertain.

RESISTANCE TO MALARIA

Innate Resistance

Individual species of malaria parasites show a high degree of host specificity. The mechanisms which determine susceptibility or innate resistance are not completely understood, but available evidence implicates the properties of host erythrocytes rather than serum (Butcher et al. 1973).

One fundamental requirement for infectivity is the presence of an appropriate red cell receptor for malaria merozoites (Butcher et al. 1973; Miller et al. 1973). Parasites are specifically orientated during attachment and adhere by the conoid end before invading the red cell (Figure 2). The nature of the merozoite receptor is uncertain, but in *P. knowlesi* it appears susceptible to the proteolytic enzymes chymotrypsin and pronase and is unaffected by neuraminidase (Miller et al. 1973). The susceptibility of human red cells to *P. knowlesi* can be correlated with the presence of the Duffy blood group Fy^a or Fy^b. The frequent absence of Duffy determinants in West Africans and American blacks may account for their well-known resistance to *P. vivax*, which contrasts with their susceptibility to the other three species of human malaria (Miller et al. 1975).

Several intraerythrocytic factors influence parasite development and contribute to innate resistance. Among these are structural modifications in hemoglobin (especially hemoglobin S), quantitative changes in hemoglobin chain synthesis (thalassaemia), glucose-6-phosphate dehydrogenase (G-6-PD) deficiency, and levels of adenosine triphosphate (ATP). Evidence that these factors influence malarial infection is based largely upon epidemiological studies, but *in vitro* analysis of the capacity of different red cell types to allow penetration and development of *P. falciparum* are beginning to provide more conclusive data (Luzzatto 1974).

Acquired Resistance

Specific Malarial Antibody

Chronic malarial infection in man provides a most potent stimulus for Ig synthesis. The reduced IgG production observed in West Africans maintained on malarial prophylactic therapy (Cohen et al. 1961) suggests that in subjects exposed to chronic infection about one third of the circulating immunoglobulin might consist of malarial antibody. Specific antibody can be demonstrated in immune sera by several serologic tests including precipitation, agglutination, opsonization, antibody fluorescence, and complement fixation. The fact that the serologic cross-reactions between malarial species revealed by these tests cannot be correlated with cross-immunity indicates that much of the specific antibody formed during infection does not have a protective function.

Protective Malarial Antibody

Acquired immunity in malaria is directed mainly against the asexual parasite cycle in the blood. Circulating gametocytes of *P. falciparum* are apparently unaffected by immune serum, although in some monkey malarias immunity may be associated with a loss of gametocyte viability in the mosquito host. Immunity to the erythrocytic stage of infection does not modify the exoerythrocytic development of malaria parasites in man, chimpanzee, or monkey (Garnham 1970) but suppresses the subsequent phase of erythrocytic development.

The role of serum antibody in acquired malarial immunity has been established by passive transfer tests in monkey and human infections and, to a lesser degree, in rodent malaria (reviewed by Brown 1969). These studies suggested that protective antibody acts against either mature schizonts or extracellular merozoites and provided some information about the classes of immunoglobulin associated with immune protection (Cohen et al. 1961). However, passive transfer tests do not provide a suitable basis for detailed investigations on the mechanism of malarial immunity.

Serum from rhesus monkeys immune to *P. knowlesi* inhibits the cyclic proliferation of the parasite maintained *in vitro* (Cohen et al. 1969). Parasite growth was assessed by incorporation of [^{3}H] leucine into parasite protein using cultures giving average multiplication rates of at least sixfold in 24 hours. Immune serum had no effect upon the growth of intracellular parasites but inhibited the cycle of development that followed schizogony. This effect was species-specific, as was shown by the failure of serum from a monkey immune to *P. cynomolgi*

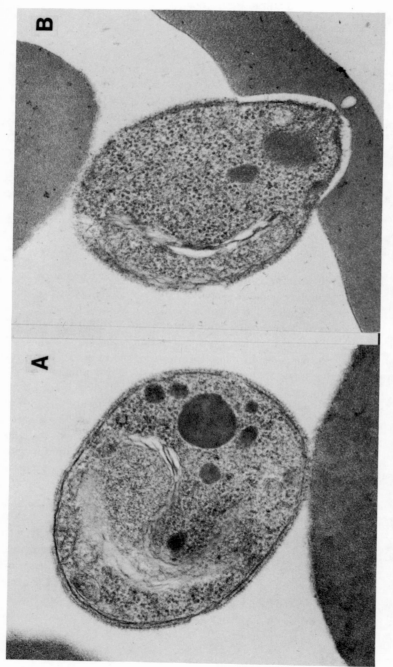

Figure 2.   Stages in the penetration of a red blood cell by a malaria parasite.   The merozoite attaches randomly to the surface of the red cell (A), becomes orientated by the conoid end (B), invaginates the red cell (C), and finally lies within the erythrocyte leaving the outer coat in the extracellular fluid (D). The process is completed within one minute.   (From Bannister et al. 1975.) X 35,000.

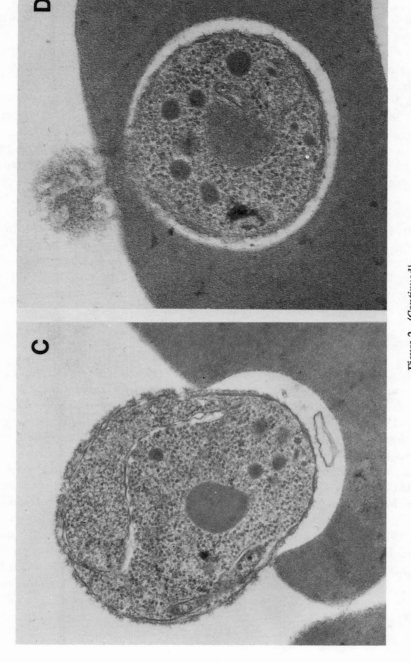

Figure 2. *(Continued)*

bastianellii to inhibit *P. knowlesi.* The action of immune serum is not complement-dependent, being unaffected either by heating at 56 C for 3 hours or by the addition of fresh normal monkey serum as a source of complement. Moreover, the bivalent fragments of immune IgG are actively antiparasitic. The degree of parasite inhibition is dose-dependent. In the sera studied, protective antibody was associated with both IgG and IgM but not with IgA or IgE (Cohen & Butcher 1970).

There has long been a need in malarial research for a dependable *in vitro* technique for the detection of protective malarial antibody. The schizont-infected red cell agglutination test (SICA) (Brown & Brown 1965) and the assay of inhibitory antibody described above (Cohen et al. 1969) have been proposed for this purpose. Comparison of these antibody activities with the clinical immune status of rhesus monkeys reveals that SICA antibody titers of appropriate specificity may be high in susceptible animals or undetectable in immune animals. On the other hand, inhibitory antibody levels correlated with immune status in all situations studied by Butcher & Cohen (1972). Repeated infection induced inhibitory antibody against variants that had never given rise to patent infections and this correlated with clinical resistance to such variants on challenge (Butcher & Cohen 1972). This indicated that merozoites, which are inactivated in the inhibitory assay, carry antigens of broad variant specificity—a prediction confirmed by cross-absorption studies (Cohen et al. 1972).

Synergistic Action of Malarial Antibody and Cells

These observations indicated that the inhibitory antibodies assayed during *in vitro* culture initiate specific protective immunity *in vivo*. This antibody is probably directed against merozoites (Cohen et al. 1961; Cohen et al. 1969; Diggs & Osler 1975; Miller et al. 1975) and its action *in vitro* is independent of complement or cells and is analogous to viral neutralizing antibody. Inhibitory antibodies are predominantly IgG. Since this class is cytophilic for macrophages and K cells, it seems certain that cell-mediated killing of parasites must occur in the living animal. The phagocytic activity of macrophages has long been recognized in malaria, and the role of specific antibody in promoting macrophage ingestion of parasites has been demonstrated *in vitro* and *in vivo* (Brown & Hills 1974; Coleman et al. 1975). Synergism between cells and antibody is suggested by the finding that immune splenic cells confer greater protection than serum when passively transferred to rats challenged with *P. berghei* (Phillips 1970). Similarly, the antimalarial action of passively transferred immune serum in rats is greatly diminished by previous splenectomy of the normal recipients (Golsener et al. 1975).

Both clinical and experimental observations suggest that antibodies may neutralize toxic malarial products but the nature of these is undefined. Damaged intracellular erythrocytic parasites (crisis forms) appear in many malarial infections during resolution of parasitemia. It is significant that this effect has never been reproduced by antibody *in vitro* and its mechanism remains unknown.

Role of Specific Cell-Mediated Immunity in Malaria

The proven role of serum antibody outlined above does not exclude the possibility that cell-mediated immunity, dependent upon actively sensitized lymphocytes of thymic origin, may play a part in specific acquired resistance to malaria. Attempts to demonstrate this have rested upon the finding that thymectomized rats are more susceptible than control animals to subsequent infection with *P. berghei* (Brown et al. 1968). Also, anti-rat thymocyte serum (ATS) raised in rabbits reduces the resistance of rats to subsequent infection with *P. berghei* (Spira et al. 1970). The interpretation of these findings solely in terms of cell-mediated responses is complicated by the fact that the majority of antigens are now known to require cooperation between thymus (T) and marrow (B) cells for induction of specific serum antibody. It follows that thymectomy or ATS may render animals susceptible to malarial infection by reducing the serum-antibody response. Lymphoid cells transferred from immune rats to inbred non-immune animals confer resistance to *P. berghei*. (Stechschulte 1969.) This finding cannot, however, be taken as evidence for cell-mediated immunity alone, since such cells are capable of producing specific antimalarial antibody (Phillips 1970).

Immune lymphocytes are not antiparasitic when tested *in vitro* (Phillips et al. 1970), even at ratios of up to 100 sensitized cells per parasitized erythrocyte (Butcher 1975). Nevertheless, it remains true that passive transfer of immunity to the erythrocytic stages of rodent malaria is much more effective with cells than with serum, since only the former can eliminate the infection, indicating that the cells do more than simply secrete antibody. Transfer of selected cell populations has produced conflicting results. Treatment of *P. berghei*-infected rats with antithymocyte serum reduced the ability of lymphoid cells from these animals to transfer immunity, whereas cell suspensions from which immunoglobulin-secreting B cells had been removed with an anti-Ig column were still capable of transferring immunity (Brown 1973, 1974). On the other hand, treatment of mice immune to *P. yoelii* with cyclophosphamide, which affects mainly B lymphocytes, reduced the ability of cells from these mice to confer protection to nonimmune recipients (Jayawardena et al. 1975). In addition, anti-θ serum treatment *in vitro* of the cells from mice that had recovered from this infection did not impair the ability of these cells to transfer immunity effectively to either intact or T-cell-deprived recipients (Jayawardena et al. 1975).

Isolation and Properties of Merozoites

Since studies on the mechanism of acquired malarial immunity suggested that merozoites have a central role in the induction of protective immunity, attempts were made to isolate blood-stage merozoites uncontaminated by other cells. Since merozoites very rapidly reinvade normal erythrocytes (Trager 1956; Dvorak et al. 1975; Bannister et al. 1975), their isolation required *in vitro* cultivation of parasitized cells relatively free of normal red cells. Under these conditions, extracellular merozoites progressively accumulate in the culture medium and a second step in their isolation requires separation from parasitized cells. In the case of *P. knowlesi*, schizont-infected erythrocytes containing fewer than 5% normal red cells can be obtained by centrifugation of highly parasitized blood from rhesus monkeys. The parasitized cells were cultured in modified medium 199 (Mitchell et al. 1973). Free merozoites present in the medium after several hours were separated from remaining intact schizonts by precipitation of the latter with antischizont antisera or, more effectively, with phytohemagglutinin (Figure 3) (Mitchell et al. 1974). The yield of merozoites with this method is about 2×10^{10} per milliliter of cultured schizonts, and contamination with normal or infected red cells is less than 0.1%. These merozoite preparations have limited viability (Mitchell et al. 1973) and are therefore of little value for studying the physiological properties of the extracellular parasite. A method for isolating merozoites as they are released from schizonts was therefore devised using polycarbonate sieves in association with a culture chamber (Figures 4 and 5). (Dennis et al. 1975).

Polycarbonate sieves with cylindrical pores of diameter 3 μm or more allow 100% transmission of human red blood cells, which have a mean diameter of 7.2 μm. This observation suggested that the normal red blood cell membrane is deformable but nonextensible, an assumption consistent with the finding that red blood cells hardened in acetaldehyde fail to pass pores 6.8 μm diameter (Gregersen et al. 1967). Rhesus cells containing schizonts have a maximum diameter similar to normal erythrocytes. The schizonts of *P. knowlesi* appear relatively nondeformable (Miller et al. 1971) and, in contrast to normal rhesus erythrocytes and those containing rings or trophozoites, are largely retained by polycarbonate membranes with 3-μm diameter pores. Free merozoites are usually ovoid with a minimum diameter of about 1.5-μm (Bannister et al. 1975) and pass freely through polycarbonate sieves with 2- or 3-μm diameter pores. These properties of the free and intracellular parasites can be exploited for the isolation of free merozoites.

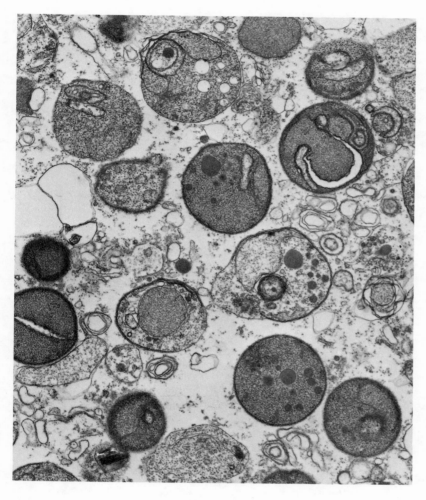

Figure 3. Electron microscopy of merozoites prepared by phytohemagglutinin (from Mitchell et al. 1974).

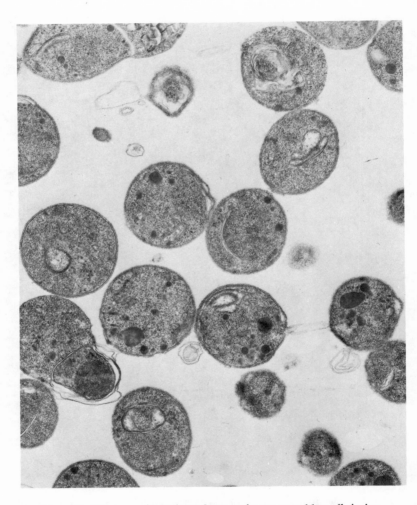

Figure 4. Electron microscopy of merozoites prepared by cell sieving. (From Dennis et al. 1975.)

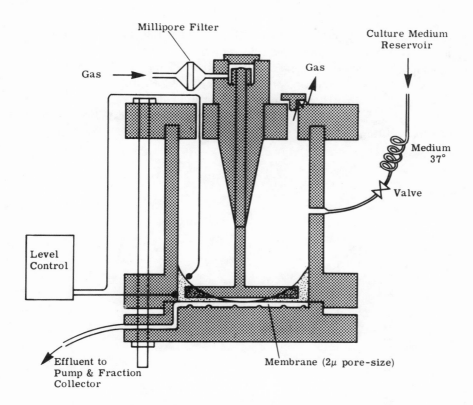

Figure 5. Diagram of culture chamber with polycarbonate sieve for isolation of merozoites. (From Dennis et al. 1975.)

Certain *Plasmodium* species (e.g., *P. falciparum*) are characterized by asynchronous parasite development and mature parasites are scanty in the peripheral circulation. Parasitized and normal cells cannot therefore be separated by centrifugation of infected blood. In such circumstances, parasites could be matured *in vitro* and the culture then continued in a 3-μm cell sieve chamber. Uninfected red cells and immature parasites would thereby be eliminated leaving a population of maturing schizonts suitable for merozoite isolation in a 2-μm sieve chamber.

For the isolation of *P. knowlesi* merozoites, the cell sieve method has proved superior to the techniques previously described. Parasite preparations are relatively free of erythrocytic membranes and other cell debris and minimally contaminated with schizonts when 2-μm sieves are used (Figure 5). The yield of merozoites is approximately 50% of the theoretical value, compared with a maximum of 15% with earlier techniques. The most significant advantage of cell sieving is that merozoites are isolated from ruptured schizonts soon after their release, when a significant proportion are viable (Dennis et al. 1975). The capacity of free merozoites to penetrate red cells and initiate a further cycle of erythrocytic development is almost completely lost within 30 minutes (Figure 6). This explains why in most experiments less than 2% of merozoites were viable after isolation by differential agglutination (Mitchell et al. 1973). The use of cell sieving for a study of *P. knowlesi* merozoite morphology and red cell attachment and penetration has been described by Bannister et al. (1975) (Figure 2).

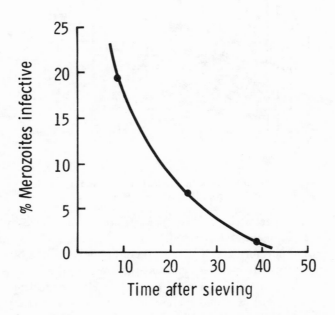

Figure 6. Percentage of *P. knowlesi* merozoites that invade normal rhesus red cells measured at intervals after merozoite release from ruptured schizonts.
(From Dennis et al. 1975.)

VACCINATION AGAINST ERYTHROCYTIC FORMS OF MALARIA

A variety of experimental methods have been used to induce immunity against erythrocytic forms of malaria species. These include drug-controlled infections and inoculation of attenuated parasites, irradiated parasites, parasitized erythrocytes in adjuvants, parasite fractions, and free merozoites (reviewed in Cohen 1975). Many studies have employed relatively avirulent infections, e.g., certain species of rodent malaria, and the significance of results was equivocal. *P. knowlesi* malaria in the rhesus monkey is invariably fatal, so that this host-parasite combination provides the most stringent of all models available for testing a malarial vaccine. The present analysis will be confined to experiments conducted with this system.

The appearance of intrastrain antigenic variants during the course of the asexual cycle of *P. knowlesi* was established by Brown & Brown (1965) on the basis of the SICA test. Subsequent experience makes it certain that this capacity to express different serotypes is an important mechanism promoting survival of *P. knowlesi* in the rhesus. Vaccination attempts carried out before 1965 and some subsequent studies have not defined the serological identity of immunizing and challenge variants. This group of experiments will be considered first.

Vaccination and Challenge Using Undefined Variants of *P. knowlesi*

Freund et al. (1948) first established the feasibility of vaccinating rhesus against *P. knowlesi*. Two injections of mature schizonts (2 or 3 g) treated overnight in 0.1% Formol and suspended in Freund's complete adjuvant (FCA) protected 17 of 18 monkeys against fatal infection. In assessing the significance of these very impressive results, the following facts are relevant. Parasites for challenge were obtained from quinine-treated donors. With strain 1 (Table 2) the course of infection in eight unvaccinated controls was relatively avirulent, since one animal survived and parasitemia in four was 6% or less on day 10 when the disease should have reached a fatal outcome. There was a high incidence of tuberculosis among experimental animals, e.g., in four out of eight control monkeys and several of the vaccinated animals. This infection is known to attenuate the course of *P. knowlesi* in the rhesus (Coggeshall & Kumm 1938; Bazaz-Malik 1973). Later experiments used a second, more virulent strain of parasite (Table 2). Five out of six animals survived challenge with this strain but three died 6 to 22 weeks after challenge with evidence of "colitis."

Table 2

Vaccination of Rhesus Monkeys Against *P. knowlesi* Malaria: Experiments In Which
Serotypes of Immunizing and Challenge Variants Were Not Defined

	Immunization				Challenge							
							Animals Surviving Infection			Duration of	Maximum	
Number of Animals	Material	Inactivation	Mass (approx.)	Adjuvant	Number of Parasites	Route	Number Negative	Positive		Parasitemia (days)	Parasitemia (%)	Fatal Infection
12	Sz[e] (strain 1)	0.1% Formol	2-3 g	FCA (2)	10^3[f]	(?)	12	4(?)	8	3-67	0.7-10	0/12[g]
6	Sz (strain 2)	0.1% Formol	3-4 g	FCA (2)	10^3[f]	(?)	5	1	4	23-31	3-5	1/6[h]

1/18

| 3 | Sz | 0.1% Formol | 2-3 g | FCA (2) | 2×10^3 | i.p.[i] | 1 | 1 | | | | 2/3 |
| 3 | Sz | red blood cell lysis | 2-3 g | FCA (2) | 2×10^3 | i.p.[i] | 1 | 1 | | | | 2/3 |

4/6

| 4 | Sz | 0.1% Formol | 1 g | FCA, FIA | 2×10^3 | i.p. | 4 | 3 | 1 | 23 | 0.5 | 0/4 |
| 3 | Sz | red blood cell lysis | 1 g | FCA, FIA | 2×10^3 | i.p. | 3 | 0 | 3 | 17-23 | 0.5-10.5 | 0/3 |

0/7

| 5 | Sz G200 fraction | pressure cell | 2 mg | FCA, FIA | 10^6 | i.v. | 3 | 2 | 1 | 9 | 6.0 | 2/5 |
| 9 | Sz Biogel fraction | pressure cell | 2 mg | FCA, FIA | 2×10^7 | i.v. | 6 | 0 | 6 | (?) | 0.5-7.5 | 3/9 |

5/14

(a) Freund et al. (1948).
(b) Targett & Fulton (1965).
(c) Schenkel et al. (1973).
(d) Simpson et al. (1974).
(e) Sz = schizonts.

(f) Parasites from quinine-treated donors. Strain 1 less virulent than strain 2 in controls.
(g) 3/12 animals died 1-36 weeks after challenge with tuberculosis or colitis.
(h) 3/6 animals died 6-22 weeks after challenge with colitis.
(i) Control monkeys show prolonged prepatent period (9-10 days).

Targett & Fulton (1965), using the same experimental protocol, could not confirm the results of Freund et al. (1948). Fatal infections occurred in two out of three animals vaccinated with Formol-treated schizonts (with FCA) and also in two out of three animals inoculated with FCA-containing schizonts lysed by anti-erythrocyte serum (Table 2). However, both these parasite preparations administered first with FCA and subsequently with Freund's incomplete adjuvant (FIA) did provide effective protection in all of seven monkeys. A relatively small challenge dose (2×10^3 parasites) was administered by the intraperitoneal route. This produced slowly developing infections in control monkeys, which became patent only on day 9 or 10 instead of on day 5 as would have been expected after intravenous inoculation. The challenge used may have influenced the favorable outcome of infections in the vaccinated animals; the challenge was certainly less testing than that employed in all other experiments (Tables 2 and 3).

The possibility of using plasmodial fractions for vaccination has been demonstrated by Schenkel et al. (1973) and Simpson et al. (1974). In their combined experiments, 9 out of 14 rhesus monkeys survived intravenous challenge with 10^6 or 2×10^7 parasites (Table 2). Many of the animals died with low levels of parasitemia associated with severe and progressive anemia of unknown cause. A notable feature of these experiments is the small mass of parasite material required for vaccination (about 0.1% of the mass used in the experiments outlined above).

Vaccination and Challenge Using Defined Variants of *P. knowlesi*

Brown et al. (1970) in a carefully controlled study vaccinated rhesus monkeys with freeze-thawed erythrocytic schizonts of known variant specificity and subsequently challenged the animals with the same or a different variant of *P. knowlesi*. Seven out of thirteen monkeys given the schizont vaccine first in FCA (containing *Mycobacterium butyricum*) and then in FIA died following challenge with the variant used for immunization (Table 3). The six surviving animals all developed parasitemia, which reached maximum levels of about 3 to 10% and lasted 8 to 15 days. Subsequent inoculation of blood from these monkeys into normal recipients showed that the parasites had been completely eliminated. Three monkeys vaccinated with schizonts in FCA and then in FIA were challenged with a variant different from that used for immunization and all suffered fatal infections. Comparable results were obtained by Mitchell et al. (1975) in two animals immunized on three occasions with mature segmenting schizonts in FCA. Homologous variant challenge produced transient parasitemia but challenge with a heterologous variant was fatal.

Table 3

Vaccination of Rhesus Monkeys Against *P. knowlesi* Using Defined Serological Variants for Immunization and Challenge

		Immunization					Challenge							
									Animals Surviving Infection			Duration Parasitemia (days)	Maximum Parasitemia (%)	Fatal Infections
Number of Animals	Material	Inactivation	Mass (approx.)	Adjuvant	Number of Parasites	Variant	Route	Number	Negative	Positive				
13 *a*	Sz[d]	frozen and thawed	1-2 g	FCA,FIA	10^3	homologous	i.v.	6	0	6	8-15	3-10	7/13
3 *a*	Sz	frozen and thawed	1-2 g	FCA,FIA	10^3	heterologous	i.v.	0					3/3
5 *b*	Mz[e]	stored 1 hour	0.1 mg	FCA(FIA) (1-3)[i]	10^4	homologous	i.v.	5	3	2	6-8	0.2	0/5
5 *b*	Mz	stored 1 hour	0.1 mg	FCA(FIA) (1-3)[i]	10^4	heterologous	i.v.	4	0	4	1-12	0.1-1.5	1/5
4[f] *c*	Mz	stored 1 hour	0.1 mg	FCA(FIA) (1-3)[i]	Spz[g]	heterologous	i.d.	4	0	4	1-6[h]	0.2	0/4

(a) From Brown et al. (1970).
(b) From Mitchell et al. (1975).
(c) From Richards et al. (1975) unpublished.
(d) Sz = schizonts.
(e) Mz = merozoites.

(f) Immunized animals previously challenged with erythrocytic forms.
(g) Each animal challenged with 10 infected *Anopheles balabacensis*.
(h) Infections in control animals reached 4% - 7% and lasted more than 7 weeks.
(i) Number of injections.

Mitchell et al. (1974, 1975) immunized ten rhesus monkeys with merozoites (10^8 to 10^9) derived from a single serological variant of *P. knowlesi*, together with FCA (Table 3). Five monkeys all survived challenge with the immunizing variant; no detectable parasitemia occurred in three animals and a transient infection (1 to 11 days) of low intensity (maximum parasitemia, 0.2%) was seen in two. Four animals inoculated at least twice with merozoites in FCA survived initial challenge with a variant of *P. knowlesi* different from that used for immunization. All these monkeys developed patent infections of brief duration (1 to 12 days) and low intensity (maximum, 1.5%). Another animal given merozoites in FCA and then in FIA died 16 days after challenge when parasitemia was 7%, the red cell count 2 X 10^6/mm^3, and blood urea above 300 mg/100 ml. Postmortem examination revealed a chronic pleural abscess infiltrating the diaphragm and upper part of the liver.

After initial challenge, merozoite-immunized animals are strongly resistant to subsequent challenge with erythrocytic parasites made at intervals of up to 8 months with several variants and a distinct strain of *P. knowlesi*. In addition, four merozoite-immunized animals were exposed 24 weeks after trophozoite challenge to 10 infected mosquitoes (*Anopheles balabacensis*). Each animal developed a transient infection lasting from 1 to 6 days with maximum parasitemia of 0.2% (Table 3). Infections in two unimmunized animals similarly challenged lasted more than 7 weeks, with maximum levels of 4%-7% (Richards et al. 1975). Merozoite-vaccinated monkeys remain susceptible to chronic infection by *P. cynomolgi bastianellii*, which demonstrates the specificity of the induced immunity (Mitchell et al. 1974, 1975). The number of merozoites (10^8 to 10^9) used for immunization was chosen arbitrarily; a smaller number might be effective. At the level used, the cell sieve *in vitro* culture method provides about 10 immunizing doses per milliliter of parasitized red cells. Each dose of vaccine contains less than 0.1 mg of parasite material.

Adjuvant Requirement for Successful Vaccination

Freund et al. (1948) clearly demonstrated that parasite material induced no protective immunity unless emulsified with FAC, and many subsequent studies in the *P. knowlesi* rhesus system have confirmed this observation. In the case of the merozoite vaccine, the following have proved ineffective: Freund's incomplete adjuvant (FIA); adjuvant 65/4 (Merck Sharp & Dohme, Pennsylvania, U.S.A.); Bacillus Calmette-Guerin (BCG) followed after 2 weeks by merozoites in FIA; aluminum hydrogel; and pertussis vaccine (Mitchell et al. 1975a). Schenkel et al. (1975) have recently reported that a freeze-dried antigen fraction administered with adjuvant 65 failed to induce immunity against *P. knowlesi*. However, this adjuvant combined with BCG and the antigen protected three out of four rhesus monkeys against challenge. The serological identity of variants used for immunization and challenge was not delineated in these experiments. The adjuvant requirements for successful merozoite vaccination are being further investigated in our laboratory.

SUMMARY AND CONCLUSIONS

Freund et al. (1948) demonstrated the feasibility of vaccinating rhesus monkeys against the normally lethal *P. knowlesi* malaria using large amounts (2 to 4g) of parasite material in FCA. The significance of their results is diminished by the use in most experiments of a *P. knowlesi* strain of low virulence, by the high incidence of tuberculosis in experimental rhesus monkeys, and by the fact that 6 out of 18 surviving monkeys died within 6 to 22 weeks after challenge. Moreover, their method of vaccination proved unsuccessful when used by Targett & Fulton (1965). When these authors administered similar parasite material first in FCA and then in FIA, immunity was induced in each of seven vaccinated monkeys. Their experiments employed a relatively low challenge dose administered by intraperitoneal injection. The course of parasitemia was prolonged in control animals and it is possible that some of the immunized monkeys would have succumbed to the intravenous challenge infections used in all other studies.

The possibility of using small quantities of plasmodial fractions to protect a proportion of monkeys against high challenge doses of *P. knowlesi* was demonstrated by Schenkel et al. (1973) and by Simpson et al. (1974). The immunizing material effectively suppressed parasite levels in most animals, but challenge was frequently associated with severe and progressive anemia.

In 1965, Brown & Brown used the SICA test to demonstrate the occurrence of intrastrain antigenic variations during the course of chronic *P. knowlesi* infections. It is clear that antigenic variation in this species is an important mechanism permitting parasite survival (Brown 1971) and complicates any attempts to achieve effective immunoprophylaxis (Cohen 1975). Thus, Brown et al. (1970) showed that vaccination with freeze-thawed schizonts protected about 50% of monkeys against homologous variant challenge but provided no protection against challenge with a variant different from that used for immunization.

Studies on the mechanism of acquired malarial immunity *in vivo* (Cohen et al. 1961) and *in vitro* (Cohen et al. 1969) indicated that protective antibody did not affect intracellular parasites but interrupted the cycle of development at the stage when merozoites were released into the plasma. In addition, immune serum agglutinated free merozoites (Butcher & Cohen 1970; Miller et al. 1975) and prevented their attachment to receptors that were demonstrated on the red cells of susceptible species (Butcher et al. 1973). These findings all indicated an important role for merozoite antigens in specific malarial immunity and prompted development of *in vitro* methods for isolating extracellular blood-stage merozoites (Mitchell et al. 1973; Dennis et al. 1975).

The results of vaccination with merozoites in FCA (two or more doses) confirm the experimentally based expectation (Cohen & Butcher 1972) that this extracellular form of the parasite carries antigens able to induce immunity with broad variant specificity. Merozoite vaccination involves injection of very small amounts of parasite material and is the only method shown unequivocally to provide protection against serologic variants different from those used for vaccination and also against sporozoite challenge. Parasitemia always follows first heterologous variant challenge but is of minor degree (maximum, 1.5%) and parasites are eliminated within 1 to 12 days. After initial challenge, merozoite-vaccinated monkeys remain resistant to subsequent challenge with erythrocytic parasites made at intervals of up to 8 months with several variants and distinct strains of *P. knowlesi*. At least 10 doses of vaccine are produced per milliliter of parasitized cells, and since successful serial cultivation of *P. falciparum* has now been achieved (Trager & Jensen 1976), the production of an effective vaccine against human malaria now appears likely.

BIBLIOGRAPHY

Bannister, L.H., Butcher, G.A., Dennis, E.D. & Mitchell, G.H. 1975. Structure and invasive behaviour of *Plasmodium knowlesi* merozoites *in vitro*. *Parasitology* 71: 483-491.

Bazaz-Malik, G. 1973. Increased resistance to malaria after Mycobacterium tuberculosis infection. *Indian J. Med. Res.* 61: 1014-1024.

Brown, I.N. 1969. Immunological aspects of malaria infection. *Adv. Immunol.* 11: 267-349.

Brown, I.N., Allison, A.C. & Taylor, R.B. 1968. *Plasmodium berghei* infections in thymectomized rats. *Nature* (Lond.) 219: 292-293.

Brown, K.N. 1971. Protective immunity to malaria provides a model for the survival of cells in an immunologically hostile environment. *Nature* (Lond.) 230: 163-167.

Brown, K.N. 1973. Antibody induced variation in malaria parasites. *Nature* (Lond.) 242: 49-50.

Brown, K.N. 1974. Antigenic variation and immunity to malaria. *In* Parasites in the Immunized Host: Mechanisms of Survival. Porter, R. & Knight, J., Eds.: 35-51. Ciba Foundation Symposium 25 (new series). Associated Scientific Publishers. Amsterdam, The Netherlands.

Brown, K.N. & Brown, I.N. 1965. Immunity to malaria: antigenic variation in chronic infections by *Plasmodium knowlesi*. *Nature* (Lond.) 208: 1286-1288.

Brown, K.N., Brown, I.N., Trigg, P.I., Phillips, R.S. & Hills, L.A. 1970. Immunity to malaria. II. Serological response of monkeys sensitized by drug-suppressed infection or by dead parasitized cells in Freund's complete adjuvant. *Exp. Parasitol.* 28: 318-338.

Brown, K.N. & Hills, L.A. 1974. Antigenic variation and immunity to *Plasmodium knowlesi:* antibodies which induce antigenic variation and antibodies which destroy parasites. *Trans. R. Soc. Trop. Med. Hyg.* 68: 139-142.

Butcher, G.A. 1975. Unpublished observations.

Butcher, G.A. & Cohen, S. 1972. Antigenic variation and protective immunity in *Plasmodium knowlesi* malaria. *Immunology* 23: 503-521.

Butcher, G.A., Mitchell, G.H. & Cohen, S. 1973. Letter: Mechanism of host specificity in malarial infection. *Nature* (Lond.) 244: 40-41.

Coggeshall, L.T. & Kumm, H.W. 1938. Effect of repeated superinfection upon potency of immune serum of monkeys harboring chronic infections of *Plasmodium knowlesi*. *J. Exp. Med.* 68: 17-27.

Cohen, S. 1975, Immunalprophylaxis of protozoal diseases. *In* Clinical Aspects of Immunology, 3rd edit. Gell, P.G.A., Coombs, R.R.A. & Lachman, P.J., Eds.: 1649-1680. Blackwell Scientific Publishing Company. Oxford, England.

Cohen, S. & Butcher, G.A. 1970. Properties of protective malarial antibody. *Immunology* 19: 369-383.

Cohen, S. & Butcher, G.A. 1972. The immunologic response to plasmodium. *Am. J. Trop. Med. Hyg.* 21: 713-721.

Cohen, S., Butcher, G.A & Crandall, R.B. 1969. Action of malarial antibody *in vitro*. *Nature* (Lond.) 223: 368-371.

Cohen, S., Butcher, G.A. & Mitchell, G.H. 1972. *In vitro* studies of malarial antibody. *Proc. Helminthol. Soc. Wash.* 39: 231-237.

Cohen, S., McGregor, I.A. & Carrington, S.P. 1961. Gamma-globulin and acquired immunity to human malaria. *Nature* (Lond.) 192: 733-737.

Coleman, R.M., Rencricca, N.J., Stout, J.P., Brissette, W.H. & Smith D.M. 1975. Splenic mediated erythrocyte cytotoxicity in malaria. *Immunology* 29: 49-54.

Dennis, E.D., Mitchell, G.H., Butcher, G.A. & Cohen, S. 1975. *In vitro* isolation of *Plasmodium knowlesi* merozoites using polycarbonate sieves. *Parasitology* 71: 475-481.

Diggs, C.L. & Osler, A.G. 1975. Humoral immunity in rodent malaria. III. Studies on the site of antibody action. *J. Immunol.* 114: 1243-1247.

Dvorak, J.A., Miller, L.H., Whitehouse, W.C. & Shiroishi, T. 1975. Invasion of erythrocytes by malaria merozoites. *Science* 187: 748-750.

Freund, J., Thomson, K.J., Sommer, H.E., Walter, A.W. & Pisani, T.M. 1948. Immunization of monkeys against malaria by means of killed parasites with adjuvants. *Am. J. Trop. Med.* 28: 1-22.

Garnham, P.C.C. 1970. Primate malaria. *In* Immunity to Parasitic Animals. Jackson, G.J., Herman, R. & Singer, I., Eds. Vol. 2: 767-791. Appleton-Century-Crofts, New York, N.Y.

Golenser, J., Spira, D.T. & Zuckerman, A. 1975. Neutralizing antibody in rodent malaria. *Trans. R. Soc. Trop. Med. Hyg.* 69: 251-258.

Gregersen, M.I., Bryant, C.A., Hammerle, W.E., Usami, S. & Chien, S. 1967. Flow characteristics of human erythrocytes through polycarbonate sieves. *Science* 157: 825-827.

Jayawardena, A.N., Targett, G.A.T., Leuchars, E., Carter, R.L., Doenhoff, M.J. & Davies, A.J.S. 1975. T-cell activation in murine malaria. *Nature* (Lond.) 258: 149.

Luzzatto, L. 1974. Genetic factors in malaria. *Bull. WHO* 50: 195-202.

Miller, L.H. 1975. Transfusion malaria. *In* Transmissable Disease and Blood Transfusion. Greenwalt, T.J. & Jamieson, G.A., Eds.: 241-266. Grune & Stratton, New York, N.Y.

Miller, L.H., Aikawa, M. & Dvorak, J.A. 1975. Malaria *(Plasmodium knowlesi)* merozoites: immunity and the surface coat. *J. Immunol.* 114: 1237-1242.

Miller, L.H., Dvorak, J.A., Shiroishi, T. & Durocher, J.R. 1973. Influence of erythrocyte membrane components on malaria merozoite invasion. *J. Exp. Med.* 138: 1597-1601.

Miller, L.H., Mason, S.J., Dvorak, J.A., McGinniss, M.H. & Rothman, I.K. 1957. Erythrocyte receptors for *(Plasmodium knowlesi)* malaria: Duffy blood group determinants. *Science* 189: 561-563.

Miller, L.H., Usami, S. & Chien, S. 1971. Alteration in the rheologic properties of *Plasmodium knowlesi*-infected red cells, a possible mechanism for capillary obstruction. *J. Clin. Invest.* 50: 1451-1455.

Mitchell, G.H., Butcher, G.A. & Cohen, S. 1973. Isolation of blood-stage merozoites from *Plasmodium knowlesi* malaria. *Int. J. Parasitol.* 3: 443-445.

Mitchell, G.H., Butcher, G.A. & Cohen, S. 1974. A merozoite vaccine effective against *Plasmodium knowlesi* malaria. *Nature* (Lond.) 252: 311-313.

Mitchell, G.H., Butcher, G.A. & Cohen, S. 1975a. Merozoite vaccination against *Plasmodium knowlesi* malaria. *Immunology* 29: 397-407.

Mitchell, G.H., Butcher, G.A. & Cohen, S. 1975b. Unpublished observations.

Phillips, R.S. 1970. *Plasmodium berghei:* passive transfer of immunity by antisera and cells. *Exp. Parasitol.* 27: 479-495.

Phillips, R.S., Wolstencroft, R.A., Brown, I.N., Brown, K.N. & Dumonde, D.C. 1970. Immunity to malaria. 3. Possible occurrence of a cell-mediated immunity to *Plasmodium knowlesi* in chronically infected and Freund's complete adjuvant-sensitized monkeys. *Exp. Parasitol.* 28: 339-355.

Richards, W.H.G., Mitchell, G.H., Butcher, G.A. & Cohen, S. 1975. Unpublished observations.

Sadun, E.H. 1976. *In* Immunity to Parasitic Diseases, Cohen, S. & Sadun, E.H., Eds.: Blackwell Scientific Publishing Company, Oxford, England.

Schenkel, R.H., Simpson, G.L. & Silverman, P.H. 1973. Vaccination of Rhesus monkeys (*Macaca mulatta*) against *Plasmodium knowlesi* by the use of non-viable antigen. *Bull. WHO* 48: 597-604.

Simpson, G.L., Schenkel, R.H. & Silverman, P.H. 1974. Vaccination of Rhesus monkeys against malaria by use of sucrose density gradient fractions of *Plasmodium knowlesi* antigens. *Nature* (Lond.) 247: 304-305.

Spira, D.T., Silverman, P.H. & Gaines, C. 1970. Anti-thymocyte serum effects on *Plasmodium berghei* infection in rats. *Immunology* 19: 759-766.

Stechschulte, D.J., 1969. Cell-mediated immunity in rats infected with *Plasmodium berghei*. *Mil. Med.* 134: 1147-1152.

Targett, G.A.T. & Fulton, J.D. 1965. Immunization of Rhesus monkeys against *Plasmodium knowlesi* malaria. *Exp. Parasitol.* 17: 180-193.

Trager, W. 1956. The intracellular position of malarial parasites. *Trans. R. Soc. Trop. Med. Hyg.* 50: 419-420.

Trager, W. & Jensen, J.B. 1976. Human malaria parasites in continuous culture. *Science* 193: 673-675.

7

A CRITIQUE OF MEROZOITE AND SPOROZOITE VACCINES IN MALARIA

Louis H. Miller

Laboratory of Parasitic Diseases
National Institute of Allergy and Infectious Diseases
National Institutes of Health
Bethesda, Maryland 20014

How can a vaccine be effective against an organism that in nature is poorly immunogenic? Children within hyperendemic areas are repeatedly infected with *Plasmodium falciparum* malaria over many years before the incidence of parasitemia, splenomegaly, and clinical disease decreases. This immunity, once acquired, may wane in the absence of repeated exposure to malaria. The theoretical problems of a malaria vaccine are further complicated by antigenic differences that exist between the different geographic strains of *P. falciparum*. James et al. (1932) observed that a patient who was resistant to challenge with the Indian strain of *P. falciparum* was susceptible to the Sardinian strain. On the other hand, gamma globulin from immune, adult West Africans suppressed falciparum parasitemia in East African children (McGregor et al. 1963). In addition, antigenic differences do not appear to exist between sporozoites of falciparum strains isolated from Asia and Panama; individuals who were immunized by irradiated sporozoites from one area of the world resisted challenge by sporozoites from other areas (Clyde et al. 1973).

Vaccines could induce a higher level of immunity than the natural infection, and immunity could be directed against forms not present in the mammalian host (e.g., gametes); vaccination against this stage could block transmission.

Sydney Cohen has presented data on vaccination with free merozoites in Freund's complete adjuvant (FCA) (Mitchell et al. 1974, 1975). The results of these studies on the feasibility of a malaria vaccine have stimulated renewed interest in *in vitro* cultivation of asexual erythrocytic parasites. In order to appreciate the significance of this work, it is necessary to compare this approach with previous attempts at vaccination and immunity after repeated infection. Discussion will be limited to the *P. knowlesi*–rhesus monkey system.

In studies of immunity after repeated infection of animals with the same stabilate, there was a progressive increase in the prepatent period (Voller &

Rossan 1969). Eventually, some animals had sufficient immunity to control an infection that would be uniformly fatal in nonimmune animals. The immune monkeys developed a mild, transient infection or remained smear-negative after challenge. However, the level of immunity was unpredictable. Four of eight animals had parasitemia above 1% after the eighth challenge. In contrast to the above, there are limited data on immunity after prolonged patent parasitemia. After drug suppression early in the infection, the parasitemia usually remains low grade. Occasionally, however, after months of low-grade and subpatent infection, parasitemia increases to levels that would cause death if untreated (Voller & Rossan 1969; Miller, unpublished data). In one monkey we observed immunity to heterologous strains after drug cure of a chronic infection (Miller et al. 1976b). Prior to the studies on free merozoite vaccines with FCA, the results of immunization with schizont-infected erythrocytes (Targett & Fulton 1965, Brown et al. 1970) and soluble antigen (Simpson et al. 1974) in FCA were not encouraging. Although mortality was reduced, parasitemia in survivors was often above 1% and severe hemolytic anemia caused death in animals with relatively low parasitemia (Freund et al. 1948; Schenkel et al. 1973). In the one study where the immunizing and infecting stabilate were determined, even homologous challenge caused death (Brown et al. 1970).

The results of merozoite vaccination are in marked contrast to the above (Mitchell et al. 1974, 1975). The immunized animals had a high degree of protection against challenge with both homologous and heterologous stabilates. Parasitemia, when present, was transient, a characteristic of immunized animals previously described by Freund et al. (1948) and Brown et al. (1970).

Before merozoite vaccines can be accepted as far superior to previous approaches, a comparative study of vaccines (e.g., merozoites, schizonts, and "soluble" antigen) against both infected erythrocyte and sporozoite challenge should be undertaken in another laboratory. Variables such as number and virulence of parasites used for challenge may make comparison among various vaccine trials in the literature unreliable. The hematocrit should be followed during all vaccine trials to detect severe hemolytic anemia after challenge.

The adjuvant is as important as the antigen in getting an immunogenic effect to asexual erythrocytic parasites (Brown et al. 1970; Desowitz 1975) or merozoites (Mitchell et al. 1975). Less toxic adjuvants than FCA should be explored for eventual human use (Schenkel et al. 1975). During discussion at the Conference, G.B. Mackaness indicated the importance of FCA in enhancing T-cell responses. He cited unpublished experiments on *P. berghei* in mice. Animals immunized by Formalin-killed blood forms developed a high level of delayed hypersensitivity if the antigen was given under the modulating influence of cyclophosphamide or Bacillus Calmette-Guerin (BCG). They were protected against intravenous challenge 28 days later only if they had been footpad-tested to demonstrate hypersensitivity. Moreover, protection was found only in animals receiving this secondary antigenic stimulus during the period of maximum hypersensitivity. Mackaness felt that induction of protective immunity under such conditions argues a role for T cells in enhancing the formation of protective antibodies.

Merozoite vaccines should also be evaluated in other malarias to ensure that the impressive results of Mitchell et al. (1975) are not limited to the *P. knowlesi*-rhesus monkey system. One possible model system of interest would be *P. coatneyi,* a falciparum-like parasite of the rhesus monkey. Producing merozoites from this system would be vastly more difficult than from *P. knowlesi*-infected monkeys. In the *P. knowlesi* system, schizont-infected erythrocytes are present in high concentrations in the peripheral circulation, are easily separated from uninfected erythrocytes because of schizonts' low density, and release merozoites into the culture system within a few hours. Merozoite collection methods during or after culture have been outlined by S. Cohen (Chapter 6). The culture of *P. coatneyi*-infected erythrocytes, on the other hand, must be initiated with immature trophozoites, as mature trophozoites and schizonts are sequestered from the peripheral circulation, attaching to venular endothelium (Desowitz et al. 1969). After a culture period of approximately 40 to 48 hours, mature parasites would have to be separated from uninfected erythrocytes so that merozoites on release would have no uninfected erythrocytes for invasion.

It may now be possible to evaluate vaccines against asexual infection with *P. falciparum* by utilizing antigens from erythrocyte culture. The continuous culture of malaria that has evaded scientists since the initial trials by Bass & Johns (1912) has finally been accomplished by Trager & Jensen (1976). This success has stimulated renewed interest in the culture field and has been a stimulus to the work on vaccine development. The culture system at present is asynchronous, can support only low parasitemia, and has no mechanism for producing merozoites.

Why is the free merozoite in FCA superior to previous antigenic preparations? Free, extracellular merozoites are surrounded by a surface coat that is absent in the intraerythrocytic forms (Miller et al. 1975a). Antibodies develop against this coat in natural infections; sera from repeatedly infected animals agglutinate the merozoites by this coat. The surface coat or some other structure on the surface of merozoites attaches to erythrocytes and initiates deformation (Dvorak et al. 1975). Theoretically, antibodies against such a group on the merozoite surface could block invasion. Isolation of the substance on the erythrocyte surface to which merozoites attach would facilitate isolation of the complementary group on the merozoite.

Recently, we have identified the receptor on the human erythrocyte for the simian parasite *P. knowlesi* (Miller et al. 1975b). Erythrocytes that lacked Duffy a and b antigens (FyFy) were resistant to invasion by *P. knowlesi* merozoites. The resistance does not appear to be caused by other associated membrane defects in Duffy-negative erythrocytes, since removal of Duffy blood group determinants [Fy(a) or Fy(b)] by chymotrypsin and specifically blocking of Fy(a) with anti-Fy(a) greatly reduce invasion. On direct observation of the merozoite/Duffy-negative-erythrocyte interaction, the merozoite markedly deformed the erythrocyte on contact, but the later sequences in invasion, the localized invagination of the erythrocyte membrane, failed to occur. Since no interaction at all occurs when *P. knowlesi* merozoites contact guinea pig or mouse erythrocytes, the Duffy-negative erythrocytes still maintain some degree of specificity.

The *P. knowlesi* resistance factor, Duffy-negative erythrocytes, occurs in high frequency in West Africa, where the people are resistant to vivax malaria. Nineteen of twenty West Africans (Bray 1958) and 70% of American blacks (Young et al. 1955) were resistant to infection by *P. vivax,* a percentage that approximates the frequency of Duffy-negative erythrocytes (FyFy) in these populations. It has now been shown that blacks who are Duffy-negative were resistant to mosquito-induced infection with *P. vivax;* Duffy-positive blacks were susceptible (Miller et al. 1976a). These studies prove that the attachment of merozoites to erythrocytes is highly specific and requires a receptor on the erythrocyte surface.

Drs. R. Gwadz and R. Carter observed that erythrocytes form a rosette around one end of a microgamete (unpublished observation). In a preliminary study we observed that microgametes of *P. gallinaceum* attached to avian erythrocytes and not to rhesus erythrocytes, whereas microgametes of *P. knowlesi* attached to rhesus erythrocytes and not to avian or rodent erythrocytes. If microgametes demonstrate the same degree of specificity in erythrocyte attachment as merozoites, then similar groups may be present on the microgamete and merozoite surface for such attachment. One could further speculate that immunization with merozoites may induce antibodies against microgametes and that these antibodies may block fertilization in the mosquito gut. Such a vaccine would not only reduce severity of disease but also reduce or eliminate transmission.

It is also probable that closely related protozoa genera such as *Theileria, Babesia,* and *Coccidia* invade cells by highly specific receptors on the host cell surface and that these receptors determine, in part, the limited host range and cell type infected (e.g., lymphocytes in *Theileria parva*). Proof of receptor specificity in these diseases might suggest new approaches to vaccine development. In addition, strains of animals may exist that lack the receptor.

Introduction of the resistant gene into a susceptible population by breeding would be another approach to disease eradication.

It is a tribute to the group at New York University that the extensive review of sporozoite immunity by Dr. R. S. Nussenzweig derives primarily from work performed by her and her colleagues. Her contribution (Chapter 5) highlights the accomplishments and identifies the problems that must be solved for vaccine development. The isolation of sporozoites free from mosquito debris and bacteria is required for kinetic studies of sporozoite distribution in the non-immune and immune host and would facilitate immunochemical studies. From such purified preparations the surface material on sporozoites that is produced in response to immune serum (Cochrane et al. 1976) could be isolated, chemically characterized, and its immunogenicity evaluated.

As a counterpoint to Dr. Nussenzweig's presentation, I will compare the relative merits of sporozoite and merozoite vaccines (Table 1). Merozoite vaccine has been under study for only a short period, experiments have been limited to one malaria (*P. knowlesi* in monkeys), and challenge has been by blood forms only. Sporozoite vaccine has been successful after sporozoite challenge in avian, rodent, monkey, and human malaria.

On challenge, merozoite-immunized monkeys usually develop patent infections of low parasitemia and of limited duration. After sporozoite vaccination the majority of rodents are solidly immune to challenge by berghei sporozoites. However, partial immunity to sporozoites will afford little or no protection to the host, since falciparum merozoites from one exoerythrocytic schizont could infect erythrocytes where no immunity exists and cause severe disease and death.

Success to date with sporozoite vaccines requires viable sporozoites, rendered noninfectious by irradiation with γ or x rays. Merozoite vaccines have the advantage of a nonviable antigen that permits storage. Merozoite vaccines, on the other hand, are only successful if combined with FCA, which is unacceptable for use in man.

Production of antigen through *in vitro* cultivation was one of the major unsolved problems in development of either vaccine. The first step towards a ready source of falciparum antigen has been accomplished by Trager & Jensen (1976) who have grown asexual erythrocytic parasites of *P. falciparum* for two months. The production of sporozoites in culture would appear to be much more difficult. One possible sequence for sporozoite production would be the culture of asexual erythrocytic parasites and the conversion of asexual development to gametocytes, gametes, ookinetes, oocysts, and infectious sporozoites in culture. Each step would require a major achievement in *in vitro* cultivation. It theoretically could be possible to circumvent this sequence by obtaining gametocytes from infected animals (extremely difficult at present) or

Table 1
Comparison of Merozoite and Sporozoite Vaccination Against Malaria

	Merozoite (*P. knowlesi* – rhesus monkey)	Sporozoite (rodent and human (malaria)
1. Functional antigen	unknown	unknown
2. Requirement for effective vaccine		
Viability	dead	live organism
Adjuvant	Freund's complete adjuvant required	not required
3. Challenge	10^4 infected red blood cells, i.v.	10^3–10^4 sporozoites, i.v.
4. Characteristics of immunity		
Stage specificity	unknown	sporozoite
Species specificity	species	species in human malaria cross-protection between rodent species
Survival	100%	90%–100% in *P. berghei*-infected rodents
Degree of immunity	low or negative parasitemia limited period of patency homologous stabilate heterologous stabilate (?) heterologous strain	immunity quantal (disease after partial immunity lethal)
Length of immunity	unknown	3 months
5. Mechanism of immunity	unknown	T-cell dependent antibody not required
6. Requirement for spleen		
Induction	unknown	not required
Effector	not required	not required
7. *In vitro* tests as indicators of immunity	inhibition of invasion (not predictive for heterologous challenge)	circumsporozoite precipitin and sporozoite-neutralizing antibody (partial correlation with immunity)
8. Culture requirements	asexual erythrocytic culture ⟶ merozoites	asexual erythrocytic culture ⟶ gametocytes ⟶ gametes ⟶ ookinetes ⟶ oocysts ⟶ infectious sporozoites

infected humans (of limited value for a large-scale program). Alternatively, a mechanism for maintaining continuously dividing cells within oocysts for indefinite sporozoite production might be developed. (No small feat!)

The inoculation of infectious sporozoites into hepatocytes or other cell lines in culture would offer another approach to *in vitro* cultivation. If successful, liberated merozoites or infected cells could act as the immunogen.

On balance, merozoite vaccine seems to me a more attainable goal, although this conclusion is based on very limited experimental data. I hope that this comment will not deter funding agencies from supporting research on sporozoite immunity and other approaches, as one suspects that a practical vaccine against malaria will be developed through methods not considered at the Conference. The momentum gained from exciting results of experiments during the last decade justifies expansion of research towards the goal of a malaria vaccine.

BIBLIOGRAPHY

Bass, C.C. & Johns, F.M. 1912. The cultivation of malarial plasmodia (*Plasmodium vivax* and *Plasmodium falciparum*) in vitro. *J. Exp. Med.* 16: 567-579.

Bray, R.S. 1958. The susceptibility of Liberians to the Madagascar strain of *Plasmodium vivax. J. Parasitol.* 44: 371-373.

Brown, K.N., Brown, I.N. & Hills, L. 1970. Immunity to malaria. I. Protection against *Plasmodium knowlesi* shown by monkeys sensitized with drug-suppressed infections or by dead parasites in Freund's adjuvant. *Exp. Parasitol.* 28: 304-317.

Clyde, D.F., McCarthy, V.C., Miller, R.M. & Hornick, R.B. 1973. Specificity of protection of man immunized against sporozoite-induced falciparum malaria. *Am. J. Med. Sci.* 226: 398-403.

Cochrane, A.H., Aikawa, M., Jeng, M. & Nussenzweig, R.S. 1976. Antibody-induced ultrastructural changes of malarial sporozoites. *J. Immunol.* 116: 859-867.

Desowitz, R.S. 1975. *Plasmodium berghei:* immunogenic enhancement of antigen by adjuvant addition. *Exp. Parasitol.* 38: 6-13.

Desowitz, R.S., Miller, L.H., Buchanan, R.D. & Permpanich, B. 1969. The sites of deep vascular schizogony in *Plasmodium coatneyi* malaria. *Trans. R. Soc. Trop. Med. Hyg.* 63: 198-202.

Dvorak, J.A., Miller, L.H., Whitehouse, W.C. & Shiroishi, T. 1975. Invasion of erythrocytes by malaria merozoites. *Science* 187: 748-750.

Freund, J., Thomson, K.J., Sommer, H.E., Walter, A.W. & Pisani, T.M. 1948. Immunization of monkeys against malaria by means of killed parasites with adjuvants. *Am. J. Trop. Med. Hyg.* 28: 1-22.

James, S.P., Nicol, W.D. & Shute, P.G. 1932. A study of induced malignant tertian malaria. *Proc. R. Soc. Med.* 25: 1153-1186.

McGregor, I.A., Carrington, S.P. & Cohen, S. 1963. Treatment of East African *P. falciparum* with West African γ-globulin. *Trans. R. Soc. Trop. Med. Hyg.* 57: 170-175.

Miller, L.H., Aikawa, M. & Dvorak, J.A. 1975a. Malaria (*Plasmodium knowlesi*) merozoites: immunity and the surface coat. *J. Immunol.* 114: 1237-1242.

Miller, L.H., Mason, S.J., Clyde, D.F. & McGinniss, M.H. 1976a. Resistance factor to *Plasmodium vivax:* Duffy genotype *FyFy*. *N. Engl. J. Med. 295: 302-304.*

Miller, L.H., Mason, S.J., Dvorak, J.A., McGinniss, M.H. & Rothman, I.K. 1975b. Erythrocyte receptors for (*Plasmodium knowlesi*) malaria: Duffy blood group determinants. *Science* 189: 561-563.

Miller, L.H., Powers, K.G. & Shiroishi, T. 1976b. *Plasmodium knowlesi:* Functional immunity and antimerozoite antibodies in Rhesus monkeys after repeated infection. *Exp. Parasitol.* In press.

Mitchell, G.H., Butcher, G.A. & Cohen, S. 1974. A merozoite vaccine effective against *Plasmodium knowlesi* malaria. *Nature* (Lond.) 252: 311-313.

Mitchell, G.H., Butcher, G.A. & Cohen, S. 1975. Merozoite vaccination against *Plasmodium knowlesi* malaria. *Immunology* 29: 397-407.

Schenkel, R.H., Cabrera, E.J., Barr, M.L. & Silverman, P.H. 1975. A new adjuvant for use in vaccination against malaria. *J. Parasitol.* 63: 549-550.

Schenkel, R.H., Simpson, G.L. & Silverman, P.H. 1973. Vaccination of Rhesus monkeys (*Maccaca mulatta*) against *Plasmodium knowlesi* by the use of nonviable antigen. *Bull. WHO* 48: 597-604.

Simpson, G.L., Schenkel, R.H. & Silverman, P.H. 1974. Vaccination of Rhesus monkeys against malaria by use of sucrose density gradient fractions of *Plasmodium knowlesi* antigens. *Nature* (Lond.) 247: 304-305.

Targett, G.A. & Fulton, J.D. 1965. Immunization of Rhesus monkeys against *Plasmodium knowlesi* malaria. *Exp. Parasitol.* 17: 180-193.

Trager, W. & Jensen, J.B. 1976. Human malaria parasites in continuous culture. *Science* 193: 673-674.

Voller, A. & Rossan, R.N. 1969. Immunological studies on simian malaria. 3. Immunity to challenge and antigenic variation in *P. knowlesi*. *Trans. R. Soc. Trop. Med. Hyg.* 63: 507-523.

Young, M.D., Eyles, D.E., Burgess, R.W. & Jeffery, G.M. 1955. Experimental testing of Negroes to *Plasmodium vivax*. *J. Parasitol.* 41: 315-318.

8

VACCINATION AGAINST BOVINE BABESIOSIS

L.L. Callow

Queensland Department of Primary Industries
Animal Research Institute
Yeerongpilly Q.4105
Australia

INTRODUCTION

Among the first to practice vaccination against babesiosis were Pound (1897) in Australia and Connaway & Francis (1899) in the United States of America. In Australia the need was to check the disastrous losses which accompanied the epizootic spread of recently introduced babesiosis (Seddon 1952), whereas in the United States the measure was adopted to protect susceptible northern cattle that were introduced to what was then the enzootic area of the South.

This chapter describes methods of vaccination against *Babesia,* but being a review it would be incomplete without some discussion of findings that have resulted from intensive studies of other aspects of babesiosis over the last 15 to 20 years. The relevance of some of these findings, particularly those of the epizootiology, to the practical protection of cattle from disease will be apparent.

BIOLOGY OF THE *BABESIA* OF CATTLE

Taxonomy and Distribution

Levine (1971) placed the class Piroplasmasida in the subphylum Apicomplexa because its members have an apical complex. Thus, the piroplasms, of which *Babesia* is one, are related to malarial parasites and *Coccidia.* He stated that there were 71 species of *Babesia* including six affecting domestic cattle. A series of studies (Simitch et al. 1955; Davies et al. 1958; Wilson 1964; Zwart et al. 1968; Brocklesby et al. 1971; Leeflang & Perie 1972; Goldman & Rosenberg 1974) support the existence of four valid species. The two temperate-zone parasites, *Babesia divergens* and *Babesia major,* which may occur only in Europe and central Asia, are transmitted by multihost ticks such as *Ixodes* and *Haemaphysalis.* The two other piroplasms that have a worldwide distribution, particularly in the warm, humid tropics, are *Babesia bovis* and *Babesia bigemina*. One-host ticks of the genus *Boophilus* are the main vectors. *Babesia bovis* is called *Babesia argentina* in Australia, Latin America, Malagasy, Sri Lanka, and several other countries. *Babesia berbera* is used for *Babesia bovis* in the Middle East, and Goldman & Rosenberg (1974) are still not convinced that *Babesia berbera* should be merged with *Babesia bovis*. A study using indirect fluorescent antibody techniques showed that the parasites of South America are serologically identical to those of Australia (Callow et al. 1976b). It is logical that *Babesia* reached widely separated environments such as South America and Australia with *Boophilus* when this vector spread from the region of its origin, perhaps southern Asia. Spread could have been via Europe to South America and via Indonesia to Australia. The degree of immunologic similarity of economically important piroplasms has considerable relevance to the application of control based on vaccination.

An interesting phylogenetic sidelight is the serologic cross-reactivity (Ludford et al. 1972) between *Babesia argentina* (= *bovis*) and two malarial parasites, *Plasmodium falciparum* and *Plasmodium vivax*. If serologic similarities reflect cross-immunity between the genera, antimalarial immunity might be induced with babesial vaccines.

Life Cycle and Transmission by Ticks

The most remarkable feature of the life cycle of *Babesia* is that organisms ingested by ticks in one generation are finally infective for cattle during a parasitic stage of the next tick generation. A cycle of development has been described (Riek 1964, 1966) but sex is not known to occur in the piroplasms (Levine 1971).

Following transmission to cattle by one or more of the three tick stages (Callow & Hoyte 1961), *Babesia* appears to invade the erythrocytes almost immediately without preerythrocytic schizogony (Hoyte 1961, 1965). The parasite grows from a small single form, and two daughter cells result from a budding process described by Nuttall & Graham-Smith (1907, 1908). Morphologic diversity occurs, leading at times to difficulty in distinguishing species. There does not appear to be an identifiable, tick-infective form equivalent to the gametocyte in other blood protozoan infections. Strains of *Babesia argentina* (= *bovis*) that lose their infectivity for *Boophilus microplus* (O'Sullivan & Callow 1966) do not undergo obvious morphologic change.

Chronic babesial infections develop in cattle that survive acute attacks. Chronic infections do not harm the host but ticks can become infected from them (Mahoney 1969). Most infections with *Babesia argentina* (= *bovis)* persist for periods of at least 1 to 4 years (Johnston & Tammemagi 1969; Mahoney et al. 1973b), whereas *Babesia bigemina* disappears from many cattle within about 6 months of initial infection (Callow et al. 1974b).

Pathological Effects

The gross effects of acute babesiosis are well documented (Seddon 1952) and further descriptions of the course of the disease, autopsy findings, histopathology, and certain hematological and biochemical changes have been given by Rogers (1971b). Clinical attacks are essentially acute hemolytic episodes lasting for about one week during which time parasites multiply rapidly. Whereas the cause of death in infections due to *Babesia bigemina* appears to be due to anemia alone, the syndrome due to *Babesia bovis* is sometimes complicated by vascular derangements. The predilection of this small babesial species for capillaries (Rees 1934) may predispose to cerebral involvement (Tchernomoretz 1943; Callow & McGavin 1963). Mahoney & Goodger (1969) suggested that the fibrinogenlike material detected in acute infections due to *Babesia argentina* (= *bovis*) was associated with intravascular clotting, and recently Dalgliesh et al. (1976) demonstrated the presence of widespread thrombus formation in certain hyperacute laboratory infections with this parasite.

There has been speculation that the anemia of babesiosis may result from a host response against uninfected as well as infected erythrocytes (Zuckerman 1964) but evidence is to the contrary. Lysis did not occur when plasma from infected calves was transferred to uninfected animals (Mahoney & Goodger 1972). In an analysis of changes occurring during the course of infection with *Babesia argentina* (= *bovis*) (Callow & Pepper 1974), strong correlations (p < 0.001) were found between values established for parasitemia and the degree of anemia.

Immunology

There is no evidence that cattle can resist babesial infection to the extent of completely inhibiting the multiplication of all strains to which they might be exposed. This applies both to cattle infected for the first time and also to cattle that have been exposed once or several times previously. Immunity to *Babesia* is relative and will depend on race, physiological state such as that due to age, and previous exposure of the cattle to infection. It will also depend on the virulence and antigenicity of the challenging parasites. Immunity is best evaluated by measuring the intensity of infection following challenge with strains whose virulence and antigenicity have been previously evaluated. Because of the variable factors that influence it, the intensity of infection recorded must be compared with that of appropriate controls exposed under identical conditions. At least seven animals per group is desirable. Methods of evaluating the intensity of infection were discussed by Callow & Pepper (1974).

Three types of immunity are relevant in deciding upon vaccination procedures. Innate or racial immunity such as that of some Zebu cattle and the nonspecific immunity exhibited by most cattle during the first year of life influence decisions on the necessity for vaccination, and also on its timing if a virulent inoculum is to be used. The third type of immunity is acquired, and is an obvious consideration in vaccination.

Innate and Nonspecific Immunity

The relatively high immunity of Zebu cattle *(Bos indicus)* to babesial infections is fairly well documented (Daly & Hall 1955; Johnston 1967; Uilenberg 1971). Innate immunity of Sahiwal cattle (Löhr 1973; Callow, L.L., unpublished data) is particularly high, and an examination of racial differences in susceptibility within Zebus would be worthwhile. All European breeds used in Australia appear equally susceptible (Callow, L.L., unpublished data).

Smith & Kilborne (1893) were the first of many observers to suggest that calves were less susceptible than adults. Although no substantial work reporting a comparison of different age groups under experimental conditions has yet been published, it appears that calves of immune mothers are protected by specific factors derived from colostrum for the first month or two of life (Hall 1960, 1963; Hall et al. 1968) and that older calves, regardless of the status of the dam, develop an enhanced, nonspecific immunity which persists for at least 6 months (Riek 1963; Callow, L.L., unpublished data).

Acquired Immunity

The concept of *prémunition* formulated by Sergent et al. (1924) and persuasively developed subsequently by this group (Sergent et al. 1934) dominated thought for many years on acquired immunity to babesiosis and immunization against the disease (Sergent et al. 1945). Nevertheless, the view that immunity depended on the animal's remaining a carrier was disputed from time to time (Thomson 1933; Coggeshall 1943; Taliaferro 1949), and a recent series of observations (reviewed by Callow et al. 1974a) has established that the immune mechanisms concerned are not basically different from those in other infections. Callow et al. (1974a) found that the degree of acquired immunity to *Babesia argentina* (= *bovis*) in drug-sterilized animals was influenced by the degree of prior exposure to the parasite. A high level of immunity was possessed by cattle that had experienced two artificially induced infections. Equally substantial was the immunity to reinfection with *Babesia bigemina* in cattle that had eliminated this parasite by means of their own immune response

(Mahoney et al. 1973b; Callow et al. 1974b). The fact that *prémunition* is not essential in protecting cattle against babesiosis widens the scope of those working to develop improved, antibabesial vaccines.

Strain differences and antigenic variation occur in *Babesia* (Callow 1964, 1967, 1968; Curnow 1968, 1973a; Uilenberg 1970; Phillips 1971a) but these qualities do not appear to be of major importance either as a cause of disease or in the preparation of vaccines. Cross-immunity tests between strains usually show that infection with one produces adequate clinical protection against others. Investigations of immunity are performed with one strain for immunization and a different one for challenge (Callow 1968).

Cross-immunity exists between certain nonbovine species (Zuckerman & Ristic 1968; Cox & Young 1969) of *Babesia*. It had been investigated for *Babesia bigemina* and *Babesia argentina* (= *bovis*) by Legg (1935) who found that carriers of the former parasite possessed some resistance to the latter although the opposite did not hold. For a short period the finding was exploited in vaccination, but the protection afforded by *Babesia bigemina* against *Babesia argentina* (= *bovis*) was not sufficiently reliable, and the practice was discontinued (Seddon 1952).

Basic mechanisms of immunity are not thoroughly understood, although evidence for an antibody-mediated response has accumulated (Hall 1960, 1963; Mahoney 1967a; Hall et al. 1968). Recently, we have investigated T-cell function in babesial immunity (Callow, L.L., unpublished data). Suppression of immunity, particularly in established infections with *Babesia argentina* (= *bovis*), followed the adminstration of antithymocyte preparations. Antigen-stimulated lymphocyte transformation was obtained during and shortly after the primary attack. No reactions suggestive of delayed hypersensitivity were produced by intradermal injections of babesial antigen. The lack of an *in vivo* correlate for the *in vitro* lymphocyte responses suggests a helper function for T cells in immunity to *Babesia*. A system of cooperating lymphocyte populations, similar to that proposed by Brown (1971) to account for the immune response and antigenic variation in chronic malarial infections, may apply in babesiosis.

Whereas the precise mechanisms by which *Babesia* is inactivated and removed from the circulation are obscure, it is clear that the spleen plays a major role in controlling the primary infection. Its role is thoroughly documented beginning with the observations by de Kock & Quinlan (1926). The effect of splenectomy in allowing overt infections to develop in abnormal hosts is reviewed by Garnham (1970). Resistant Sahiwal cattle became very susceptible after being splenectomized (Löhr 1973). Splenectomy of cattle with established infections regularly causes nonfatal parasitemias with *Babesia bigemina,* but relapses to *Babesia argentina* (= *bovis*) following this procedure occur less frequently (Legg 1935; Uilenberg 1969).

THE NEED FOR VACCINATION

Losses from babesiosis in unvaccinated cattle occur during epizootic spread of the parasite and its vector, in cattle imported to an enzootic area, and in environments or under systems of management allowing the development of enzootic instability (Mahoney & Ross 1972; Mahoney 1973). When losses occur due to epizootic spread and importation of cattle they may be spectacular, but frequently involve relatively small groups of animals and occur over a short period of time. The insidious losses from enzootic instability in large beef herds established in subtropical and temperate regions of the world are of greater economic importance.

Epizootic Spread

A spectacular example of epizootic spread occurred in Australia between 1880 and 1900 (Seddon 1952) when *Boophilus microplus* spread rapidly from a focus in northwest Australia to areas south of Brisbane on the eastern coast, a distance of over 3,000 km. Mortality has been estimated in millions, and in many susceptible herds from 50% to 80% of the cattle died. These losses are much higher than those observed when susceptible cattle are exposed under the enzootic conditions that prevail today, suggesting that an escalation of virulence may occur during epizootic spread.

Boophilus has colonized most areas that are ecologically favorable for its propagation and where cattle are grazed. In Australia the regions infested by *Boophilus microplus* have varied little in 60 to 70 years (Seddon 1968). Occasionally ticks make short incursions into uninfected areas. Whether these are accompanied by outbreaks of babesiosis or not depends on the incidence of babesial infection in the ticks (Mahoney & Mirre 1971). Under field conditions this infection rate can be so low (Mahoney 1973) that clinical babesiosis is not observed. Recently, however, reports of losses of 1,000 to 3,000 cattle have been received from districts in northern Australia following the spread of ticks.

Epizootic babesiosis is a hazard in tick eradication schemes. Unsuccessful eradication schemes create susceptible herds that are at risk, and no country should attempt to eradicate *Boophilus* unless a reliable vaccination method for babesiosis is available. Despite the existence of effective vaccination and of extensive technical data on tick control in Australia, sociopolitical, economic, and management factors are considered to preclude the early eradication of *Boophilus microplus* from this country (Anon. 1975).

Cattle Imported to an Enzootic Area

Losses due to babesiosis may result when susceptible cattle are introduced into an enzootic area. The most serious losses occur when temperate-breed cattle are imported into tropical regions highly favorable for *Boophilus*. High inoculation rates (Mahoney & Ross 1972) under these conditions predispose to acute attacks shortly after the arrival of the cattle.

Enzootic Instability

The epizootiological studies of Mahoney and his coworkers (Mahoney 1962, 1969, 1973; Mahoney & Mirre 1971; Mahoney & Ross 1972; Mahoney et al. 1973b; Ross & Mahoney 1974) explain why there is an incidence of babesiosis in the indigenous cattle of an enzootic area, and indicate how the risk to cattle in this situation can be estimated. Enzootic instability defines the situation in which some animals in the herd fail to become infected for a considerable period after birth despite being constantly exposed to the vector. With the alternative condition of stability, infection of all cattle with *Babesia* occurs within the period that young animals are protected by passively acquired and nonspecific factors. At this time acquired immunity develops without the host becoming obviously sick. If initial infection is delayed until cattle have passed out of their resistant stage, clinical cases are usually seen.

The level of stability depends on the inoculation rate, which is the product of the number of ticks attaching and the percentage of these infected with *Babesia*. According to Mahoney (1973) there is a risk of clinical babesiosis when the inoculation rate is below 0.005 (one infective tick bite every 200 days). An inoculation rate of 0.005 would result from about 12 ticks biting each day from a population in which the proportion of infected tick larvae is 0.0004.

In defining risk it is not necessary to measure the inoculation rate. A relationship exists between inoculation rate and the infection rate in the cattle, that is, the percentage of the group that has been exposed to babesial infection at any time (Mahoney & Ross 1972). In Australia infection rates are determined by applying one of the serologic tests developed there (Mahoney 1967c; Goodger 1971, 1973; Curnow 1973b; Johnston et al. 1973; Goodger & Mahoney 1974a, 1974b). Tests developed for other environments have been summarized and described by Todorovic & Kuttler (1974). It is obvious that if infection is present in less than 100% of a group the uninfected segment is likely, sooner or later, to contract babesiosis. Thus, in a study of infection rates in five commercial herds in South Queensland (latitude 24.5 to 27.5 degrees S.) it was found that an average of 43.1% of yearling cattle had not been infected with *Babesia argentina* (= *bovis*) (Callow et al. 1976a). Subsequent losses due to this infection were highest on the property recording the lowest infection rate.

APPROACHES TO VACCINATION

Prémunition or the Carrier Donor System

As well as being the terminology of Sergent et al. (1924) for their concept of the immune state in babesiosis, *prémunition* and anglicized variations such as "premunize" are sometimes used to describe the procedure of vaccinating susceptible cattle with the blood of an animal clinically recovered from an attack of babesiosis. The method has been used for almost 80 years with varying degrees of care and efficiency. The greatest control has operated where special government laboratories and staff have been maintained to provide a service, such as in colonial Algeria (Sergent et al. 1945) and Queensland (Seddon 1952). At these two centers vaccine donors were prepared by obtaining previously unexposed cattle and inoculating them with parasitized blood. Vaccine strains passaged for this purpose were kept "pure" by keeping donors and recipients in tick-free quarters and avoiding mechanical transmission with contaminated needles and instruments. Collection of blood began at least several weeks after the donor's acute attack had subsided. In Australia vaccine donors ("bleeders") were either used at the laboratory or sold to farmers who bled them when vaccine was required. Although this system was changed in Australia in 1964, it is still used in some countries such as Israel, Sri Lanka, and Uruguay. A more rudimentary method used when laboratory facilities are not available is to choose tick-infested, indigenous animals as donors.

Carriers were used as donors because their blood produces less severe reactions in recipients than blood from clinical cases (Tidswell 1899; Callow & Tammemagi 1967). In Israel, although it was found that carriers were not always infective (Kemron et al. 1964), subsequent investigations (Pipano 1969a, 1969b) indicated that a satisfactory level of infectivity with *Babesia berbera* (= *bovis*) was provided by splenectomized and nonsplenectomized carrier calves. Other modern workers (Löhr 1969; Uilenberg 1971) used carriers but selected only those showing parasites in blood films at the time of collection.

In Australia an attempt was made to counteract the lack of infectivity of vaccine provided by carrier donors by collecting vaccine within 6 weeks of the termination of the primary attack. The incidence of vaccination failure fell but there was an increased mortality due to severe vaccination reactions. In one instance, 58 of 130 cattle died as a result of vaccination (Dalgliesh 1968).

The selection of a herd animal as a vaccine donor or the use of a bleeder that has become tick-infested on the farm creates similar hazards. Active transmission of virulent *Babesia* from ticks to the donor may occur during periods when vaccine is collected. Such donors may become infected with anaplasmosis. However, during the period when bleeders were popular in Australia (Seddon

1952), there were few reports of fatal infections being transmitted regularly from field donors. This may have been a result of low tick inoculation rates in temperate, tick-infested areas where bleeders were generally used. By contrast, in tropical areas severe losses have followed the use of indigenous cattle as donors of vaccine for imported, exotic cattle.

Surveillance and Treatment

When babesicides are used at adequate dose rates and before the disease is well advanced, even very acute babesiosis can be controlled. Close inspection of vaccinated cattle with the treatment of obviously reacting cattle is a recommended procedure in more than one vaccination system (Dalgliesh 1968; Pipano 1969b; Uilenberg 1971). Use of virulent blood with the treatment of all animals in the group a specified time after inoculation is a method that could be used (Todorovic et al. 1975). However, when cattle industries are practiced under very extensive and primitive conditions and the numbers to be vaccinated are measured in hundreds and even thousands, surveillance and treatment are at times difficult.

In some tropical countries no vaccination method is available. When susceptible cattle have to be imported, the procedure is to allow them to become tick-infested, observe them for clinical signs of babesiosis, and treat those affected. The results are frequently unsatisfactory. Wide variations in the time taken for cattle to show clinical signs and lack of experience in dealing with acute attacks combine to make the operation hazardous.

Chemoprophylaxis

The advantages of chemoprophylaxis against babesiosis (Newton & O'Sullivan 1969) led to the development of a depot compound based on the well-known babesicide, quinuronium sulphate. Encouraging results against *Babesia divergens* (Ryley 1964) and *Babesia argentina* (= *bovis*) (Newton & O'Sullivan 1969; Callow & McGregor 1969) were obtained, but commercial production did not proceed because toxic nephritis occurred in some calves.

Prophylactic qualities were observed (Callow & McGregor 1970) during early testing of a recently synthesized babesicide (Schmidt et al. 1969) now known as imidocarb. The usefulness of these properties under field conditions was confirmed by Roy-Smith (1971) and the drug was marketed. Its main prophylactic application at the present time is in certain developing countries where effective vaccines may not be available. Thus, it has been tested successfully in Colombia (Todorovic et al. 1975) and also in Bolivia where previously most imported cattle died (McCosker 1975).

Chemoprophylaxis as a method of controlling babesiosis does not now have the strong appeal it did several years ago. Apart from the general objection that resistant strains of organisms may emerge following prophylactic use of a drug, there are two other disadvantages applying specifically to bovine babesiosis. First, long-lasting protection following a prophylactically controlled primary attack is dependent on infection occurring during the period the drug is exerting its effect. Because of variations in the inoculation rate (Mahoney & Ross 1972) there is no assurance that the primary attack will occur at the appropriate time. Second, an increased social sensitivity to the effect of residues in products for human consumption has resulted in restrictive regulations governing the use of drugs having depot effects.

Stimulation of Nonspecific Immunity

The recent demonstration that high levels of nonspecific protection can be induced against murine species of *Babesia* when the host is injected several weeks earlier with Bacillus Calmette-Guerin (BCG) and *C. parvum* vaccines (Clark et al. 1976; Clark & Allison 1976) has obvious relevance in bovine babesiosis. If the principle can be established in cattle, its exploitation might provide another approach, similar to chemoprophylaxis, in the control of the disease. Factors such as duration of activity, chemical or microbial residual effects, cost, and convenience of use would determine the applicability of vaccines promoting nonspecific immunity.

Experimental Approaches to Antigen Production

Before dealing in some detail with a method used in Australia of preparing a highly infective vaccine of reduced virulence, several alternative experimental approaches should be mentioned. New approaches might, if successful, reduce the danger to recipients from severe reactions and undesirable contaminants of whole blood vaccine and, in other instances, avoid the establishment in the field of reservoirs of infection from which disease could spread.

Dead Parasites, Their Products and "Exoantigens"

This has been thoroughly explored for *Babesia argentina* (= *bovis*) by Mahoney and his collaborators in Australia (Mahoney 1967b, 1971; Mahoney & Goodger 1972). Immune responses were stimulated by freeze-dried suspensions of infected erythrocytes, by a complement-fixing antigen, and by whole and fractionated plasma from acute cases. These responses protected satisfactorily against the strain from which the antigens were prepared but were not so successful against a different antigenic strain. The greatest species-specific protection was produced by "exoantigen" from infected plasma. Todorovic et al. (1973), using a similar approach, obtained more encouraging results in calves vaccinated with products of *Babesia argentina* (= *bovis*) and *Babesia bigemina* and then exposed to field challenge. Again the greatest protection was provided by antigens derived from the plasma of acute cases. The studies are important in that they show that cattle might be immunized with nonliving material that could be sterilized. Future development should be towards purification and potentiation of the immunogen. Because a hemolytic syndrome in newborn calves has been a consequence of the use of some blood vaccines (Dimmock & Bell 1970), ways and means of eliminating contaminating blood group substances and avoiding the use of powerful adjuvants should be sought.

Irradiated Parasites

The principle of irradiating *Babesia* to inhibit its multiplication either partially or totally has been applied by several workers. Phillips (1971b) concluded that irradiated *Babesia rodhaini* were more immunogenic than killed parasites. Brocklesby et al. (1972) studied the effect of different levels of irradiation on *Babesia major*. Mahoney et al. (1973a) attenuated *Babesia argentina* (= *bovis*) by this approach and produced immunity only with replicating parasites, whereas Bishop & Adams (1974) found that immunity to *Babesia bigemina* resulted even if the irradiated parasites were incapable of multiplying in the host.

These are interesting findings that could solve the problem of virulence in some babesial vaccines. In the future, if strains other than the immunogen are used for challenge, it should be possible to make a better evaluation of the method than at present. A limitation may be the large numbers of parasites that may have to be irradiated to produce an effective inoculum. This could cause production difficulties in a large-scale operation and also might result in a bulky inoculum with a high content of blood group substances. The massive loss of infectivity that occurs during irradiation could pose practical problems in providing a vaccine that would still be infective after transport and throughout its period of use in the field.

Infective Forms From Ticks

The recent success of workers in isolating infective *Theileria parva* from *Rhipicephalus appendiculatus*, beginning with the study by Purnell & Joyner (1967), no doubt stimulated attempts to produce infective babesial suspensions from ticks. This was achieved recently by Mahoney & Mirre (1974) for *Babesia argentina* (= *bovis*), Potgieter & van Vuuren (1974) for *Babesia bovis*, and by Morzaria et al. (1974) for *Babesia major*. Difficulties in applying the findings to vaccine production could be those of producing sufficient material and of controlling the virulence of the unmodified parasites. An advantage of this approach over others is the certainty that the tick forms would produce species-specific immunity. It should also be possible to prepare an inoculum relatively free of erythrocytes and other possible contaminants of bovine origin.

In Vitro Culture

For some years we have pursued the aim of *in vitro* culture of *Babesia* with a view to providing antigenic material that could be used in approaches using dead or irradiated parasites as described above. An empirical approach has met with little success, and it appears that a method must be built on findings that result from studies of the basic biochemistry and physiology of the parasites. Very few studies of these aspects have been performed, particularly for *Babesia* occurring in domestic animals.

VACCINATION AGAINST *BABESIA ARGENTINA* (= *BOVIS*) IN AUSTRALIA

The carrier donor system used in Australia until 1964, described earlier and reviewed in detail by Seddon (1952), was changed because of an appreciable incidence of natural babesiosis in vaccinated cattle. Vaccine failure was found to be due to variable infectivity of the blood of donors (Callow & Tammemagi 1967).

Apart from two reports (Callow & Mellors 1966; Callow 1971) there has been no formal documentation of the research that led to the introduction of the new vaccine. Many of the experiments will never be reported in detail. I propose to use this review to outline an approach to the problem of producing effective vaccination against *Babesia argentina* (= *bovis*) and to summarize the more significant findings which allowed development to proceed. Current methods of production and use will be described and an evaluation of these methods given.

Research, Development, and Production

Defining the Problem

The finding that 5 ml of blood from carriers did not always contain sufficient parasites to infect recipients brought an awareness of the importance of infectivity in babesial vaccines. Much subsequent research has been directed towards improving infectivity. There were two problems. One was to provide sufficient parasites to allow large-scale production of a highly infective vaccine, and the other was to maintain the viability of the parasites *in vitro* by providing an optimal physical and chemical environment for them.

Dose Rate Studies

Infectivity titrations were a necessary preliminary to fixing an appropriate dose for vaccine. Starting with highly parasitized blood from splenectomized calves, infectivity was titrated by inoculating groups of steers with various dilutions of the blood. Infectivity became variable with dilutions containing 10^5 parasites given subcutaneously. It was also found that there was an inverse linear relationship between the number of parasites inoculated and the time taken for an animal to react. A dose of 10^7 was chosen for vaccine because it was approximately 100 times the minimum infective dose and usually produced a reaction 8 to 9 days after inoculation. It was anticipated that the highly infective vaccine would produce acute reactions and that the predictable response time would allow mass treatment to be given to the vaccinated groups.

Diluent Studies

Many diluent experiments have been completed (Farlow, G.E. & Callow, L.L., unpublished data). These are performed by incubating parasites for 24 hours at 37 C in the diluent being investigated and then testing infectivity by inoculating groups of animals intravenously. Because of the linear dose-response relationship, the mean period between the time of inoculation and the detection of parasitemia gives an estimate of the parasite survival. At least seven animals per group should be used, and because up to six groups are included in any one experiment, the work is expensive and laborious. Some saving can, however, be effected by performing preliminary experiments using a rodent piroplasm, *Babesia rodhaini,* in laboratory mice and rats.

An initial series of experiments showed that citrated blood and plasma were less detrimental to parasites than a number of synthetic diluents including Alsever's solution and Tyrode's solution. As a result whole blood from uninfected donors was initially used as the diluent. Further experimentation led to the development of cell-free diluents incorporating bovine plasma. At the present time the diluent is composed of 25% bovine plasma and 75% balanced salt solution, the composition of which is based on the electrolyte concentrations of bovine plasma. Osmolality, pH, and glucose values are adjusted to physiological levels. The final aim of this work (which is continuing) is to identify plasma factors aiding the survival of parasites.

Parasites Used in Vaccine

<u>Production</u>. Splenectomized calves inoculated with *Babesia argentina* (= *bovis*) collected from acutely infected donors invariably experience acute infections themselves. Parasitemias usually range from 5×10^7 to 5×10^8 parasites per ml, and blood collected from them for vaccine has to be diluted to limit the number of organisms in a 2-ml dose to 10^7.

In the beginning parasites were produced for vaccine by infecting a splenectomized calf each week and collecting about 1 liter of blood from the jugular vein. As demand for vaccine increased, calves were utilized more efficiently by performing exchange transfusions (Callow & Mellors 1966). This involved canulating the carotid artery, and allowed collections to be made on two or three consecutive days. The development of the parasitemia was not inhibited by the removal of the calf's blood, and yields on the second and third day frequently exceeded that on the first day of collection.

At the present time, two or three calves are infected each week. At least 10^9 parasites are given intravenously, and collection starts 3 or 4 days later. Parasites for infection are from the previous donor so that, in effect, vaccine strains are serially passaged every few days.

In an attempt to maximize production of parasites, calves were immuno-suppressed by treating them with a corticosteroid (Callow & Parker 1969). The use of this drug was discontinued when it appeared to be causing sudden death of calves from disseminated intravascular coagulation (Dalgliesh et al. 1976).

<u>Handling and Use</u>. Approximately 4 liters of blood are collected into a sterile plastic bag containing heparin. This is taken immediately to the laboratory; samples are removed for parasite counting and, at times, for bacteriological examination; an antibacterial agent is added; and the blood is chilled to 2-4 C. The parasite content, established by a direct counting method (Parker 1973), determines the dilution at which the blood is initially used. Because of loss of infectivity during storage, the dilution is decreased each day by a factor of 1.5 and the concentrate is not used for more than 1 week after collection. Vaccine is dispensed into plastic bags, packed in ice, and dispatched from the laboratory in insulated containers.

<u>Strains Used in Vaccine</u>. Five different strains of *Babesia argentina* (= *bovis*) have been used for vaccine. Four of these were isolated in the last 15 years and used experimentally before being processed for vaccine. The fifth has been used for vaccine production for many years and is believed to be one isolated over 40 years ago (Legg 1935). Although slight immunologic differences amongst them can be shown by methods described by Callow (1968) and

Curnow (1968), there is no obvious difference in their capacity to protect cattle in the field.

All five strains changed their character during passage in splenectomized calves. After about 10 passages infections in this host became more intense, allowing considerably more parasites to be collected from each calf. As this change was taking place, virulence for nonsplenectomized recipients decreased appreciably. As a result, expected severe vaccine reactions did not eventuate and postvaccination surveillance of cattle is now frequently not undertaken. A return to passaging vaccine strains in nonsplenectomized hosts reverses these effects.

Repeated passage by blood inoculation has induced a more permanent biological change in four of the vaccine strains. The original vaccine strain when tested was found to have lost its infectivity for ticks (O'Sullivan & Callow 1966). This change has since been observed to occur in three of the more recent isolates (Dalgliesh, R.J. & Stewart, N.P., unpublished data). Strains not transmissible by ticks are now used in vaccine in preference to transmissible ones to avoid spread of disease from vaccinated to unvaccinated cattle.

Control of Contamination

A major disadvantage of a living vaccine grown in an animal host is the possibility of contamination. In Australia there is a risk of animals used in vaccine production becoming infected with *Anaplasma marginale, Eperythrozoon, Theileria mutans, Trypanosoma theileri,* and *Borrelia theileri* as well as "wild" strains of *Babesia.* Measures taken to avoid these infections are the purchase of cattle from districts not enzootically affected by tick-borne diseases, serologic testing of vaccine animals for *Babesia* and *Anaplasma* and monitoring of blood films and rectal temperatures of animals prior to use. The use of young calves that have had little opportunity to become infected with *Eperythrozoon, Theileria mutans, Trypanosoma theileri,* and *Borrelia theileri* reduces the risk of including these organisms in vaccine. Strict quarantine prevents *Boophilus microplus* from becoming established in areas where vaccine animals are kept. Because of the possibility of transmission by biting flies, precautions are taken not to house animals being used for vaccine production close to those with *A. marginale* infections.

Of the blood infections listed above, only contamination with *A. marginale* and a wild strain of *Babesia* could have serious consequences. The other four parasites do not normally cause disease, are widely distributed in Australia and, in fact, regularly contaminated vaccine supplied from the carrier donors used before 1964.

An important concern is to avoid contamination with the agent of bovine leukosis. This condition was apparently spread by the use of a blood vaccine against babesiosis in Sweden (Olson 1961; Bodin et al. 1961). In Australia, calves are purchased from an area where enzootic leukosis has not been diagnosed. The adult animals that are used to provide blood for transfusions and for separation to produce the plasma-based diluent are checked hematologically every 3 months. They are observed for approximately 1 year after purchase and before use. To date, no animal with a lymphocytosis or any other sign of leukosis has been detected.

From time to time vaccine animals have become infected with ephemeral fever and salmonellosis. Vaccine is not prepared from cattle suffering from any infection or suspected of being infected. The absence in Australia of many major animal diseases such as bluetongue, rinderpest, and foot and mouth disease makes the task of preparing a "clean" vaccine less difficult. It is obvious that the specific infections in the environment should be taken into account in planning vaccine production in other countries.

Contamination with skin and air-borne organisms has proved difficult to prevent. Measures to reduce infection include sterile technique where possible, hygienic precautions at all stages of production, and the addition of an anti-biotic to vaccine. Bacterial contamination of vaccine is undesirable on two counts. Apart from the risk of causing localized or generalized infections in recipients, babesial infectivity of the vaccine may be adversely affected by growth of the bacteria.

Evaluation of the Method

Effectiveness of Vaccination

The protective capacity of the vaccine was not exhaustively tested before its introduction in 1964. There was, however, immediate strong field evidence that it was much more effective than the carrier donor vaccine it replaced. More recently, laboratory evaluation has resulted from ancillary immunologic investigations. These have concerned such questions as the immunogenicity of different strains, the duration of immunity, the value of using more than one strain in a vaccination program, the effect of age on the persistence of immunity, and the effect of complete cure on immunity. Because many laboratory challenges are not lethal, other responses were measured (Callow & Pepper 1974). These included parasitemia, febrile response, and depression of the hematocrit. Almost all vaccinated cattle have proved considerably less susceptible than previously unexposed controls (Callow, L.L. & McGregor, W., unpublished data). Although challenged animals usually experience parasitemia and mild fever, they seldom appear sick. An exception was the experiment of Rogers (1971a) in which a group of vaccinated cattle were as susceptible as controls. This experiment is of additional interest because a second group given the same vaccination as the first group but not challenged until after a further 12 months had elapsed then showed considerable resistance.

A critical appraisal of field vaccination was begun 6 years ago on farms in southeast Queensland. Groups were left unvaccinated and subjected to the same field challenge as vaccinated cattle. Observations were made on approximately 1,000 cattle, three quarters of which were vaccinated. Just over 1% of vaccinated cattle were clinically affected during field attacks, but the incidence in controls was almost 18% (Emmerson et al. 1976).

Over the last 3 years there has been a sporadic occurrence of very acute babesiosis in herds that have been vaccinated once, twice, or even three times (Callow, L.L., unpublished data). Although it has not been possible to make controlled observations, it has appeared that some outbreaks have been more sudden and severe than if the cattle had not been previously infected. The cause is not apparent and may be complex, involving an abnormal or incomplete immune response to the primary inoculation, and the eventual natural exposure of the cattle to an antigenically extreme ("breakthrough") strain. The possibility of immunologic blocking is being considered. The occurrence of the syndrome under different circumstances is described below.

Hazards of Vaccination

As stated in an earlier section, an anticipated increase in the incidence of acute reactions following vaccination with highly infective material did not result. Cattle vaccinated in the field experience febrile responses (Dalgliesh 1968), but generally control their infections without treatment. There have been few reports of abortion attributable to vaccination of pregnant females.

Very severe reactions were observed in the field when cattle were revaccinated with a strain that had been recently isolated and processed for use in vaccine (Callow, L.L. & McGregor, W., unpublished data). The reactions usually occurred 2 to 4 weeks after inoculation instead of 1 to 2 weeks, as is the general rule. Farmers were caught unawares by the unexpected response, and mortalities of up to 10% were recorded. Fortunately, a relatively small proportion of herds being revaccinated was affected. The effect was reproduced in the laboratory, and it was concluded that a breakthrough strain had been inadvertently selected for vaccine production. Immunologic blocking was suggested by the fact that cattle receiving a primary inoculation reacted much less acutely than superinfected cattle developing the syndrome. Similar responses have been rarely observed with other vaccine strains.

An unexpected difficulty resulted from the use of whole blood as the diluent for the parasites when this was combined with the practice of vaccinating cattle repeatedly. Towards the end of the 1960s a low incidence of hemolytic anemia in newborn calves was observed (Dimmock & Bell 1970; Langford et al. 1971). This resulted from sensitization of the dam with blood group antigens. Hemolytic anemia occurred when the calf had inherited from its sire the same blood group as one occurring in vaccine used for the dam. Ingestion of lytic antibodies in colostrum by the calf shortly after birth caused acute hemolysis. The development of cell-free diluents and a reduction in the number of vaccinations to one or two per beast has eliminated hemolytic anemia as a problem.

The possibility of various types of contamination occurring at the laboratory has been dealt with in an earlier section. To date there is no evidence that this has led to the transmission of a harmful agent in the field. It is possible, however, that anaplasmosis is transmitted within a herd from time to time as vaccinators do not usually sterilize needles between animals.

Organization of a Vaccine Service

Vaccine is prepared and supplied in Australia by a government laboratory. Most is used in Queensland with a small demand from the Northern Territory, Western Australia, New Guinea, Indonesia, Malaysia, and Sri Lanka. Cattle being exported to Asia are frequently vaccinated before leaving Australia.

Orders are placed directly with the laboratory by cattle owners or their agents and vaccine is supplied, if necessary, within 24 hours. Because it does not store well, vaccine is produced continuously.

Serious consideration has been given to the preparation of frozen vaccine, and basic studies to determine conditions allowing optimal recovery of *Babesia* have been completed (Dalgliesh 1971, 1972a, 1972b; Dalgliesh & Mellors 1974). Even now that optimal conditions such as type and concentration of cryoprotectant, cooling and thawing rates, and dimensions of the container have been defined, the yield of viable *Babesia* is estimated at less than 10% (Dalgliesh, R.J. & Mellors, L.T., unpublished data). This relatively poor recovery is a limiting factor when it is necessary to provide large quantities of highly infective vaccine. Based on an annual demand for 1,200,000 doses, and the fact that the weekly demand has not been less than 18,000 doses in recent years, it was calculated that weekly production of fresh vaccine is cheaper than batch production followed by cryopreservation. However, in situations in which either suitable donor animals may be difficult to obtain, hazardous conditions for production exist, or demand is low and infrequent, a frozen vaccine system or one combined with intermittent production of fresh vaccine may be the correct approach and, in fact, is the method adopted in Bolivia (McCosker 1975).

Field Use of Vaccine

Cattle are usually vaccinated by the owner of the herd or his manager. Most vaccinations are prophylactic but, at times, vaccine is supplied to counteract an outbreak in an unvaccinated herd. The farmer usually receives it within 24 hours of dispatch from the laboratory. Ideally, the vaccine is chilled in the refrigerator on arrival and used within the following week. When large mobs are vaccinated, repeating syringes are used to give a 2-ml dose.

The relatively long duration of immunity following infection (see section on immunology) means that, for practical purposes, only one or two vaccinations are necessary. Farmers are advised to begin vaccinating within the first year of life (Emmerson et al. 1974). If vaccinations are spaced 6 months apart, cattle automatically receive a different strain of *Babesia argentina* (= *bovis*) at their second vaccination because strains are varied by the laboratory every 5 months. An increasing demand for protection against anaplasmosis has led to the incorporation of *Anaplasma centrale* in about 30% of babesial vaccine.

Varying degrees of surveillance are applied to vaccinated cattle. Farmers are told to anticipate a reaction 7 to 14 days after inoculation, but this advice is frequently ignored without serious consequences. Prophylaxis with imidocarb (Callow & McGregor 1970) is sometimes used, especially when heavily pregnant cattle are to be vaccinated.

VACCINATION AGAINST *BABESIA BIGEMINA*

The foregoing has dealt mainly with protection against *Babesia argentina* (= *bovis*) in Australia. The routine use of *Babesia bigemina* in vaccine was discontinued in 1964 when production of highly infective *Babesia argentina* (= *bovis*) vaccine began. Legg (1939) remarked that *Babesia bigemina* rarely caused outbreaks of babesiosis in Australia, and recent examinations of diagnostic records indicate that this situation had not changed (Johnston 1968; Rogers 1971c). A confirmation of the low pathogenicity of *Babesia bigemina* was obtained before omitting it from vaccine by observing the exposure to natural infection of 32 animals in three groups in different tick-infested environments. These animals developed parasitemias with *Babesia bigemina* but were not clinically affected (Callow, L.L., unpublished data).

On the rare occasions that *Babesia bigemina* is incriminated in serious outbreaks of babesiosis, a vaccine may be supplied. Virulence of this parasite has not been appreciably reduced by rapid passage in splenectomized calves, and laboratory-maintained *Babesia bigemina* tends to be more virulent than most naturally occurring strains. To reduce the risk of severe reactions associated with rapidly passaged *Babesia bigemina,* relapse parasitemias provoked by splenectomy of calves carrying infection for at least 2 months are utilized. Parasites collected from these can be used immediately, but usually are frozen in liquid nitrogen until vaccine is required. Then a splenectomized calf is inoculated with stabilate material, and vaccine prepared from the resultant parasitemia (Dalgliesh, R.J. & Callow, L.L., unpublished data).

FUTURE REQUIREMENTS AND DEVELOPMENTS

In certain countries other than Australia, there is a need to determine the epizootiology of babesiosis before considering vaccination. Areas of enzootic stability and instability should be defined using methods described by Mahoney and his coworkers (see Mahoney 1973) and reviewed in an earlier section of this paper. It is equally important to determine by means of careful studies of disease incidence and accurate diagnosis the relative economic effects of the tick-borne parasites occurring in a region, so that an appropriate vaccine can be prepared. For example, observations on natural infections in cattle imported to Malaysia have indicated that *Babesia bigemina* is more pathogenic there than in Australia (Rajamanickam 1970) although, as in Australia, *Babesia argentina* (= *bovis*) is the more dangerous parasite.

The performance in the future of large-scale vaccination such as that practiced in Australia will depend on several factors. First, vaccination must be economically worthwhile. A current, sharp decrease in demand for vaccination in Australia reflects a marketing situation in which many beef cattle are almost unsaleable. Second, there is a growing impetus amongst beef producers in a number of countries to incorporate a substantial Zebu component into their herds. It is likely that this will reduce the need for vaccination. Third, new approaches to tick control or eradication may alter requirements for vaccination. The suggestion of Mahoney and Ross (1972) that lowering the vector density could lead to a gradual disappearance of *Babesia* from the environment deserves credence. Vector density will decrease as the Zebu component of herds increases and also if more cattle owners reduce tick numbers by using methods presently available. The present practice in Australia of using vaccine strains that are not transmissible by ticks could lead to a decrease in the infection rates with *Babesia* in ticks. A situation could develop in which cattle but not ticks are infected, making eradication by sterilizing drug treatment (Callow & McGregor 1970) a practical proposition.

Whereas requirements may change for the large beef herds established in the enzootic areas of the world, there will be a continuing need for vaccination for susceptible cattle imported to tropical, developing countries. Because of the severity of the challenge to be faced by such cattle in their new environment, methods may have to be more stringent than those described in this review as being effective under Australian conditions. There is no obvious reason why the same principles should not apply, and there is already evidence that the immunogenicity of the vaccine is not limited to Australia (Rajamanickam 1970; McCosker 1975). To achieve the best results, however, it may be necessary to vaccinate against *Babesia bigemina* and also to use appropriate combinations of strains of *Babesia argentina* (= *bovis*) to broaden and enhance the immune response. Experience with Australian cattle proceeding to Southeast Asia has indicated it is far better for cattle to be immune when they arrive than to undergo the immunization process after introduction. Stress, management difficulties, and lack of expertise in dealing with tick-borne disease combine to take toll of unprotected cattle following importation to some tropical countries (McCosker 1975; Callow, L.L., unpublished data). Unless effective protection against vectors and a stable environment can be provided for several months in the importing country, immunization should be performed before departure from the country of origin.

ACKNOWLEDGMENTS

I wish to acknowledge the efforts of present and past staff of the Department of Primary Industries, Tick Fever Research Centre, in the accumulation of information that has not yet been formally published and which is recorded here as "unpublished data." I also thank Mr. R.J. Dalgliesh and Mrs. Gail Farlow for access to their unpublished material.

BIBLIOGRAPHY

Anon. 1975. Cattle Tick in Australia. Cattle Tick Control Commission Inquiry Report 1973. Australian Government Publishing Service, Canberra, pp. 108.

Bishop, J.P. & Adams, L.G. 1974. *Babesia bigemina:* immune response of cattle inoculated with irradiated parasites. *Exp. Parasitol.* 35: 35-43.

Bodin, S., Enhorning, G., Olson, H. & Winqvist, G. 1961. Die Anzahl der Lymphozyten im Blut von Rinder bei lymphatischer Leukose und Piroplasmose. *Acta Vet. Scand.* 2 (Supp. 2): 47-54.

Brocklesby, D.W., Purnell, R.E. & Sellwood, S.A. 1972. The effect of irradiation on intra-erythrocytic stages of *Babesia major*. *Brit. Vet. J.* 128: iii-v.

Brocklesby, D.W., Zwart, D. & Perie, N.M. 1971. Serological evidence for the identification of *Babesia major* in Britain. *Res. Vet. Sci.* 12: 285-287.

Brown, K.N. 1971. Protective immunity to malaria provides a model for the survival of cells in an immunologically hostile environment. *Nature* (Lond.) 230: 163-167.

Callow, L.L. 1964. Strain immunity in babesiosis. *Nature* (Lond.) 204: 1213-1214.

Callow, L.L. 1967. Sterile immunity, coinfectious immunity and strain differences in *Babesia bigemina* infections. *Parasitology* 57: 455-465.

Callow, L.L. 1968. A note on homologous strain immunity in *Babesia argentina* infections. *Aust. Vet. J.* 44: 268-269.

Callow, L.L. 1971. The control of babesiosis with a highly infective attenuated vaccine. *In* Proceedings of the 19th World Veterinary Congress. 1: 357-360.

Callow, L.L., Emmerson, F.R., Parker, R.J. & Knott, S.G. 1976a. Infection rates and outbreaks of disease due to *Babesia argentina* in unvaccinated cattle on five beef properties in Southeast Queensland. *Aust. Vet. J.* 52: 446-450.

Callow, L.L. & Hoyte, H.M.D. 1961. Transmission experiments using *Babesia bigemina, Theileria mutans, Borrelia* sp. and the cattle tick, *Boophilus microplus. Aust. Vet. J.* 37: 381-390.

Callow, L.L. & McGavin, M.D. 1963. Cerebral babesiosis due to *Babesia argentina. Aust. Vet. J.* 39: 15-21.

Callow, L.L. & McGregor, W. 1969. Vaccination against *Babesia argentina* infection in cattle during chemoprophylaxis with a quinuronium compound. *Aust. Vet. J.* 45: 408-410.

Callow, L.L. & McGregor, W. 1970. The effect of imidocarb against *Babesia argentina* and *Babesia bigemina* infections of cattle. *Aust. Vet. J.* 46: 195-200.

Callow, L.L., McGregor, W., Parker, R.J. & Dalgliesh, R.J. 1974a. The immunity of cattle to *Babesia argentina* after drug sterilization of infections of varying duration. *Aust. Vet. J.* 50: 6-11.

Callow, L.L., McGregor, W., Parker, R.J. & Dalgliesh, R.J. 1974b. Immunity of cattle to *Babesia bigemina* following its elimination from the host, with observations on antibody levels detected by the indirect fluorescent antibody test. *Aust. Vet. J.* 50: 12-15.

Callow, L.L. & Mellors, L.T. 1966. A new vaccine for *Babesia argentina* infection prepared in splenectomised calves. *Aust. Vet. J.* 42: 464-465.

Callow, L.L. & Parker, R.J. 1969. Cortisone-induced relapses in *Babesia argentina* infections of cattle. *Aust. Vet. J.* 45: 103-104.

Callow, L.L. & Pepper, P.M. 1974. Measurement of and correlations between fever, changes in the packed cell volume and parasitaemia in the evaluation of the susceptibility of cattle to infection with *Babesia argentina. Aust. Vet. J.* 50: 1-5.

Callow, L.L., Quiroga, Q.C. & McCosker, P.J. 1976b. Serological comparison of Australian and South American strains of *Babesia argentina* and *Anaplasma marginale. Int. J. Parasitol.* 6: 307-310.

Callow, L.L. & Tammemagi, L. 1967. Vaccination against bovine babesiosis. Infectivity and virulence of blood from animals either recovered from or reacting to *Babesia argentina. Aust. Vet. J.* 43: 249-256.

Clark, I. & Allison, A. 1976. Immune defences against blood parasites. *New Sci.* 69: 668-669.

Clark, I.A., Allison, A.C. & Cox, F.E.G. 1976. Protection of mice against *Babesia* and *Plasmodium* with BCG. *Nature* (Lond.) 259: 309-311.

Coggeshall, L.T. 1943. Immunity in malaria. *Medicine* (Balt.) 22: 87-102.

Connaway, J.W. & Franics, M. 1899. Texas fever. Experiments made by the Missouri experiment station and the Missouri state board of agriculture in cooperation with the Texas experiment station in immunizing northern breeding cattle against Texas fever for the southern trade. *Mo. Agric. Exp. Stn. Bull.* 48: 1-64.

Cox, F.E.G. & Young, A.S. 1969. Acquired immunity to *Babesia microti* and *Babesia rodhaini* in mice. *Parasitology* 59: 257-268.

Curnow, J.A. 1968. *In vitro* agglutination of bovine erythrocytes infected with *Babesia argentina. Nature* (Lond.) 217: 267-268.

Curnow, J.A. 1973a. Studies on antigenic changes and strain differences in *Babesia argentina* infections. *Aust. Vet. J.* 49: 279-283.

Curnow, J.A. 1973b. Studies on the epizootiology of bovine babesiosis in northeastern New South Wales. *Aust. Vet. J.* 49: 284-289.

Dalgliesh, R.J. 1968. Field observations on *Babesia argentina* vaccination in Queensland. *Aust. Vet. J.* 44: 103-104.

Dalgliesh, R.J. 1971. Dimethyl sulphoxide in the low-temperature preservation of *Babesia bigemina. Res. Vet. Sci.* 12: 469-471.

Dalgliesh, R.J. 1972a. Theoretical and practical aspects of freezing parasitic protozoa. *Aust. Vet. J.* 48: 233-239.

Dalgliesh, R.J. 1972b. Effects of low temperature preservation and route of inoculation on infectivity of *Babesia bigemina* in blood diluted with glycerol. *Res. Vet. Sci.* 13: 540-545.

Dalgliesh, R.J., Dimmock, C.K., Hill, M.W.M. & Mellors, L.T. 1976. Disseminated intravascular coagulation in acute *Babesia argentina* infections in splenectomized calves. *Exp. Parasitol.* 40: 124-131.

Dalgliesh, R.J. & Mellors, L.T. 1974. Survival of the parasitic protozoan, *Babesia bigemina*, in blood cooled at widely different rates to $-196°C$. *Int. J. Parasitol.* 4: 169-172.

Daly, G.D. & Hall, W.T.K. 1955. A note on the susceptibility of British and some Zebu-type cattle to tick fever (babesiosis). *Aust. Vet. J.* 31: 152.

Davies, S.F.M., Joyner, L.P. & Kendall, S.B. 1958. Studies on *Babesia divergens* (M'Fadyean and Stockman, 1911). *Ann. Trop. Med. Parasitol.* 52: 206-215.

Dimmock, C.K. & Bell, K. 1970. Haemolytic disease of the newborn in calves. *Aust. Vet. J.* 46: 44-47.

Emmerson, F.R., Knott, S.G. & Callow, L.L. 1976. Vaccination with *Babesia argentina* in 5 beef herds in Southeast Queensland. *Aust. Vet. J.* 52: 52: 451-454.

Emmerson, F.R., Knott, S.G. & McGregor, W. 1974. Tick fevers - - and how to prevent them. *Queensl. Agric. J.* 100: 405-415.

Garnham, P.C.C. 1970. The role of the spleen in protozoal infections with special reference to splenectomy. *Acta Trop.* 27: 1-14.

Goldman, M. & Rosenberg, A.S. 1974. Immunofluorescence studies of the small *Babesia* species of cattle from different geographical areas. *Res. Vet. Sci.* 16: 351-354.

Goodger, B.V. 1971. Preparation and preliminary assessment of purified antigens in the passive haemagglutination test for bovine babesiosis. *Aust. Vet. J.* 47: 251-256.

Goodger, B.V. 1973. Further studies of haemagglutinating antigens of *Babesia bigemina. Aust. Vet. J.* 49: 81-84.

Goodger, B.V. & Mahoney, D.F. 1974a. Evaluation of the passive haemagglutination test for the diagnosis of *Babesia argentina* infection in cattle. *Aust. Vet. J.* 50: 246-249.

Goodger, B.V. & Mahoney, D.F. 1974b. A rapid slide agglutination test for the herd diagnosis of *Babesia argentina* infection. *Aust. Vet. J.* 50: 250-254.

Hall, W.T.K. 1960. The immunity of calves to *Babesia argentina* infection. *Aust. Vet. J.* 36: 361-366.

Hall, W.T.K. 1963. The immunity of calves to tick-transmitted *Babesia argentina* infection. *Aust. Vet. J.* 39: 386-389.

Hall, W.T.K., Tammemagi, L. & Johnston, L.A.Y. 1968. Bovine babesiosis: the immunity of calves to *Babesia bigemina* infection. *Aust. Vet. J.* 44: 259-264.

Hoyte, H.M.D. 1961. Initial development of infections with *Babesia bigemina. J. Protozool.* 8: 462-466.

Hoyte, H.M.D. 1965. Further observations on the initial development of infections with *Babesia bigemina. J. Protozool.* 12: 83-85.

Johnston, L.A.Y. 1967. Epidemiology of bovine babesiosis in northern Queensland. *Aust. Vet. J.* 43: 427-432.

Johnston, L.A.Y. 1968. The incidence of clinical babesiosis in cattle in Queensland. *Aust. Vet. J.* 44: 265-267.

Johnston, L.A.Y., Pearson, R.D. & Leatch, G. 1973. Evaluation of an indirect fluorescent antibody test for detecting *Babesia argentina* infection in cattle. *Aust. Vet. J.* 49: 373-377.

Johnston, L.A.Y. & Tammemagi, L. 1969. Bovine babesiosis: duration of latent infection and immunity to *Babesia argentina. Aust. Vet. J.* 45: 445-449.

Kemron, A., Hadani, A., Egyed, M., Pipano, E. & Neuman, M. 1964. Studies on bovine piroplasmosis caused by *Babesia bigemina.* III. The relationship between the number of parasites in the inoculum and the severity of the response. *Refu. Vet.* 112-108.

de Kock, G. & Quinlan, J.B. 1926. Splenectomy in domesticated animals and its sequelae, with special reference to anaplasmosis in sheep. *In* 11th and 12th Reports of the Director of the Veterinary Education and Research, Department of Agriculture, South Africa; Pretoria, South Africa. 369-480.

Langford, G., Knott, S.G., Dimmock, C.K. & Derrington, P. 1971. Haemolytic disease of newborn calves in a dairy herd in Queensland. *Aust. Vet. J.* 47: 1-4.

Leeflang, P. & Perie, N.M. 1972. Comparative immunofluorescent studies on 4 *Babesia* species of cattle. *Res. Vet. Sci.* 13: 342-346.

Legg, J. 1935. The occurrence of bovine babesiellosis in Northern Australia. Council for Scientific and Industrial Research of Australia, Pamphlet No. 56: 1-48.

Legg, J. 1939. Recent observations on the premunization of cattle against tick fevers in Queensland. *Aust. Vet. J.* 25: 46-53.

Levine, N.D. 1971. Taxonomy of the piroplasms. *Trans. Am. Microsc. Soc.* 90: 2-33.

Löhr, K.F. 1969. Immunisierung gegen Babesiose und Anaplasmose von 40 nach Kenya importierten Charollais-Rindern und Bericht über Erscheinungen der Photosensibilität bei diesen Tieren. *Zentralbl. Veterinaermed.* B16: 40-46.

Löhr, K.F. 1973. Susceptibility of non-splenectomized and splenectomized Sahiwal cattle to experimental *Babesia bigemina* infection. *Zentralbl. Veterinaermed.* B20: 52-56.

Ludford, C.L., Hall, W.T.K., Sulzer, A.J. & Wilson M. 1972. *Babesia argentina, Plasmodium vivax,* and *P. falciparum:* antigenic cross-reactions. *Exp. Parasitol.* 32: 317-326.

Mahoney, D.F. 1962. The epidemiology of babesiosis in cattle. *Aust. J. Sci.* 24: 310-313.

Mahoney, D.F. 1967a. Bovine babesiosis: the passive immunization of calves against *Babesia argentina* with special reference to the role of complement fixing antibodies. *Exp. Parasitol.* 20: 119-124.

Mahoney, D.F. 1967b. Bovine babesiosis: the immunization of cattle with killed *Babesia argentina. Exp. Parasitol.* 20: 125-129.

Mahoney, D.F. 1967c. Bovine babesiosis: preparation and assessment of complement-fixing antigens. *Exp. Parasitol.* 20: 232-241.

Mahoney, D.F. 1969. Bovine babesiasis: a study of factors concerned in transmission. *Ann. Trop. Med. Parasitol.* 63: 1-14.

Mahoney, D.F. 1971. Immunization against *Babesia argentina* (Lignieres, 1903). Proceedings of the 19th World Veterinary Congress. 1: 351-356.

Mahoney, D.F. 1973. Babesiosis of cattle. *Aust. Meat Res. Comm. Rev.* 23: 1-21.

Mahoney, D.F. & Goodger, B.V. 1969. *Babesia argentina:* serum changes in infected calves. *Exp. Parasitol.* 24: 375-382.

Mahoney, D.F. & Goodger, B.V. 1972. *Babesia argentina:* immunogenicity of plasma from infected animals. *Exp. Parasitol.* 32: 71-85.

Mahoney, D.F. & Mirre, G.B. 1971. Bovine babesiasis: estimation of infection rates in the tick vector *Boophilus microplus* (Canestrini). *Ann. Trop. Med. Parasitol.* 65: 309-317.

Mahoney, D.F. & Mirre, G.B. 1974. *Babesia argentina:* the infection of splenectomized calves with extracts of larval ticks *(Boophilus microplus). Res. Vet. Sci.* 16: 112-114.

Mahoney, D.F. & Ross, D.R. 1972. Epizootiological factors in the control of bovine babesiosis. *Aust. Vet. J.* 48: 292-298.

Mahoney, D.F., Wright, I.G. & Ketterer, P.J. 1973a. *Babesia argentina:* the infectivity and immunogenicity of irradiated blood parasites for splenectomized calves. *Int. J. Parasitol.* 3: 209-217.

Mahoney, D.F., Wright, I.G. & Mirre, G.B. 1973b. Bovine babesiasis: the persistence of immunity to *Babesia argentina* and *Babesia bigemina* in calves *(Bos taurus)* after naturally acquired infection. *Ann. Trop. Med. Parasitol.* 67: 197-203.

McCosker, P.J. 1975. Control of piroplasmosis and anaplasmosis in cattle. A practical manual. Food and Agriculture Organisation, Santa Cruz, Bolivia. pp. 64.

Morzaria, S.P., Brocklesby, D.W., Harradine, D.L. & Barnett, S.F. 1974. *Babesia major* in Britain: infectivity of suspensions derived from ground-up *Haemaphysalis punctata* nymphs. *Int. J. Parasitol.* 1: 437-438.

Newton, L.G. & O'Sullivan, P.J. 1969. Chemoprophylaxis in *Babesia argentina* infection in cattle. *Aust. Vet. J.* 45: 404-407.

Nuttall, G.H.F. & Graham-Smith, G.S. 1907. Studies on the morphology and life-history of the parasite. (Canine piroplasmosis 6). *J. Hyg.* 7: 232-272.

Nuttall, G.H.F. & Graham-Smith, G.S. 1908. The mode of multiplication of *Piroplasma bovis, P. pitheci* in the circulating blood compared with that of *P. canis* with notes on other species of *Piroplasma. Parasitology* 1: 134-142.

Olson, H. 1961. Studien über das Auftreten und die Verbreitung der Rinderleukose in Schweden. *Acta Vet. Scand.* 2 (Supp. 2) 13-46.

O'Sullivan, P.J. & Callow, L.L. 1966. Loss of infectivity of a vaccine strain of *Babesia argentina* for *Boophilus microplus*. *Aust. Vet. J.* 42: 252-254.

Parker, R. 1973. A direct counting technique for estimating high parasitaemias in infections of *Babesia argentina, Babesia bigemina,* and *Plasmodium berghei. Ann. Trop. Med. Parasitol.* 67: 387-390.

Phillips, R.S. 1971a. Evidence that piroplasms can undergo antigenic variation. *Nature* (Lond.) 231: 323.

Phillips, R.S. 1971b. Immunity of rats and mice following injection with ^{60}Co-irradiated *Babesia rodhaini* infected red cells. *Parasitology* 62: 221-231.

Pipano, E. 1969a. Immunization of cattle against *Babesiella berbera* infection. I. Infection of cattle with blood from patent and latent carriers. *Refu. Vet. 26: 11-18.*

Pipano, E. 1969b. Immunization of cattle against *Babesiella berbera* infection. II. Immunization of calves in the field with blood from latent carriers. *Refu. Vet.* 26: 113-117.

Potgieter, F.T. & Van Vuuren, A.S. 1974. The transmission of *Babesia bovis* using frozen infective material obtained from *Boophilus microplus* larvae. *Onderstepoort J. Vet. Res.* 41: 79-80.

Pound, C.J. 1897. Tick fever. Notes on the inoculation of bulls as a preventive against tick fever at Rathdowney and Rosedale. *Queensland Agric. J.* 1: 473-477.

Purnell, R.E. & Joyner, L.P. 1967. Artificial feeding technique for *Rhipicephalus appendiculatus* and the transmission of *Theileria parva* from the salivary secretion. *Nature (Lond.)* 216: 484-485.

Rajamanickam, C. 1970. Blood protozoan diseases of imported temperate breeds of cattle in West Malaysia. *Kajian Vet.* 2: 145-152.

Rees, C.W. 1934. Characteristics of the piroplasms *Babesia argentina* and *Babesia bigemina* in the United States. *J. Agric. Res.* 48: 427-438.

Riek, R.F. 1963. Immunity to babesiosis. *In* Immunity to Protozoa, P.C.C. Garnham, Pierce, A.E. & Roitt, I., Eds.: 160-179. Blackwell Scientific Publications. Oxford, England.

Riek, R.F. 1964. The life cycle of *Babesia bigemina* (Smith and Kilborne 1893) in the tick vector *Boophilus microplus* (Canestrini). *Aust. J. Agric. Res.* 15: 802-821.

Riek, R.F. 1966. The life cycle of *Babesia argentina* (Lignières 1903) (Sporozoa: Piroplasmidea) in the tick vector *Boophilus microplus* (Canestrini). *Aust. J. Agric. Res.* 17: 247-254.

Rogers, R.J. 1971a. The acquired resistance to *Babesia argentina* of cattle exposed to light infestation with cattle tick *(Boophilus microplus). Aust. Vet. J.* 47: 237-241.

Rogers, R.J. 1971b. Observations on the pathology of *Babesia argentina* infections in cattle. *Aust. Vet. J.* 47: 242-247.

Rogers, R.J. 1971c. An evaluation of tick fever outbreaks in Northern Queensland in recent years. *Aust. Vet. J.* 47: 415-417.

Ross, D.R. & Mahoney, D.F. 1974. Bovine babesiosis: computer simulation of *Babesia argentina* parasite rates in *Bos taurus* cattle. *Ann. Trop. Med. Parasitol.* 68: 385-392.

Roy-Smith, F. 1971. The prophylactic effects of imidocarb against *Babesia argentina* and *Babesia bigemina* infections of cattle. *Aust. Vet. J.* 47: 418-420.

Ryley, J.F. 1964. A chemoprophylactic approach to babesiosis. *Res. Vet. Sci.* 5: 411-418.

Schmidt, G., Hirt, R. & Fischer, R. 1969. Babesicidal effect of basically substituted carbanilides. I: Activity against *Babesia rodhaini* in mice. *Res. Vet. Sci.* 10: 530-539.

Seddon, H.R. 1952. Diseases of domestic animals in Australia, Part 4. Protozoan and viral diseases. Service Publication No. 8. Commonwealth Department of Health, Canberra, pp. 214.

Seddon, H.R. 1968. Diseases of domestic animals in Australia, Part 3 (Rev. by H.E. Albiston). Arthropod infestations (Ticks and mites). *Service Publication* No. 7. Commonwealth Department of Health, Canberra, pp. 170.

Sergent, E., Donatien, A., Parrot, L. & Lestoquard, F. 1945. Études sur les piroplasmoses bovines. Institut Pasteur d'Algérie, Alger, pp. 816.

Sergent, E., Parrot, L. & Donatien, A. 1924. Une question de terminologie: immuniser et premunir. *Bull. Soc. Pathol. Exot.* 17: 37-38.

Sergent, E., Sergent, Et. & Catanei, A. 1934. Un type de maladie à prémunition: le paludisme des passeraux à *Plasmodium relictum. Ann. Inst. Pasteur* (Paris). 53: 101-119.

Simitch, T., Petrovitch, Z. & Rakovec, R. 1955. Les espèces de *Babesiella* du boeuf d'Europe. *Arch. Inst. Pasteur Alger.* 33: 310-314.

Smith, T. & Kilborne, F.L. 1893. Investigations into the nature, causation and prevention of Texas or Southern cattle fever. *U.S. Dept. Agric. Bur. Anim. Ind. Bull.* 1: 1-301.

Taliaferro, W.H. 1949. Immunity to the malaria infections. *In* Malariology. M.F. Boyd, Ed. Vol. 2: 935-965. W.B. Saunders Co., Philadelphia and London.

Tchernomoretz, I. 1943. Blocking of the brain capillaries by parasitized red blood cells in *Babesiella berbera* infections in cattle. *Ann. Trop. Med. Parasitol.* 37: 77-79.

Thomson, J.G. 1933. Immunity in malaria. *Trans. R. Soc. Trop. Med. Hyg.* 26: 483-514.

Tidswell, F. 1899. Report on Protective Inoculation Against Tick Fever. New South Wales Department of Public Health. Sydney, Australia. 16 pp.

Todorovic, R.A., Gonzalez, E.F. & Adams, L.G. 1973. Bovine babesiosis: sterile immunity to *Babesia bigemina* and *Babesia argentina* infections. *Trop. Anim. Health Prod.* 5: 234-245.

Todorovic, R.A. & Kuttler, K.L. 1974. A babesiosis card agglutination test. *Am. J. Vet. Res.* 35: 1347-1350.

Todorovic, R.A., Lopez, L.A., Lopez, A.G. & Gonzalez, E.F. 1975. Bovine babesiosis and anaplasmosis: control by premunition and chemoprophylaxis. *Exp. Parasitol.* 37: 92-104.

Uilenberg, G. 1969. Notes sur les babésioses et l'anaplasmose des bovins à Madagascar. II. Influence de la splénectomie. *Rev. Élevage Méd. Vét. Pays Trop.* 22: 237-248.

Uilenberg, G. 1970. Notes sur les babésioses et l'anaplasmose des bovins à Madagascar. V.A. Immunité et prémunition. B. Epizootologie. *Rev. Élevage Méd. Vét. Pays Trop.* 23: 439-454.

Uilenberg, G. 1971. Notes sur les babésioses et l'anaplasmose des bovins à Madagascar. VI. Prémunition artificielle. *Rev. Élevage Méd. Vét. Pays Trop.* 24: 23-35.

Wilson, S.G. 1964. Babesiasis in cattle in the Netherlands. I. Identification of *Babesia major* and *B. divergens. Tijdschr. Diergeneesk.* 89: 1783-1790.

Zuckerman, A. 1964. Autoimmunization and other types of indirect damage to host cells as factors in certain protozoan diseases. *Exp. Parasitol.* 15: 138-183.

Zuckerman, A. & Ristic, M. 1968. Blood parasite antigens and antibodies. *In* Infectious Blood Diseases of Man and Animals. D. Weinman and M. Ristic Eds., Vol. 1: 79-122. Academic Press, Inc. New York, N.Y.

Zwart, D., Van den Ende, M.C., Kouwenhoven, B. & Buys, J. 1968. The difference between *B. bigemina* and a Dutch strain of *B. major. Tijdschr. Diergeneesk.* 93: 126-140.

Part IV. Anaplasmosis

9

METHODS OF IMMUNOPROPHYLAXIS AGAINST BOVINE ANAPLASMOSIS WITH EMPHASIS ON USE OF THE ATTENUATED *ANAPLASMA MARGINALE* VACCINE*

Miodrag Ristic and C.A. Carson

Department of Veterinary Pathology and Hygiene
College of Veterinary Medicine
University of Illinois at Champaign-Urbana
Urbana, Illinois 61801

INTRODUCTION

One of the major obstacles to the development of methods for immunoprophylaxis against hemotropic diseases has been the lack of techniques for *in vitro* propagation of the causative agents (*Anaplasma, Babesia*), or the availability of similar systems for laboratory production of arthropod-associated "prototype" antigens (trypanosomes). A recent accomplishment in this direction has been the development of cell culture methods for *Theileria parva,* the causative agent of East Coast fever. While this step is considered an important breakthrough providing incentive for more optimistic future endeavors in the entire field, the accomplishment must not be viewed as an indication that this technique can be directly applied to other hemotropic agents. *Theileria parva* actively invades cellular elements of both the erythrocytic and lymphocytic series, the latter being adapted to *in vitro* propagation. *Anaplasma, Babesia,* and *Plasmodium* are considered to primarily affect the more inert circulating erythrocyte which, rather than offering replication ability in cell culture, continues its *in vivo* destiny of degeneration.

Anaplasmosis is a worldwide tick-borne disease of cattle and some wild ruminants caused by the rickettsia *Anaplasma marginale.* The organism is extremely host-specific and the mature erythrocyte constitutes the only cell known to support growth and development of the agent in an infected animal. Premunition, which consists of infecting and subsequently treating an animal to establish a carrier infection, is the oldest preventive method. It is, however, hazardous, time-consuming, and costly.

*Supported in part by Research Grant RF-44-40-30-362 from The Rockefeller Foundation, New York, N.Y. 10036.

Research toward the development of an *A. marginale* immunogen may utilize the blood of an animal in the acute phase of infection or infected arthropod vectors (tick) as possible sources of the antigen. In view of the limited knowledge regarding development of the organism in the tick, the latter source must presently be considered as theoretical. A degree of transient protection has been . induced by inoculation of susceptible cattle with inactivated *Anaplasma* derived from the blood of infected animals and introduced in oil adjuvant. The method, however, caused development of isoimmunity in vaccinated animals followed by often fatal erythroblastosis in calves of vaccinated dams. Moreover, the procedure is laborious and expensive, since the two initial doses of vaccine must be followed by yearly revaccination to maintain a level of protection.

In view of the aforementioned information as well as other data, our laboratory developed an attenuated *A. marginale* vaccine by adapting *A. marginale* to growth in sheep, an atypical host. After 10 years of research, a strain of *Anaplasma* was derived which was safe for susceptible cattle yet sufficiently immunogenic to protect inoculated animals against laboratory and field challenge with the virulent organism. Although not original in concept, the method signifies the first successful adaptation of an erythrocytic parasite to solution of the disease problem.

BIOLOGIC PROPERTIES OF *ANAPLASMA MARGINALE*

The Organism and Related Species

In *Bergey's Manual* (8th edition), *A. marginale* is the representative species of the genus *Anaplasma,* family Anaplasmataceae, order Rickettsiales (Ristic & Kreier 1974) (Figure 1). The organism (initial body) was shown to enter the erythrocyte by invagination of the cytoplasmic membrane with subsequent formation of a vacuole (Ristic & Watrach 1961). Thereafter, the initial body multiplies by binary fission and forms an inclusion body which consists generally of four to eight initial bodies (Ristic & Watrach 1963) (Figure 2). Inclusion bodies are numerous during the acute phase of the infection; however, low-level infections persist for several years thereafter. Of the three *Anaplasma* species, *A. marginale* is the most pathogenic for cattle. *Anaplasma centrale* causes a relatively "mild" form of bovine anaplasmosis in Africa and *Anaplasma ovis* is the cause of ovine and caprine anaplasmosis.

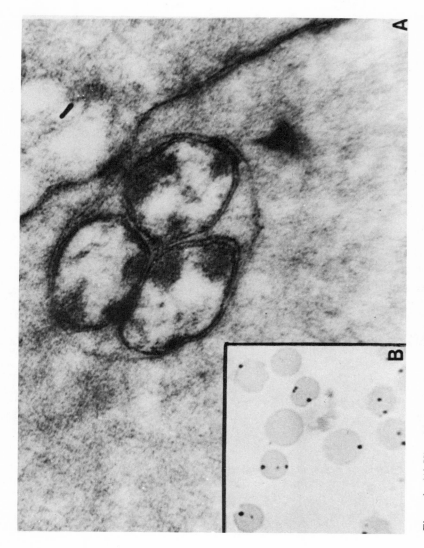

Figure 1. (A) Ultrathin section of an erythrocyte containing marginal *Anaplasma* body with 3 initial bodies. X 118,000. (B) Blood film from a cow in the acute phase of anaplasmosis stained by Giemsa method. X 1,400

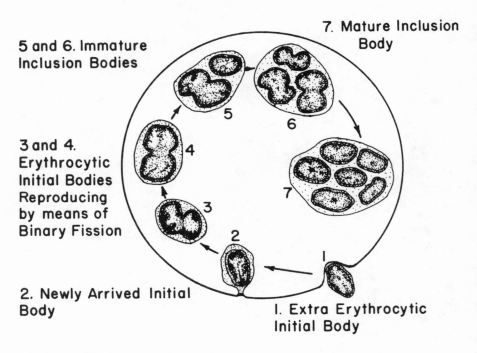

7. Mature Inclusion Body

5 and 6. Immature Inclusion Bodies

3 and 4. Erythrocytic Initial Bodies Reproducing by means of Binary Fission

2. Newly Arrived Initial Body

I. Extra Erythrocytic Initial Body

Figure 2. Proposed developmental cycle of *Anaplasma marginale* based on static evidence obtained from electron microscopic studies.

Paranaplasma caudatum (genus *Paranaplasma*) (Kreier & Ristic 1963a, 1963b, 1963c) was initially found in Oregon cattle in a mixed infection with *A. marginale*. Inclusion bodies of *P. caudatum* have appendages usually in the form of a tapering tail, a loop, or a ring, demonstrated only by use of special techniques. A recent study by Carson et al. (1974) showed that manifestation of *P. caudatum* appendages is a function of bovine host erythrocytes and does not occur in infected deer erythrocytes.

The various anaplasma organisms have at least one species-specific antigen and they are sensitive to the tetracycline group of antibiotics. Anaplasmas morphologically resemble other hemotropic rickettsiae, i.e., *Haemobartonella* and *Eperythrozoon* and share common antigens with these agents (Kreier & Ristic 1972). Ristic (1960, 1968) has compiled general reviews on anaplasmosis, the parasite itself, and the host response.

Intraerythrocytic Behavior, Transfer, and Circulatory Clearance of Infected Erythrocytes

According to Moulder (1974) a successful intracellular parasite must avoid its demise by regulating its growth rate so that demands on the host do not exceed tolerable limits. It appears that the kinetics of *Anaplasma* initial body movement between erythrocytes occurs in a manner that avoids irreparable damage of the host cell membrane. Incubation of *A. marginale* in an *in vitro* system showed that the decrease of observable marginale bodies equalled twice the degree of hemolysis, indicating that the organism may leave the erythrocyte without concomitant host cell lysis (Erp & Fahrney 1975). Since the organism is rarely observed extracellularly, the transit may occur through intercellular tissue bridges. The consequence of organismal interaction with erythrocytic membrane is indicated by a decrease in the concentration of phospholipids in erythrocytic stroma and a high serum sialic acid concentration (Rao & Ristic 1963). The removal of the organism from the circulation takes place by phagocytosis of entire infected erythrocytes. Phagocytosis of apparently noninfected erythrocytes, as frequently observed, may be caused by stimulation of an autoimmune response due to erythrocytic membrane alterations by anaplasma.

Glycine incorporation into protein by *Anaplasma*-infected erythrocytes *in vitro* has been the only available metabolic information associated with anaplasma infection of the host cell (Mason & Ristic 1966). The finding of a food-vacuole-like structure inside an erythrocytic "matrix" harboring initial bodies suggested possible means of metabolism by *Anaplasma* (Amerault et al. 1975, Simpson et al. 1967). Concurrent studies in our laboratory confirmed these findings (Figure 3).

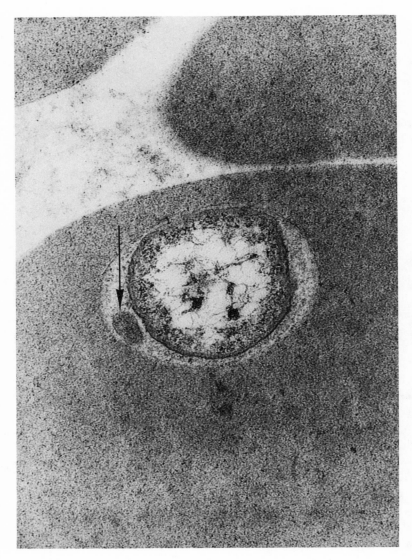

Figure 3. Ultrathin section of an erythrocyte containing marginal *Anaplasma* body with one initial body. Note the presence of a food vacuole in the erythrocytic vacuole surrounding the organism (arrow). X 122,000

Thus, a partial analogy of food intake among *Plasmodium, Babesia,* and *Anaplasma* may exist. Unlike *Plasmodium* and *Babesia,* however, the phagotrophy leading to formation of the food vacuole in *Anaplasma* is extraparasitic and the underlying mechanism not understood.

ANTIGENIC AND SEROLOGIC STUDIES OF *A. MARGINALE*

As a prelude to the development of immunoprophylactic measures, a complete understanding of the antigen structure of *Anaplasma* becomes necessary. Subsequent use of information related to the organism's antigenic profile can then support immunogenic studies based on biochemically defined constituents.

Intraerythrocytic Antigens

Anaplasma marginale antigens precipitated by soluble HC1 and protamine sulfate (PS) have been found to be lipoproteins. The antigens were reacted with antibody in the agar gel precipitation test (Ristic et al. 1963; Ristic & Mann 1963). Chemical resemblance of the PS antigen to a similar preparation made from *Anaplasma*-free erythrocytes incriminated it as a possible antigen responsible for the autoimmune state observed in anaplasmosis. A soluble proteinaceous *A. marginale* antigen has been derived from lysed erythrocytes and its reactivity studied in agar gel diffusion (Amerault & Roby 1967).

No antigenic differences were found between two virulent *A. marginale* isolates and the attenuated *A. marginale* when soluble antigens and specific antisera were reacted in agar gel and immunoelectrophoresis tests (Carson et al. 1970).

Various particulate antigens for diagnostic tests have been prepared from infected erythrocytes (Franklin et al. 1963; Ristic 1962; Amerault & Roby 1968). The active component of the complement fixation (CF) antigen was found to be a lipoprotein (Franklin et al. 1963). Capillary tube agglutination (CA) antigen consists of structures resembling initial *Anaplasma* bodies which reacted specifically with sera from infected animals (Ristic 1962).

Serum Antigens

Sera from animals in the acute phase of anaplasmosis have been found to contain soluble antigens of *A. marginale* (Amerault & Roby 1964). Cyclic emission of soluble parasite antigen was indicated by fluctuation of test results. The presence of detectable intraerythrocytic *A. marginale* bodies did not always coincide with the presence of soluble antigens in serum. It also appeared that a soluble component of the CF antigen and the exoantigen found in serum of infected cattle were antigenically identical.

Serology and Kinetics of the Humoral Response

Serum protein changes occurring during anaplasmosis, particularly with respect to globulins, have been studied extensively (Murphy et al. 1964; Murphy et al. 1966). Prior to the appearance of *A. marginale* bodies, the concentration of all serum proteins decreased. As the number of parasitized erythrocytes diminished, the albumin-globulin ratio decreased. It was determined that early CF antibody arising in response to experimental inoculation of *A. marginale* consisted exclusively of gamma M (19S) globulin, but within 4 to 5 days this was augmented by an electrophoretically fast gamma G globulin (6.2S). Agglutinating antibodies moved from the gamma M to the gamma G globulins much later in the disease (Murphy et al. 1966).

The serologic relationship of *A. marginale* and *A. centrale* has been compared using the CF and CA tests. Significantly higher titers were obtained with homologous antigen (Kuttler 1967a). The indirect Coomb's test also showed quantitative differences in antibody titers produced in response to infections with the above agents (Schindler et al. 1966).

PERSISTENCE OF THE ORGANISM IN THE IMMUNOLOGICALLY HOSTILE HOST

It is apparent from our current knowledge of anaplasmosis that an affected animal is fully capable of developing humoral and cell-mediated immune responses to the etiologic agent. While induction of an immune response is essential for the survival of the host, it also provides for continuous survival and transmission of the parasite. This state of biological host-parasite balance has been described as a "tolerant symbiosis" which allows the parasite to persist and, in exchange, the host develops lasting protection against homologous organisms in the environment (Jones 1974). Obviously there are different mechanisms which the parasite may use to avoid destruction by the immunologically hostile host. The nature of these escape mechanisms in plasmodias, trypanosomes, babesias and certain other species was the subject of the recent symposium (Porter & Knight 1974).

Without evidence of intravascular hemolysis, *Anaplasma* appears to be a strict intracellular obligate parasite. Under the circumstances the organism is well protected against direct antibody effects. Antibodies arising in response to *Anaplasma* infection are of two types: specific and nonspecific. The latter, characterized as autohemagglutinins and opsonins, were shown to react with nonparasite antigenic determinants such as trypsin-treated and intact erythrocytes of *Anaplasma*-free animals (Ristic 1968). In addition, some of these immunoglobulins were shown to be antinuclear (anti-DNP), anticardiolipin (anti-Wasserman antigen), and antihuman gamma globulin reminiscent of the rheumatoid factors (Gewurz 1975). Greenwood (1974) proposed that the appearance of such nonspecific antibodies suggests their synthesis occurs in a disorganized way. It is thus possible that the nonspecific immune response may benefit the parasite by "swamping" a specific immunologic response aimed at its destruction.

Evidence for antigenic variation of *Anaplasma* is not available. Clinical and hematologic observations, however, indicate that the primary parasitemia may be followed by milder recrudescence. If these relapses are triggered by antigenic dissociation of the organism, this could be a primary factor whereby the *Anaplasma* evades the host's lethal immune effect.

Free serum antigens were shown to be *Anaplasma*-specific, thus, antigen-antibody complexes are expected to occur. Such complexes may induce immunologic injuries to the host while serving as a protective shield for the parasite.

IMMUNOGENS OF *ANAPLASMA*

Naturally Occurring *A. marginale* and *A. centrale*

Early use of field isolates of *Anaplasma* for premunization consisted of injecting blood from known carriers into susceptible cattle (Schmidt 1937). This procedure presented a risk, since it was necessary to control the initial infection with drugs so recovery and development of the carrier state can occur. A method of premunization using a small inocula to induce protection has also been reported (Franklin & Huff 1967) but later results indicated that severe disease and mortality can result from even very small doses of *A. marginale* (Kliewer et al. 1973).

Prior infection with *A. centrale* did not prevent infection with *A. marginale* but reduced the severity of the superimposed disease. On this basis, Theiler (1910) developed the method of *A. centrale* vaccination which is still used in several countries. Variable resistance to *A. marginale* resulting from vaccination with *A. centrale* was later described (Legg 1936). Furthermore, it was observed in Australia that cattle inoculated with South African *A. centrale* strain developed severe symptoms of the disease. *Anaplasma marginale* and *A. centrale* have more recently been compared on a clinical, hematologic, and serologic basis (Kuttler 1967a; Kuttler 1966). Heterologous challenge in all cases produced a definite hematologic reaction, but an initial infection with *A. centrale* usually reduced the severity of a subsequent *A. marginale* challenge.

Inactivated *A. marginale* of Bovine and Ovine Origin

Use of a vaccine containing inactivated *Anaplasma* organisms has been described in Africa (McHardy & Simpson 1973) and the United States (Brock et al. 1965). The U.S. vaccine presently used commercially, "Anaplaz,"* was prepared from blood of infected animals derived at the peak of parasitemia. Erythrocytes were washed, lysed, and lyophilized. The dessicated material was reconstituted with an oil adjuvant. Two doses of the vaccine were given subcutaneously at 4- to 19-week intervals. A degree of protection from the clinical signs of anaplasmosis has been reported to be afforded 2 weeks after the second injection but the vaccine reportedly sensitizes cattle to bovine erythrocyte histocompatibility antigens stimulating production of isoantibodies. Calves nursing vaccinated dams, which have a high concentration of colostral isoantibody, are at risk in the potential development of neonatal isoerythrolysis. Vaccinated animals became carriers after field challenge. An annual booster injection is also recommended.

A preparation similar to Anaplaz was developed in our laboratory using ovine erythrocytes infected with the attenuated *A. marginale.* This modified preparation was aimed at the induction of an adequate degree of protection against *Anaplasma* development after challenge but without the concurrent development of isoantibodies directed against bovine erythrocytes. The Anaplaz adjuvant has been used to reconstitute the lyophilized material and the aforementioned vaccination regimen followed. A degree of resistance to development of clinical signs of anaplasmosis has similarly been detected after challenge with virulent *A. marginale,* although the development of postchallenge anemia has not been controlled.

*Anaplaz, Fort Dodge Laboratories, Fort Dodge, Iowa.

Laboratory-Attenuated A. marginale

Research toward development of the attenuated anaplasmosis vaccine started at the University of Illinois in 1959 with the following objectives in mind: (1) the strain should be A. *marginale*; (2) the attenuated organism should be sufficiently immunogenic to confer complete protection against challenge with the virulent strain; (3) the attenuated organism should not revert to virulence when transmitted by means of ticks or subinoculation of blood from vaccinated to susceptible cattle; and (4) the vaccine should be produced in a nonbovine host due to the hazards of transmitting other bovine infectious agents in the process of vaccination.

The Development of the Strain

The A. *marginale* isolate was a pooled blood sample termed the Florida *Anaplasma* * isolate collected from naturally infected cattle in various sections of Florida. Detailed description of the development of the vaccine strain is reported elsewhere (Ristic et al. 1968). The basic methodology used for attenuation of the Florida isolate has been: (1) induction of an apparently accelerated rate of mutation of the organism by exposure to irradiation; (2) selection of an avirulent A. *marginale* strain by serial passage of irradiated organisms in splenectomized deer (2 passages) and sheep (138 passages). Lots of sheep-blood-derived seed material of established immunogenicity, growth pattern, and safety were preserved by storage in liquid nitrogen. For vaccine production, the seed material is reactivated in splenectomized sheep, using four to five passages at 7- to 9-day intervals. The vaccine is dispensed in liquid nitrogen and inoculated intramuscularly in 1- to 2-ml doses. The prepatent period in inoculated animals varies between 4 and 5 weeks, after which the organism may be detected in approximately 0.5% to 8% of the peripheral blood erythrocytes. A slight hematocrit decrease, usually not exceeding 5% to 10% of the preinoculation value, generally occurs. These manifestations are transitory and are in evidence for 1 to 2 weeks. Inoculated animals are not clinically affected.

*Isolated in 1955 by Dr. D.A. Sanders, Department of Veterinary Science, University of Florida, Gainesville, Florida.

Effects of Adaptation to an Atypical Host

Adaptation of the organism to sheep resulted in the loss of certain traits apparently not essential for immunogenicity and intracellular existence of the organism. The loss of virulence is the principal and the most important of these. The incubation period of the attenuated agent does not differ greatly from that of the virulent organism. Thus, the speed of growth and replication does not seem to be a factor in altered virulence. Attenuation appears to be a stable property as indicated by failure of the organism to revert to virulence after several consecutive passages (5 to 12) in highly susceptible mature cattle, pregnant cattle, and splenectomized calves (Welter & Ristic 1969). The mechanism of altered virulence probably is biochemically based and arises from the organismal dependency on the new intracellular habitat.

An extensive study with *Dermacentor andersoni* (Popovic 1968) showed that the vaccine strain cannot be transmitted by natural tick feeding or inoculation of cattle with various tick tissue homogenates. These findings were further substantiated by the results obtained from examination of tick tissues by means of the fluorescent antibody method and electron microscopy. Conversely, *Anaplasma* was found in tissues of ticks fed on calves inoculated with the field strain of the organism, and the infection was then transmitted to cattle using these ticks and their tissues. More information is needed to substantiate these findings, but prolonged maintenance of hemotropic and other tick-borne agents by needle passage in natural hosts has been shown to result in a loss of organismal propensity toward growth and development in the tick vector (Holbrook et al. 1968; Price 1954).

Finally, the attenuated *A. marginale* is more easily destroyed by tetracyclines than is the virulent counterpart (Welter & Ristic 1969). For example, daily administration of 8.5 mg tetracycline per pound of body weight to vaccinated cattle for 4 days completely destroyed the attenuated agent as contrasted with 10 mg tetracycline per pound of body weight for 7 days to completely destroy the virulent organism.

IMMUNE RESPONSES TO INACTIVATED
A. MARGINALE VACCINES

Humoral and Cell-Mediated Responses

A study in our laboratory using both Anaplaz, the commercial inactivated *A. marginale* vaccine of bovine origin, and ovine origin counterpart (attenuated

A. marginale) indicated that the CA response remains mildly positive for at least 6 weeks after the second vaccine dose. We further compared the cell-mediated immune responses induced by the two vaccines. The leukocyte migration inhibition test (LMIT) and the lymphocyte transformation test (LTT) were used as *in vitro* correlates of cell-mediated immunity (CMI). The LMIT response in normal cattle ranged between 25% and 35% (baseline) and a significant elevation in the response was determined to be at least 18.6%. The baseline for the LTT stimulation index indicated that normal values for cattle ranged between 1.0 and 1.3, whereas specifically increased values were at least 1.3—an increase above the baseline of 21.3%. One group of cattle was vaccinated with two doses of Anaplaz administered 4 weeks apart. A second group of cattle received a lyophilized preparation of *A. marginale* produced by exposing ovine erythrocytes containing the attenuated *A. marginale* to an extraction process similar to that used for commercial preparation of Anaplaz. The immunogen was reconstituted in the Anaplaz oil adjuvant and administered as recommended for the commercial preparation. Both vaccines elicited a low-level and transient (1 to 3 weeks) LMIT response (Figure 4). Lymphocyte transformation studies using [^{14}C]-labeled thymidine revealed a lack of correlation between test results and clinical protection. Stimulation indices after vaccination, defined as the ratio of incorporated activity in antigen stimulated cell cultures compared with control cultures, were in the order of 2 to 8 or higher (Table 1). Indices of 1.2 to 1.6 were evident in leukocytes collected from cattle inoculated with live-attenuated *A. marginale* vaccine (Table 2). Since cattle inoculated with the attenuated *A. marginale* are clinically protected against challenge by homologous strains of *Anaplasma*, there seems to be no direct correlation between stimulation indices and protection.

Development of Isoimmunity and Delayed Cutaneous Hypersensitivity

Neonatal isoerythrolysis has been associated with the use of the commercial Anaplaz vaccine (Dennis et al. 1970). Hemolytic inhibition tests have indicated the presence of bovine blood group antigens in Anaplaz (Hines et al. 1973). Blood group isoantibodies identified in cow sera and colostrum (in addition to natural anti-J) were anti-A, anti-H, anti-F, and anti-V. Their concentration in colostrum was 10 to 15 times greater than in serum (Hines et al. 1973). Our studies, which compared inactivated *A. marginale* preparations containing bovine erythrocytic components (Anaplaz) with similar preparations containing ovine erythrocytic stroma (attenuated *A. marginale*), demonstrated that isoantibodies to bovine erythrocytes developed only (Table 3) in response to inoculation with Anaplaz (Carson et al. 1976). Intradermic skin testing with antigens prepared

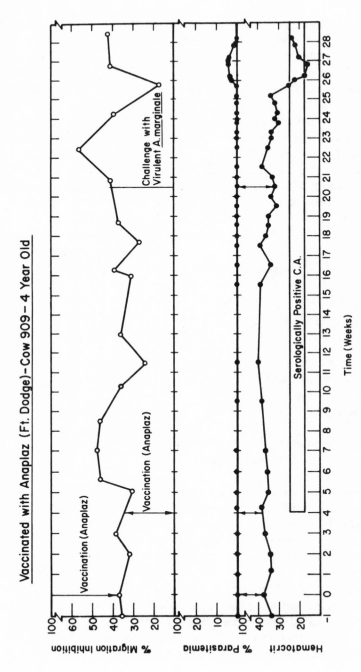

Figure 4. Leukocyte migration inhibition, parasitemia, hematocrit, and capillary tube agglutination (CA) results for cow 909 vaccinated with Anaplaz and challenged with virulent *A. marginale* approximately 17 weeks after the second vaccinal injection. Severe anemia in the presence of relatively mild parasitemia was observed.

Table 1
Leukocyte Transformation Studies, [^{14}C] Thymidine Incorporation,
in Cattle Vaccinated with Inactivated *Anaplasma marginale* of Ovine Origin[a]

Cow Number	Days Postvaccination	Stimulant		Stimulation Index
		CA Ag[b]	None	
908	0	322.7[c]	288.4	1.1
	8	1830.7	361.9	5.1
	30	2070.0	1281.0	1.6
912	0	387.8	362.3	1.1
	14	1253.6	214.7	5.8
	25	1873.1	1593.7	1.2
	38	3981.3	1810.4	2.2
	52	1530.2	716.9	2.1

(a) Vaccinated on days 0 and 28.
(b) CA Ag = *A. marginale* capillary tube agglutination antigen.
(c) Average counts per minute of three or four cultures.

Table 2
Leukocyte Transformation Studies, [^{14}C] Thymidine Incorporation,
in Cattle Vaccinated with Attenuated *Anaplasma marginale*[a]

Cow Number	Days Postvaccination	Stimulant		Stimulation Index
		CA Ag[b]	None	
834	-1	419.5[c]	405.9	1.0
	20	769.6	599.6	1.3
	34	830.0	501.7	1.6
	57	473.9	297.9	1.6
	88	810.7	842.5	1.0
	109	123.3	133.3	1.0
845[d]	50	665.0	457.1	1.4
	70	611.0	429.7	1.4
	113	362.7	361.4	1.0
	144	986.5	770.5	1.3
	164	1732.9	1285.0	1.3

(a) Vaccinated on day 0.
(b) CA Ag = *A. marginale* capillary tube agglutination antigen.
(c) Average counts per minute of three or four cultures.
(d) Challenged with virulent *A. marginale* on day 108.

Table 3
Hemagglutination (HA) Titers Using Sera from Cattle Injected with
Inactivated *A. marginale* Contained in Bovine or Ovine Erythrocytes

Serum Donor	Treatment: Strain in *Anaplasma* Erythrocytes in Vaccine	Erythrocyte Used in HA Test				
		Bovine 1	Bovine 2	Bovine 3	Bovine 4	Ovine
1	Virulent *A. marginale*[a] bovine	16[b]	16	64	8	32
2	Virulent *A. marginale* bovine	4	4	4	2	64
3	Attenuated *A. marginale* ovine	0	0	0	0	32
4	Attenuated *A. marginale* ovine	0	0	0	0	128

(a) Inactivated *A. marginale* vaccine produced by Fort Dodge Laboratories,
Fort Dodge, Iowa.
(b) Maximum titers reached during 3-month period after exposure.

from normal bovine and ovine erythrocytes showed that cattle which had been vaccinated with Anaplaz of bovine origin were skin-test positive to both bovine and ovine erythrocytic components, whereas those which had received the ovine origin anaplasma reacted only to ovine origin erythrocytes (Table 4). The skin reactions appeared prior to 24 hours, indicating an immediate or Arthus-type response involving humoral antibody. This response increased over the 72-hour surveillance period, indicating a delayed cutaneous hypersensitivity limb of the response.

Protection and Immunologic Injury Following Challenge

Studies in our laboratory showed that cattle vaccinated with inactivated *A. marginale* of either bovine or ovine origin developed on challenge a low-level parasitemia with a greatly reduced hematocrit (Figure 4). Since the degree of parasitemia which resulted from challenge of these animals was very low compared to parasitemia expected in unprotected susceptible control cattle, there appeared to be some protection afforded by use of the inactivated vaccine preparations administered in adjuvant.

Table 4

Skin Reactions Following Intradermal Exposure with Normal Bovine and Ovine Erythrocytes of Cattle Vaccinated with Inactivated Preparations of Virulent *A. marginale* in Bovine Erythrocytes and Attenuated *A. marginale* in Ovine Erythrocytes

Cow Number	Treatment	Normal Bovine Erythrocytes[a]				Ovine Erythrocytes[a]
		1	2	3	4	
1	Inactivated *A. marginale* in adjuvant[b]	0,7,9,10[c]	0,4,9,10	3,15,12,14	0,5,9,10	0,3,0,7
2	Inactivated *A. marginale* in adjuvant	–	–	3,8,0,10	0,0,2,7	0,8,12,9
3	Inactivated attenuated *A. marginale*	–	–	–	–	3,15,28,23
4	Inactivated attenuated *A. marginale*	–	–	–	–	4,10,16,15

(a) Test antigen.
(b) Vaccines were mixed with an oil adjuvant (commercial Anaplaz) and injected.
(c) Gross measurement in millimeters of skin reaction at 6, 24, 48, and 78 hours, respectively.

The severe anemic syndrome which developed following challenge may be related to an autohemolytic mechanism in view of the fact that abnormal erythrocyte components are included in the vaccinal inocula and have definite immunogenic properties. Subsequent infection of host erythrocytes changes membranous constituents which the host may not distinguish from the original vaccinal components. This situation may lead to an accelerated autoimmune antierythrocytic host response.

The apparent protection against parasitemia resulting from challenge assessed in association with the absence of production of bovine erythrocyte-directed isoantibodies could allude to the potentially beneficial effect of the inactivated attenuated *A. marginale* in ovine erythrocytes. It would remain necessary to modify this preparation to avoid induction of immunogenic mechanisms prone to the production of anemia after challenge exposure.

IMMUNE RESPONSES TO LIVE ATTENUATED AND VIRULENT *A. MARGINALE*

Hematology and Serology

Hematologic responses in adult cattle to vaccination with the attenuated *A. marginale* have been extensively studied in our laboratory. This agent produces a mild infection with a concomitant low parasitemia and a generally imperceptible hematocrit variation at approximately 4 to 5 weeks after inoculation. Serologic responses measured by the CA or CF tests are detected between 3 and 4 weeks postvaccination. These serologic responses persist for 2 to 3 years in the absence of reinfection (Welter & Ristic 1969). Cattle which survive infection with virulent *A. marginale* develop similar serologic responses.

In Vitro Measurement of Cell-Mediated Immunity

Following vaccination of susceptible adult cattle with attenuated *A. marginale*, the LMIT becomes positive after approximately 2 to 4 weeks and either remains at a moderately high level or fluctuates between prevaccination levels and positive response values (Figure 5). Cattle inoculated with virulent *A. marginale* developed positive LMIT values either prior to or after the onset of parasitemia which generally occurred at 4 weeks postinfection (Figure 6). The clinical severity of the disease depended on the time of appearance of parasitemia with reference to the LMIT; when the parasitemia preceded development of a positive LMIT, the chance of mortality was increased (Figure 7). The specificity of the response

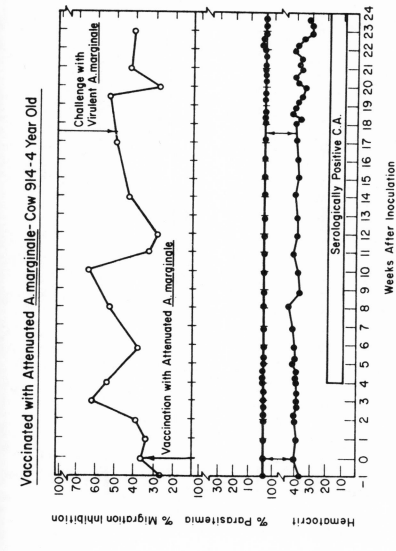

Figure 5. Leukocyte migration inhibition, parasitemia, hematocrit, and capillary tube agglutination (CA) results for cow 914 injected with the attenuated *A. marginale* vaccine and challenged with virulent *A. marginale* approximately 17 weeks later. The animal demonstrated full clinical resistance.

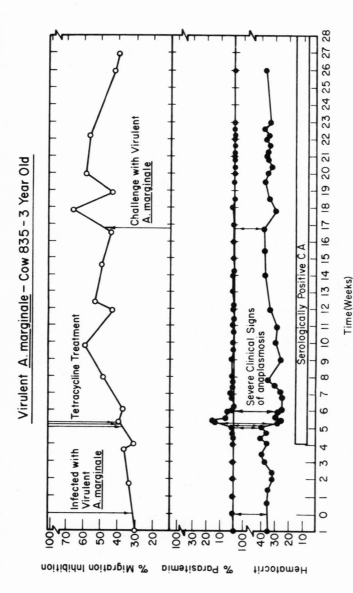

Figure 6. Leukocyte migration inhibition, parasitemia, hematocrit, and capillary tube agglutination (CA) results for cow 835 injected with the virulent *A. marginale*. The animal developed severe signs of anaplasmosis and was treated three times with oxytetracycline at approximately 5 weeks after exposure. On challenge at 17 weeks after initial exposure, the animal demonstrated full clinical resistance. Note that this animal failed to develop appreciable LMIT response until recovered from the acute phase of the disease.

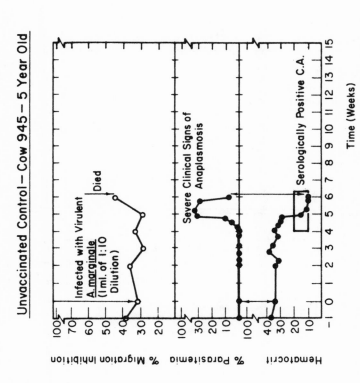

Figure 7. Leukocyte migration inhibition, parasitemia, hematocrit, and capillary tube agglutination (CA) results for cow 945 infected with virulent *A. marginale* but not treated. Note that the animal developed severe parasitemia and anemia but failed to develop a LMIT response before expiring 6 weeks after infection.

has also been proven by use of test antigens containing normal erythrocyte stroma, CA antigen containing attenuated *Anaplasma*, CA antigen containing virulent *Anaplasma*, tuberculin (purified protein derivative) and nonspecific mitogens such as phytohemagglutinin and concanavalin A (Table 5). Evidence supporting the concept that the test is largely dependent on T-lymphocyte activity has also been determined using antilymphocyte IgG labeled with ^{125}I and measurement of residual radioactive leukocyte populations before and after antigenic stimulation. Challenge of vaccinated cattle with virulent strains of *A. marginale* appears either to elicit a decreased measurable LMIT response followed by an elevated response (if LMIT values are high at the time of challenge) or an anamnestic elevation in the LMIT response.

The lymphocyte transformation test using [^{14}C]-labeled thymidine has also been related in our laboratory to vaccination of adult cattle with attenuated *A. marginale* or premunization with virulent *A. marginale*. Stimulation indices recorded after inoculation with either agent are comparable and range in the area of approximately 1.3 to 2.5.

Table 5
Effect of Various Antigens in Leukocyte Migration Inhibition Test Using Cells
Presensitized with Various *A. marginale* Immunogens

Experiment Number	Source of Leukocytes	*A. marginale* Immunogen	Antigens			
			CA[a]	NCA[b]	PHA[c]	PPD[d]
1	130 days PI[f]	virulent	55.2[e]	28.1[e]	63.9[e]	22.6[e]
2	127 days PI	attenuated	61.4	39.1	67.6	32.2
3	42 days PI	inactivated	30.8	34.6	70.4	34.2
4	C 846	uninfected control	28.6	31.5	66.7	30.4

(a) CA = *A. marginale* capillary tube agglutination antigen derived from bovine erythrocytes infected with virulent *A. marginale*.
(b) NCA = antigen derived from normal bovine erythrocytes using the method for preparation of *A. marginale* capillary tube agglutination antigen.
(c) PHA = tuberculin-purified protein derivative.
(d) PPD = phytohemagglutinin.
(e) Results expressed as percentage migration inhibition.
(f) PI = Postinoculation.

Correlation Between Cell-Mediated Immunity and Protection

The level of LMIT responsiveness recorded after vaccination with attenuated *A. marginale* or premunization with virulent *A. marginale* seems to be directly proportional to the level of clinical protection induced against challenge with virulent *A. marginale*. Following challenge, either a low-level or negligible parasitemia was recorded and the hematocrit either did not vary or was transiently reduced. There has been no evidence of clinical illness related to anaplasmosis after challenge (Figures 6 and 8).

Stimulation indices recorded in lymphocyte transformation test (LTT) of mixed leukocytes collected from vaccinated or premunized cattle were not related to the degree of clinical protection afforded by either *Anaplasma* inoculum. Much higher indices were elicited by the inactivated *Anaplasma* in oil adjuvant while these cattle were not clinically protected as were animals which received live *Anaplasma*.

The classical concept of protection in anaplasmosis has been that maintenance of protective immunity depended on maintenance of the carrier state. Recently, Roby et al. (1974) reported that *Anaplasma* carriers which were freed from virulent *Anaplasma* by chemotherapy demonstrated considerable protection to challenge at 12 months after sterilization. To further examine this observation, we subjected two 4-year-old cows, which were previously vaccinated with the attenuated agent and subsequently resisted challenge of the virulent organism, to systemic therapy. The animals received ten daily doses of oxytetracycline at 5 mg/lb administered intravenously. Subinoculation of 100 ml of whole blood from these cows into two splenectomized calves failed to produce an infection in the recipient animals. Approximately 10 weeks after treatment, the cows were rechallenged with virulent *A. marginale*. A prompt LMIT response was noted after the challenge and the animals demonstrated full clinical resistance (Figure 9).

VACCINATION STUDIES WITH THE ATTENUATED *A. MARGINALE*

A series of laboratory and field experiments conducted in the United States (Ristic et al. 1968; Welter & Ristic 1969; Taylor 1969; Welter & Woods 1963), Peru (Lora 1971; Lora & Koechlin 1969; Castillo, 1968), Venezuela (Welter & Ristic 1969; Schroeder et al. 1971), Colombia (Kuttler 1967b; Kuttler 1972), and Mexico (Osorno et al. 1973; Vizcaino et al. 1976; Osorno et al. 1975) have shown that the immune response induced by the attenuated *A. marginale* vaccine protects adult susceptible cattle against challenge with virulent endemic strains.

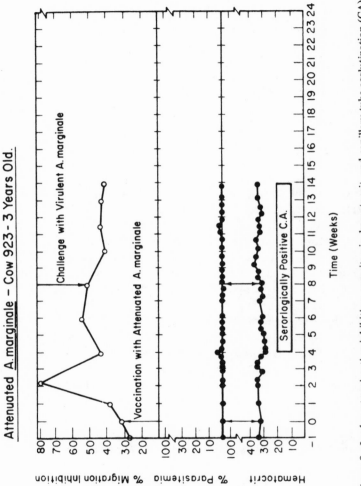

Figure 8. Leukocyte migration inhibition, parasitemia, hematocrit, and capillary tube agglutination (CA) results for cow 923 injected with the attenuated *A. marginale* vaccine and challenged with virulent *A. marginale* 8 weeks later. The animal fully resisted the challenge. Note a prominent LMIT response with maximal values reached 2 to 3 weeks after vaccination.

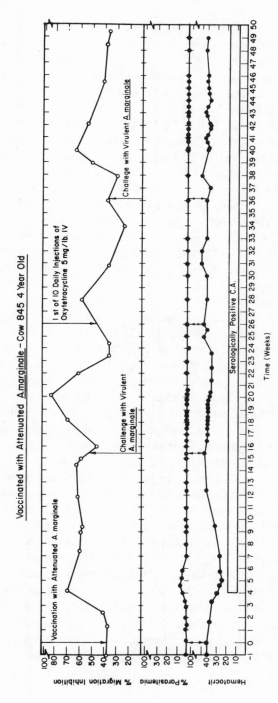

Figure 9. Leukocyte migration inhibition, parasitemia, hematocrit, and capillary tube agglutination (CA) results for cow 845. This animal was initially injected with the attenuated vaccine, resisted challenge with virulent A. marginale, was treated with oxytetracycline to destroy the Anaplasma and rechallenged with the virulent organism approximately 10 weeks after treatment. Note the rapid LMIT response following challenge. The animal fully resisted challenge.

Most of the studies conducted in the United States were designed to test specificity (Taylor 1969), safety (Ristic et al. 1968; Welter & Ristic 1969), and immunogenicity (Ristic et al. 1968; Welter & Ristic 1969; Welter & Woods 1963) of the vaccine using highly susceptible cattle (older animals, pure breeds, and pregnant animals) and challenging them with field isolates from various regions. Results showed that the single dose of the vaccine conferred solid protection to challenge with field isolates. As judged by the persistence of the serologic reaction in vaccinated animals, the protection is expected to last for at least 3 years. The largest experiment involved 2,700 beef cattle of mixed breeds which were vaccinated en route from the United States to Venezuela (Welter & Ristic 1969; Schroeder et al. 1971). On arrival all animals were found to be serologically positive, presumably as a result of vaccination. The losses in this herd were reduced from 9.5% in 1967, when nonvaccinated cattle were imported, to 2.5%, when vaccinated cattle were imported. On arrival in Venezuela the animals were exposed to a tropical climate and blood-sucking arthropods known to be carriers of *Anaplasma* and other blood parasites. In spite of this unfavorable environment, no side effects, spontaneous reversion to virulence, or any other adverse effects were noted.

As an example of the efficacy of the vaccine, four controlled experiments conducted by veterinary government scientists in Peru (Lora & Koechlin 1969) and Mexico (Osorno et al. 1973; Osorno et al. 1975; Osorno 1975) will be cited. In Peru (Lora & Koechlin 1969) 18 Brown Swiss cattle, 5 to 6 years old and free of *A. marginale,* were divided into 2 groups: vaccinated (13 cattle) and nonvaccinated (5 cattle). Forty-eight days later, the 18 cattle were each challenged subcutaneously with 5 ml of carrier blood containing a virulent Peruvian isolate of *A. marginale.* All control cattle developed typical signs of anaplasmosis and died within 44 days after challenge. Clinical signs of disease were not observed in any of the vaccinated animals following challenge inoculation.

In Mexico (Osorno et al. 1973) 20 two-and-one-half-year-old Herefords originating from *Anaplasma*-free regions were housed in isolation units of the National Institute for Animal Studies in Mexico City. Prior to use in the experiment the animals were examined clinically, their hematocrit level established, Giemsa-stained blood films examined microscopically, and blood serum subjected to the capillary tube agglutination (CA) test (Ristic 1962). The animals were divided into two equal groups and each animal of the first group was inoculated intramuscularly with 1.0 ml of the vaccine. Animals of the second group served as nontreated controls. Following vaccination the temperature was recorded daily and the hematocrit determinations, microscopic blood film examinations, and the CA tests were performed three times a week. Six months later all animals were inoculated subcutaneously with 1.0 ml of the challenge strain. The strain was isolated from field outbreaks of anaplasmosis in Mexico and had a standard potency sufficient to kill 80% of adult susceptible cattle. The organism was maintained in liquid nitrogen. After challenge, clinical, hematologic, and blood microscopic examinations were made daily. The experiment was considered terminated when the surviving animals regained their prechallenge hematologic and clinical condition.

Hematocrit levels, temperature, and general clinical condition of vaccinated animals remained unaltered during the postvaccination period. The average post-vaccinal parasitemia was 2.2%. Agglutinating serum antibody detected by the CA test was first noticed in these animals approximately 6 weeks following adminis-tration of the vaccine. The antibody persisted throughout the duration of the experiment. Animals of the control group, maintained in the proximity of the vaccinated animals, retained good clinical condition and showed no hematologic and serologic abnormalities.

A slight hematocrit drop, followed by parasitemia averaging 20%, and a temp-erature averaging 40.5 C, were first noted in animals of the control group during the 25 to 30 days after challenge. Thereafter, parasitemia rose sharply, reaching an average of 58% at 37 days postchallenge. The parasitemia was followed by a decrease in hematocrit and persistently high temperature, with a maximum aver-age of 41.5 C at the 34th day after challenge. Thereafter, the temperature de-creased and oscillated at subnormal levels during 37 to 41 postchallenge days. All control animals developed severe clinical signs and anaplasmosis manifested by anorexia, anemia, icterus, severe weakness, emaciation, and dehydration. The first two animals of the control group died on days 35 and 37 postchallenge, respectively. At the time of death, the hematocrit levels of these animals were 30% and 23%, respectively. The remaining animals died during 38 to 41 days postchallenge. The hematocrit levels of these animals ranged between 17% and 11% (Figure 10).

The parasitemia in the vaccinated group occurred between days 34 and 40 postchallenge, reaching the maximum average peak of 15% on day 38. The maxi-mum average hematocrit drop in vaccinated animals was 10% and occurred on day 42 postchallenge. Three of the vaccinated animals developed clinical signs of the disease as measured by the following criteria: the first animal had a temperature of 40.2 C for one day; the second two animals had hematocrit re-cordings of less than 20% during a period of 2 to 6 days, respectively.

In Colombia (Vizcaino et al. 1976), anaplasmosis is reported to cause severe losses not only in mature cattle but also in young calves 3 to 8 months of age. An experiment in which the vaccine was administered to young calves, who were later challenged with the virulent Colombian A. marginale strain, was recently completed by scientists of the Instituto Colombiano Agropecuario (ICA) in Bogota, Colombia.

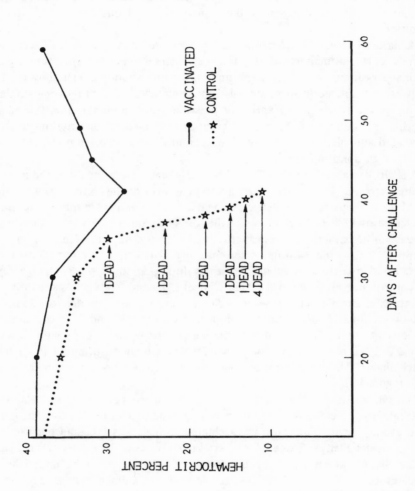

Figure 10. Average hematocrit of vaccinated and control cattle and mortality sequences among the animals of the latter group following challenge with a virulent Mexican *Anaplasma* strain.

Eight Holstein-Friesian calves approximately 4 months old were procured on the Bogota Savannah of Colombia, South America, and determined to be free of anaplasmosis by the capillary agglutination (CA) test. The calves were randomly divided into four groups of two calves. Group 1 (calves 1 and 2) were injected intramuscularly with 1 ml of vaccine containing approximately 3.5×10^9 organisms; group 2 (calves 3 and 4) received 2 ml of vaccine; group 3 (calves 5 and 6) received 3 ml of vaccine; and group 4 remained as unvaccinated control animals. Blood was collected in sodium and potassium oxalate twice weekly for hematocrit determinations and Giemsa-stained blood films were examined for parasitemia. Serum samples were also collected twice weekly for the CA test. Temperature and general clinical appearance were also recorded. After the 63rd day of the postvaccination observation period, all calves were challenge-inoculated subcutaneously with 1 ml of virulent Colombian Monteria isolate of *A. marginale* (approximately 2.6×10^8 anaplasma organisms) stored in liquid nitrogen at -176 C for 2 months prior to use. Blood samples were collected as previously described during the 51-day postchallenge (PC) observation period.

Regardless of the vaccine dose used, calves of all three groups showed very mild postvaccinal hematologic and serologic responses, with no indication of clinical illness. The maximum postvaccinal parasitemia ranged between 0.1% and 0.3%. There was, however, a difference in the average of postvaccinal patent period between animals inoculated with 1 ml (51 days) and those that received 2 ml and 3 ml doses (36.5 and 31 days, respectively).

Challenge exposure revealed the most marked differences between vaccinated and control calves. Vaccinated animals of all three groups showed complete clinical protection as compared to animals of the control group which developed acute anaplasmosis accompanied by low hematocrit and high parasitemia. Postchallenge results and statistical analysis are shown in Table 6.

In the field experiments (Osorno et al. 1975), the cattle, which were raised in isolation units free of arthropods, consisted of ten Brown Swiss calves (1 to 13 months of age) and eight Holstein calves (5 to 7 months of age). They were paired by breed, age, and body weight and allotted to two equal groups. Calves in one group were vaccinated and 6 weeks after vaccination calves in both groups were placed in the field where they were raised for approximately one year. Two Holstein and three Brown Swiss calves of the nonvaccinated group developed clinical anaplasmosis, and the remaining calves of this group had hematologic evidence of the disease during the 2 to 4 months after introduction to the field. The vaccinated group, which remained free of anaplasmosis, showed consistently greater weight gain than did the controls. Among the Holstein calves the maximum weight difference in favor of the vaccinated group was 50 kg/head at 5.5 months after field exposure, and among the Brown Swiss calves the difference in weight gain in favor of vaccinated calves at the end of the 12-month period was between 11% and 30%.

Table 6
Response of Vaccinated and Nonvaccinated Calves to Virulent
Anaplasma marginale Challenge in Bogota, Colombia

	Groups				Significance of Group Differences[a]
	1[a]	2[b]	3[c]	4[a,b,c]	
Average prechallenge packed all volume (PCV)	28.5%	29.5%	28.5%	31%	N.S.[d]
Average low PCV	21.5%	24.5%	22.0%	14.5%	p = 0.01
Average time (days) required for onset of parasitemia	28	27	25.5	25.5	NS
Average maximum percentage parasitized erythrocytes	3	1	1.5	25	p = 0.01

(a) Significance of groups 1 and 4: p = 0.01 (low PCV); p < 0.01 (maximum parasitemia).
(b) Significance groups 2 and 4: p = 0.01 (low PCV); p < 0.01 (maximum parasitemia).
(c) Significance groups 3 and 4: p = 0.01 (low PCV); p < 0.01 (maximum parasitemia).
(d) N.S. = not significant.

Finally, a larger experiment recently completed in Mexico (Osorno 1975) involved movement of vaccinated and nonvaccinated animals from the northern tick-free portion of the country (Sonora) to the southern endemic region of Tabasco. There were 383 vaccinated and 42 nonvaccinated yearling cattle of mixed breeds. After 6 months residence in the endemic area, there were no losses due to anaplasmosis among vaccinated cattle, whereas 23 of the controls (54%) died of the disease. More recently, the efficacy of the vaccine was confirmed in field experiments involving more than 2,000 cattle vaccinated upon introduction from *Anaplasma*-free regions into endemic areas (Osorno 1975).

PROPOSED MECHANISM OF PROTECTION INDUCED BY THE ATTENUATED *A. MARGINALE* VACCINE

It has been shown that similarly to the virulent organism the attenuated vaccine induces both humoral and cell-mediated immune responses (Ristic & Nyindo 1973; Carson 1975). Sera from convalescing animals are active in precipitation, agglutination, complement fixation, and fluorescent antibody tests. Transfer of sera from immune cattle to susceptible animals, however, did not confer protection against anaplasmosis.

Cell-mediated immunity (CMI), as indicated by *in vitro* tests, developed 2 to 4 weeks following vaccination with the attenuated *A. marginale* (Figures 5 and 8). These cattle were protected when challenged with the virulent *A. marginale*. When susceptible animals were first inoculated with the virulent organism, a significantly elevated CMI response (see statistical analysis below) usually coincided with the development of clinical signs of the disease (Figure 6). Once these animals were treated and recovered from the acute phase of the infection, a strong CMI response became evident and they were then clinically protected. This finding indicates a correlation between CMI and protection, as well as the need for a gradual or balanced host-parasite interaction before protective immunity may be achieved.

Leukocyte migration inhibition and lymphocyte transformation tests using peripheral blood leukocytes were employed for *in vitro* measurement of CMI. In view of the fact that the LT but not LMI test rendered positive results following inoculation of inactivated antigens, and such animals on challenge showed a limited degree of protection, we concluded that the LMIT is a more accurate indicator of protective immunity. Animals inoculated with attenuated and virulent agents failed to develop cutaneous delayed hypersensitivity, while less protected animals inoculated with inactivated, adjuvant-fortified *Anaplasma* developed a delayed cutaneous hypersensitivity. The above-described studies indicated that such cutaneous reactions were due to erythrocytic antigenic determinants rather than to *Anaplasma* antigens.

While there is no indication of protection by antibody per se, opsonins of the IgG type were eluted from erythrocytes of infected animals and shown to sensitize autologous and homologous bovine erythrocytes to phagocytosis by an *in vitro* test. The period of maximal opsonic activity coincided with the time of anemic crisis and erythrophagocytosis in the bone marrow (Ristic et al. 1972). Preliminary results in our laboratory indicate a cytophilic macrophage-bound antibody may exert an enhancement of phagocytosis of infected erythrocytes. Thus, the participating role of antibodies for *in vivo* protection is indicated. Under the circumstances, one could visualize that the protective immunity in anaplasmosis is an expression of participation of humoral and cell-mediated immunity, with the latter possibly assuming the principal role. Upon contact with antigens of the virulent organism, sensitized lymphocytes of vaccinated animals would induce activation of phagocytic macrophages and these, in turn, aided by effects of opsonizing and cytophilic antibodies, rapidly remove infected erythrocytes from the circulation (Figure 11).

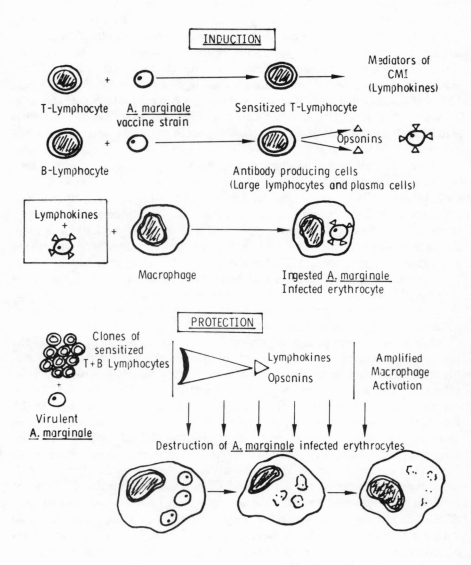

Figure 11. Proposed mechanism of protection induced by the attenuated *A. marginale*.

STATISTICAL ANALYSIS

Combined analysis of variance and t-tests on LMIT data representing 0 to week 8 postinjection (PI) for 4 cattle in each of the treatment groups (attenuated vaccine, premunized, inactivated vaccine, and susceptible controls) generated the following information: The highly significant ($p = 0.01$) interaction of times with treatments makes it necessary to compare treatments at specific times rather than without regard to changes with time; the effect of the various treatments and associated changes with time were highly significant ($p = 0.01$).

The following comparisons are based on t-tests using the error-means square from the general analysis of variance and the appropriate numbers of observations per mean: (1) In cows immunized with the attenuated vaccine LMIT values increased slightly by the week 4 PI and exceeded baseline levels during weeks 6 through 8 PI to a highly significant extent ($p = 0.01$). (2) There was no significant change in LMIT values during the first 8 weeks PI in cattle which received the inactivated vaccine. The slight rise in inhibition levels for different cows occurring at various times established no general trend. (3) Cattle infected with the virulent organism, i.e., premunized (treated) and controls (not treated) showed no significant ($p = 0.05$) increase in LMIT values until week 7 PI. (4) Percentage inhibition (LMIT) for cows having received the attenuated vaccine exceeded that of cows immunized with the inactivated vaccine by a highly significant ($p = 0.1$) degree in the 6th through 8th weeks PI, although earlier differences are not significant ($p = 0.05$). (5) In the 7th and 8th weeks PI, premunized cows and those which received the attenuated *A. marginale* had similarly high levels of inhibition.

APPLICATION OF THE ATTENUATED *A. MARGINALE* VACCINE FOR PREVENTION OF ANAPLASMOSIS

Throughout tropical and semitropical regions of the world, anaplasmosis is considered one of the most important diseases of cattle. Although the mortality rate due to anaplasmosis is staggering, it is minor as compared to weight, milk, and calf losses. In addition, expense of treatment, special management, and palliative convalescent care further add to the economic burden caused by anaplasmosis. Based on reports submitted by practicing veterinarians, a recent publication of the U.S. Department of Agriculture estimates that 50,000 to 100,000 annual cattle losses can be attributed to anaplasmosis. These losses, combined with morbidity effects, are estimated at $100 million a year (McCallon 1973).

In the southern United States and throughout Latin America, the economic impact of anaplasmosis is much greater. There are numerous enzootic areas in which losses due to the disease are experienced throughout the year. Cattle raised in these areas develop anaplasmosis during early calfhood and those transported from tick-free areas become ill shortly after introduction. Based upon our preliminary observation of the effect of anaplasmosis on cattle brought from northern Mexico (Sonora) into southern endemic regions (Yucatan, Tabasco, or Veracruz), we estimated that translocation of 100,000 cattle will produce losses in excess of $20 million.

In other Latin American countries, the situation is similar, as evidenced during the recent International Hemoparasite workship at CIAT,* Cali, Colombia, in which the participants unanimously agreed that anaplasmosis is the most important cattle disease of Latin America. Apart from the Western Hemisphere, anaplasmosis is spread throughout Africa, the Middle East, and Southeast Asia. However, the incidence may vary from country to country.

Although effective chemotherapeutic compounds for treatment of anaplasmosis are now available, field experience has shown that immunoprophylaxis is the only feasible means of controlling the disease in enzootic areas. In these areas, application of the attenuated *A. marginale* vaccine would augment the development of the livestock industry.

ACKNOWLEDGMENT

The authors acknowledge the assistance of Dr. A.J. Lee, Department of Dairy Science, University of Illinois, in the statistical analysis of data.

BIBLIOGRAPHY

Amerault, T.E. & Roby, T.O. 1964. An exo-antigen of *A. marginale* in serum and erythrocytes of cattle with acute anaplasmosis. *Am. J. Vet. Res.* 25: 1642-1647.

Amerault, T.E. & Roby, T.O. 1967. Preparation and characterization of a soluble *Anaplasma marginale* antigen. *Am. J. Vet. Res.* 28: 1067-1072.

Amerault, T.E. & Roby, T.O. 1968. A rapid card agglutination test for bovine anaplasmosis. *J. Am. Vet. Med. Assoc.* 153: 1828-1834.

*Centro Internacional de Agricultura Tropical (International Center for Tropical Agriculture).

Amerault, T.E., Roby, T.O. & Sealock, R.L. 1975. Ultrastructure of *Anaplasma marginale* after freeze-fracture. *Am. J. Vet. Res.* 36: 1515-1519.

Brock, W.E., Kliewer, I.O. & Pearson, C.C. 1965. A vaccine for anaplasmosis. *J. Am. Vet. Med. Assoc.* 147: 948-951.

Buening, G.M. 1973. Cell-mediated immune responses in calves with anaplasmosis. *Am. J. Vet. Res.* 34: 757-763.

Carson, C.A. 1975. Measurement of cell-mediated immune response in cattle induced by virulent and attenuated strains of *Anaplasma marginale* introduced in both live and killed form and correlation with protective immunity. Ph.D. thesis, University of Illinois at Champaign-Urbana.

Carson, C.A., Adams, L.G. & Todorovic, R.A. 1970. An antigenic and serologic comparison of two virulent strains and an attenuated strain of *Anaplasma marginale. Am. J. Vet. Res.* 31: 1071-1078.

Carson, C.A., Weisiger, R.M., Ristic, M., Thurmon, J.C. & Nelson, D.R. 1974. Appendage-related antigen production by *Paranaplasma caudatum* in deer erythrocytes. *Am. J. Vet. Res.* 35: 1529-1531.

Castillo, A.G. 1968. Laboratory and field trails of attenuated *Anaplasma marginale* vaccine in Peru. *In* Proceedings of the 5th National Anaplasmosis Conference: 88-96. Stillwater, Okla.

Dennis, R.A., O'Hara, P.J., Young, M.F. & Dorris, K.D. 1970. Neonatal immunohemolytic anemia and icterus of calves. *J. Am. Vet. Med. Assoc.* 156: 1861-1869.

Erp, E. & Fahrney, D. 1975. Exit of *Anaplasma marginale* from bovine red blood cells. *Am. J. Vet. Res.* 36: 707-709.

Franklin, T.E., Heck, F.C. & Huff, J.W. 1963. Anaplasmosis-complement-fixation antigen production. *Am. J. Vet. Res.* 24: 483-487.

Franklin, T.E. & Huff, J.W. 1967. A proposed method of premunizing cattle with minimum inocula of *Anaplasma marginale. Res. Vet. Sci.* 8: 415-418.

Gewurz, H. 1975. School of Medicine, Presbyterian-St. Luke's Hospital, Chicago, Illinois. Personal communication.

Greenwood, B.M. 1974. Possible role of a B-cell mitogen in hypergammaglobulinemia in malaria and trypanosomiasis. *Lancet* 1: 435-436.

Hines, H.C., Bedell, D.M., Kliewer, I.O. & Hayat, C.S. 1973. Some effects of blood antigens on *A. marginale* and other vaccines. *In* Proceedings of the 6th National Anaplasmosis Conference: 82-85. Las Vegas, Nevada.

Holbrook, A.A., Anthony, D.W. & Johnson, A.J. 1968. Observations on the development of *Babesia caballi* (Nuttall) in the tropical horse tick *Dermacentor nitens* Neumann. *J. Protozool.* 15: 391-396.

Jones, T.C. 1974. Macrophages and intracellular parasitism. *J. Reticuloendothel. Soc.* 15: 439-450.

Kliewer, I.O., Richey, E.J., Jones, E.W. & Brock, W.E. 1973. The preservation and minimum infective dose of *A. marginale*. *In* Proceedings of the 6th National Anaplasmosis Conference: 39-41. Las Vegas, Nevada.

Kreier, J.P. & Ristic, M. 1963a. Anaplasmosis. X. Morphologic characteristics of the parasite present in the blood of calves infected with the Oregon strain of *Anaplasma marginale*. *Am. J. Vet. Res.* 24: 676-687.

Kreier, J.P. & Ristic, M. 1963b. Anaplasmosis. XI. Immunoserologic characteristics of the parasites present in the blood of calves infected with the Oregon strain of *Anaplasma marginale*. *Am. J. Vet. Res.* 24: 688-696.

Kreier, J.P. & Ristic, M. 1963c. Anaplasmosis. XII. The growth and survival in deer and sheep of the parasites present in the blood of calves infected with the Oregon strain of *Anaplasma marginale*. *Am. J. Vet. Res.* 24: 697-702.

Kreier, J.P. & Ristic, M. 1972. Definition and taxonomy of *Anaplasma* species with emphasis on morphologic and immunologic features. *Z. Tropenmed. Parasitol.* 23: 88-98.

Kuttler, K.L. 1966. Clinical and hematologic comparison of *Anaplasma marginale* and *Anaplasma centrale* infections in cattle. *Am. J. Vet. Res.* 27: 941-946.

Kuttler, K.L. 1967a. Serological relationship of *Anaplasma marginale* and *Anaplasma centrale* as measured by the complement-fixation and capillary tube agglutination tests. *Res. Vet. Sci.* 8: 207-211.

Kuttler, K.L. 1967b. A study of the immunological relationship of *Anaplasma marginale* and *Anaplasma centrale*. *Res. Vet. Sci.* 8: 467-471.

Kuttler, K.L. 1972. Comparative response to premunization using attenuated *Anaplasma marginale*, virulent *A. marginale*, and *A. centrale* in different age groups. *Trop. Anim. Health Prod.* 4: 197-203.

Legg, J. 1936. Anaplasmosis cross-immunity tests between *Anaplasma centrale* (South Africa) and *Anaplasma marginale* (Australia). *Aust. Vet. J.* 12: 230-233.

Lora, C.O. 1971. Enfermedades por hematozoarios del ganado bovino del Peru: *Rev. Inst. Zoonosis Invest. Pecu., Lima* 1: 15-19.

Lora, C.O. & Koechlin, A. 1969. An attenuated *Anaplasma marginale* vaccine in Peru. *Am. J. Vet. Res.* 30: 1993-1998.

Mason, R.A. & Ristic, M. 1966. *In vitro* incorporation of glycine by bovine erythrocytes infected with *Anaplasma marginale*. *J. Infect. Dis.* 116: 335-342.

McCallon, B.R. 1973. Prevalence and economic aspects of anaplasmosis. *In* Proceedings of the 6th National Anaplasmosis Conference: 1-3. Las Vegas, Nevada.

McHardy, N. & Simpson, R.M. 1973. Attempts at immunizing cattle against anaplasmosis using a killed vaccine. *Trop. Anim. Health Prod.* 5: 166-173.

Moulder, J.W. 1974. Intracellular parasitism: life in an extreme environment. *J. Infect. Dis.* 130: 300-306.

Murphy, F.A., Aalund, O. & Osebold, J.W. 1964. Physical heterogeneity of bovine gamma globulins: Gamma-1M globulin electrophoretic heterogeneity. *Proc. Soc. of Exp. Biol. Med.* 117: 513-517.

Murphy, F.A., Osebold, J.W., & Aalund, O. 1966. Kinetics of the antibody response to *Anaplasma marginale* infection. *J. Infect. Dis.* 116: 99-111.

Osorno, B.M. 1975. Unpublished data: Instituto Nacional de Investigaciones Pecuarias, Mexico, D.F., Mexico.

Osorno, B.M., Solana, P.M., Perez, J.M. & Trujillo, R.L. 1975. Study of an attenuated *Anaplasma marginale* vaccine in Mexico -- natural challenge of immunity in an enzootic area. *Am. J. Vet. Res.* 36: 631-633.

Osorno, B.M., Solana, P. & Ristic, M. 1973. Study of an attenuated *A. marginale* vaccine in Mexico: I. Challenge of immunity by a virulent endemic anaplasma strain. *In* Proceedings of the 6th National Anaplasmosis Conference: 113-116. Las Vegas, Nevada.

Popovic, N.A. 1968. Pathogenesis of two strains of *Anaplasma marginale* in *Dermacentor andersoni* tick. Ph.D. thesis, University of Illinois, Urbana, Illinois.

Porter, R. & Knight, J. eds. 1974. Parasites in the Immunized Host: 1-280. Mechanisms of Survival. Ciba Foundation Symposium 25 (new series). Associated Scientific Publishers. Amsterdam, The Netherlands.

Price, W.H. 1954. Variation in virulence of *"Rickettsia rickettsii"* under natural and experimental conditions. *In* The Dynamics of Virus and Rickettsial Infection, Hartman, F.W., Horsfall, F.L., Jr. & Kidd, J.G., Eds.: 164-183. Blakiston, New York.

Rao, P.J. & Ristic, M. 1963. Serum sialic acid levels in experimental anaplasmosis. *Proc. Soc. Exp. Biol. Med.* 114: 447-452.

Ristic, M. 1960. Anaplasmosis. *Adv. Vet. Sci.* 6: 111-192.

Ristic, M. 1962. A capillary tube-agglutination test for anaplasmosis - a preliminary report. *J. Am. Vet. Med. Assoc.* 141: 588-594.

Ristic, M. 1968. Anaplasmosis. *In* Infectious Blood Diseases of Man and Animals, Weinman D. & Ristic, M., Eds. 2: 478-542. Academic Press, Inc. New York, New York.

Ristic, M. & Kreier, J.P. 1974. Family Anaplasmataceae. *In* Bergey's Manual of Determinative Bacteriology, Buchanan, R.E. & Gibbons, N.E., Eds. 8: 906-908. William & Wilkins. Baltimore, Maryland.

Ristic, M., Lykins, J.D. & Morris, H.R. 1972. Anaplasmosis: opsonins and hemagglutinins in etiology of anemia. *Exp. Parasitol.* 31: 2-12.

Ristic, M. & Mann, D.K. 1963, Anaplasmosis IX. Immunologic properties of soluable anaplasma antigen. *Am. J. Vet. Res.* 24: 478-482.

Ristic, M., Mann, D.K. & Kodras, R. 1963. Anaplasmosis VIII. Biochemical and biophysical characterization of soluble anaplasma antigens. *Am. J. Vet. Res.* 24: 472-477.

Ristic, M. & Nyindo, M.B.A. 1973. Mechanisms of immune response to an attenuated *Anaplasma marginale* vaccine. *In* Proceedings of the 6th National Anaplasmosis Conference: 66-70. Las Vegas, Nevada.

Ristic, M., Sibinovic, S. & Welter, C.J. 1968. An attenuated *Anaplasma marginale* vaccine. *Proc. U.S. Livestock Sanit. Assoc.* 72: 56-69.

Ristic, M. & Watrach, A.M. 1961. Studies in anaplasmosis: II Electron microscopy of *Anaplasma marginale* in deer. *Am. J. Vet. Res.* 22: 109-116.

Ristic, M. & Watrach, A.M. 1963. Anaplasmosis. VI. Studies and a hypothesis concerning the cycle of development of the causative agent. *Am. J. Vet. Res.* 24: 267-277.

Roby, T.O., Amerault, T.E., Mazzola, V., Rose, J.E. & Ilamobade, A. 1974. Immunity in bovine anaplasmosis after elimination of *Anaplasma marginale* infections with imidocarb. *Am. J. Vet. Res.* 35: 993-995.

Schindler, R., Ristic, M. & Wokatsch, R. 1966. Vergleichende Untersuchungen mit *Anaplasma marginale* und *A. Centrale. Z. Tropenmed. Parasitol.* 17: 337-360.

Schmidt, H.E. 1937. Anaplasmosis in cattle. *J. Am. Vet. Med. Assoc.* 90: 723-736.

Schroeder, W.F., Rivas, C.E.L., Benitez, M.T. & Lopez, B.R. 1971. Anaplasmosis prevencion y control. Ministerio de Agricultura y Cria, Centro de Investigaciones Veterinarias: 129. Maracay, Venezuela.

Simpson, C.F., Kling, J.M., Love, J.N. 1967. Morphologic and histochemical nature of *Anaplasma marginale. Am. J. Vet. Res.* 28: 1055-1065.

Taylor, Robert L. 1969. Immunogenic differences between two *Anaplasma marginale* isolates. *Am. J. Vet. Res.* 30: 1999-2002.

Theiler, A. 1910. *Anaplasma marginale.* The marginal points in the blood of cattle suffering from specific disease. *In* Report of the Veterinary Bacteriologist, Dept. of Agriculture, Union of South Africa, Pretoria, 1908-1909: 6-64.

Vizcaino, O.G., Carson, C.A., Lee, A.J. & Ristic, M. 1976. Response of calves to various doses of attenuated *Anaplasma marginale* vaccine and effect of challenge. (In preparation)

Welter, C.J. & Ristic, M. 1969. Laboratory and Field Trials with an attenuated *Anaplasma marginale* vaccine. *Proc. U.S. Anim. Health Assoc.* 73: 122-130.

Welter, C.J. & Woods, R.D. 1963. Preliminary evaluation of an attenuated *Anaplasma marginale* vaccine in cattle. *Vet. Med. Small Anim. Clin.* 63: 798-802.

10

IMMUNIZATION OF CATTLE AGAINST *THEILERIA PARVA* *

M.P. Cunningham

Food and Agriculture Organization
United Nations Development Program
Immunological Research on Tick-borne Cattle
Diseases and Tick Control Project
East African Veterinary Research Organization
Muguga, Kikuyu
Kenya

INTRODUCTION

Throughout its distribution in East and Central Africa, East Coast fever (ECF) is considered to be the most important of the tick-borne diseases which inhibit the development of the livestock industry. At present, the only method of controlling the disease is by close-interval application of acaricides to cattle, in dips or sprays, to kill the tick vector. Susceptible cattle not so protected have a morbidity and mortality approaching 100%.

The disease is caused by a protozoan parasite, *Theileria parva,* which is transmitted by ticks, the most important of which is *Rhipicephalus appendiculatus.* Although only cattle and closely related species are susceptible to infection with *Theileria parva,* other species of *Theileria* are commonly observed in wild African bovidae. *Theileria lawrencei,* a common parasite of African buffalo (*Syncerus caffer*) is also pathogenic for cattle, causing a syndrome known as Corridor disease. Because of the many similarities observed between these two parasites, some investigators consider that *Theileria parva* and *Theileria lawrencei* are different biological strains of the same parasite (Barnett & Brocklesby 1966; Uilenberg 1976; Young & Purnell 1973).

*Project supported by the United Nations Development Program with the Food and Agriculture Organization of the United Nations as the Executing Agency, in cooperation with the East African Community. The Project is also supported by the Ministry of Overseas Development of the United Kingdom (Research Projects R 2396, R 2494, and R 2845 A & B), the United States Department of Agriculture, The Rockefeller Foundation, the International Atomic Energy Agency, and the Pfizer Corporation, Inc.

Theileria parva in the salivary gland of the unfed tick is not infective for cattle, but when the tick attaches and feeds on an animal the parasite undergoes a cycle of maturation. Maximum numbers of the mature infective stage are excreted by the tick between 3 and 5 days (Purnell & Joyner 1968) after attachment. After a latent period of at least 4 days, the macroschizont stage of the parasite is found intracellularly in lymphoblastoid cells obtained from a lymph node adjacent to the site of attachment of the tick. The macroschizont appears to stimulate the host cell to divide, producing two schizont-infected daughter cells. This process continues until more than 50% of lymphoid cells contain parasites. In the early stages the division of the infected cell and the growth of the macroschizont appear to be synchronous. Approximately 12 days after infection, a proportion of the infected cells are no longer capable of responding to stimulation, and the macroschizont increases in size. At this stage the macroschizont switches to microschizont, the host cell is disrupted, and micromerozoites are released to invade the red blood cells as piroplasms. It is this stage of the parasite, the piroplasm, which is considered to be infective for the tick vector.

It is well established that in ECF-enzootic areas where no tick control methods are practiced a proportion of cattle naturally acquire an immunity against the disease. Therefore, vaccination should be possible. Based on this information, many attempts have been made to produce a method for vaccinating cattle. Three main approaches have been used.

INOCULATION OF MACROSCHIZONT-INFECTED LYMPHOID CELLS HARVESTED FROM ANIMALS DYING OF EAST COAST FEVER INTO SUSCEPTIBLE CATTLE

This method was used on a large scale in South Africa at the beginning of this century (Theiler 1912; Spreull 1914). Between 200,000 and 300,000 cattle were inoculated with suspensions prepared from spleens and lymph nodes taken from infected cattle. Approximately 25% of the inoculated cattle died, and approximately 75% of those surviving the inoculation withstood natural challenge. Comparable results were obtained by later workers using smaller numbers of cattle, although some workers, for example Walker & Whitworth (1930), reported 100% success with suspensions obtained from particular cattle. Jarrett et al. (1969) at the Veterinary Faculty, Nairobi, Kenya, estimated that 10^{10} schizont-infected lymphoid cells were required to immunize cattle and confirmed their estimates in a small number of cattle.

CONCURRENT INFECTION OF CATTLE AND TREATMENT WITH TETRACYCLINE DRUGS

Neitz (1953) found that when infected ticks were applied to cattle that were simultaneously treated with Aureomycin the cattle underwent mild reactions and were immune on challenge. The drug was administered intravenously at a dosage rate of 10 mg/kg, starting 24 hours after tick infestation and continuing on approximately alternate days for 2 to 3 weeks. Neitz also reported the efficacy of Terramycin used in the same manner. This was confirmed by Jezierski et al. (1959) in Zaire. Brocklesby & Bailey (1965) found that daily oral administration of Aurofac (and other related drugs) to infected tick-infested cattle for 28 days produced immunity comparable to that produced in cattle naturally recovered from ECF.

Jarrett et al. (1969), using Aureomycin orally at a dosage rate of 16 mg/kg, found that 10 daily treatments to infected tick-infested cattle markedly suppressed the reaction, whereas 14 daily treatments gave complete suppression and subsequent immunity.

Other workers (Robson et al. 1961; Roe 1962, 1962a; Stobbs 1964) treated cattle exposed to natural infection orally with Aurofac. Since the attachment of infected ticks was random and unpredictable, continuous daily treatment for as long as 3 months was required to produce immunity.

QUANTUM OF INFECTION HYPOTHESIS

The "quantum of infection" hypothesis was put forward by Wilde et al. (1968). It is based on the observations of Lowe (1933) in enzootic areas in Tanzania that under climatic conditions unfavorable to tick survival there was a reduced calf mortality to ECF. Lowe thought that the reduced mortality could be attributed to the small numbers of ticks feeding on the calves. Lewis (1950) reported that infection rates in ticks became reduced with age and that old ticks were more likely to produce mild reactions in cattle. Wilson (1950, 1950a, 1951) found that when the number of infected ticks applied to cattle was limited, increased numbers of mild reactions with recovery and subsequent immunity were observed. Barnett (1957) suggested a direct relationship between numbers of parasites inoculated and the severity of the ensuing reaction but decided that, since one infected tick could kill a susceptible animal, this approach had no practical application. Wilde et al. (1968), however, found that the infective stage of the parasite could be obtained in suspension from the salivary glands of partially fed ticks, that cattle could be infected by inoculation, and that the parasite survived freezing to approximately -70 C and retained its infectivity for cattle.

Based on the above observations, we considered that to investigate any or all of the three approaches it was first necessary to achieve two objectives:
1. Obtain suspensions of protozoites from prefed ticks which would regularly infect cattle by inoculation, which could be preserved alive at low temperature, and whose infectivity could be established by titration in cattle.
2. Grow schizont-infected lymphoid cells *in vitro*.
If this were possible, we would then be in a position to:
1. Investigate the quantum of infection hypothesis.
2. Improve on the infection and treatment approach.
3. Investigate the effects of irradiation of protozoites.
4. Investigate the possibility of vaccinating cattle by inoculation of schizonts grown in tissue culture.

SUMMARY OF RESULTS

The objectives outlined above have been achieved.

Stabilates

Suspensions of the infective stage of the parasite can be harvested from ticks that will regularly and reproducibly infect cattle by inoculation. These suspensions can be viably preserved at low temperatures as stabilates without loss of infectivity for at least 600 days (Cunningham et al. 1973a).

Tissue Culture

Using the method developed by Malmquist et al. (1970), macroschizont-infected cell lines can be regularly isolated from infected cattle and established *in vitro*. The cell lines can be grown in both static and suspended culture, yielding 1 to 3 $\times 10^6$ cells/ml, approximately 95% of which contain macroschizonts of the *Theileria* species and strain isolated. With a $\log_{10}$ growth rate of 3 days, cultures up to 4 liters in volume can be harvested twice weekly, making mass suspension cultures a conceivable prospect.

Recently, Brown (1973) has been able to establish protozoites from infected ticks in primary cell lines of thymus, bone marrow, spleen, and lymph nodes from embryo cattle, as well as spleen and lymph nodes from young and adult cattle. After a dormant stage of 5 to 8 weeks, lymphoblastoid cells begin to proliferate, the majority containing macroschizonts.

ATTEMPTS TO VACCINATE CATTLE

Investigation of Quantum of Infection Hypothesis

By serial dilution of stabilates and inoculation into groups of cattle we have shown a direct relationship between the numbers of parasites inoculated and the severity of the ensuing infections. Large numbers of parasites cause acute, severe reactions, while small numbers cause mild, transient reactions, thus supporting Barnett's prediction and Wilde's hypothesis (Cunningham et al. 1974a).

Irradiation of Protozoites Harvested from Ticks

In a series of experiments we found that increasing doses of gamma irradiation caused increasing mortality of the parasites, so that irradiation merely produced a dilution effect as with the serial dilution of stabilates (Cunningham et al. 1973).

Infection and Treatment

Four different drugs in the tetracycline series have been shown to be active in inducing immunity when used at a dosage rate of 5 mg/kg administered as a daily dose on the day of inoculation of the stabilate and on the following 3 days. The drugs used are n-pyrrolidinomethyl tetracycline (Reverin), chlortetracycline (Aureomycin), oxytetracycline (two formulations: PVP Terramycin and PG Terramycin), and tetracycline. More than 200 cattle have been immunized by this method, all of them solidly immune to lethal homologous challenge (Radley et al., in preparation).

Depending on the drug used, the duration of its administration, and the magnitude of the infecting dose a proportion of cattle develop patent transient infections, with small numbers of macroschizonts in the local drainage lymph node and small numbers of piroplasms in the red cells.

Further investigations indicated that cattle can be immunized by the infection and treatment method, using Terramycin at a dosage rate of 10 mg/kg administered on days 0 and 4 following a sublethal stabilate challenge (Radley et al., in preparation).

Recently, a long-acting formulation of oxytetracycline (Terra ECF) has been produced by Pfizer Corporation which will immunize cattle when inoculated at a dosage rate of 20 mg/kg simultaneously with stabilate (Radley et al., in preparation).

More recently, improved formulations have been produced, increasing the concentration and reducing the volume of drug to be inoculated.

Tissue Culture

At present, approximately 90% of cattle can be immunized by inoculation of tissue culture material (Brown et al. 1971). Of the remaining 10%, a proportion die and some fail to be immunized. An attempt is being made to attenuate the tissue culture material so that larger doses can be inoculated into cattle without fatalities, hopefully with enhanced immunogenicity.

DURATION OF IMMUNITY

Cattle immunized against *Theileria parva* (Muguga) retain their immunity for at least 3.5 years against lethal stabilate challenge (Burridge et al. 1972).

CROSS-IMMUNITY

Unfortunately there are no serological tests which can be used to identify the immunogenic specificity of theilerial parasites involved in the ECF syndrome. It is therefore necessary to carry out cross-immunity tests in cattle, tests which are costly and time consuming. Tables 1 to 7 give results of some of the cross-immunity tests which have been carried out (Radley et al. 1975a, 1975b, 1975c). As a result of this work, three strains were identified that can be used as a combination to immunize cattle. Aliquots of stabilates of the three strains are pooled and inoculated into cattle simultaneously with Terra ECF. Cattle so immunized have withstood stabilate challenge with 15 strains available at the East African Veterinary Research Organization and obtained from Uganda, Tanzania, and Kenya.

FIELD TRIALS

Two trials have been carried out where reactions in susceptible control cattle indicated presence of a lethal ECF challenge. In both trials it is probable that *Theileria lawrencei* challenge occurred. In the first trial, at Aitong in Kenya Masai land, susceptible cattle and cattle immunized against *Theileria parva* (Muguga) all died (Snodgrass et al. 1972).

Table 1

The Reactions of ECF-Susceptible Cattle During Immunization Against Theileria parva (Muguga) and Subsequent Challenge With Various Theilerial Strains[a]

| | Reactions During T. parva (M) Immunization | | | | | Reactions to Various Challenge Strains | | | | | |
| | | Severity | | | | Mean Time (days) | | | | Severity | |
Number of Animals	No Reaction	Mild	Severe	Strain	Group	Prepatent Period	Febrile Response	Death	No Reaction	Mild	Severe
5	–	3	2	T. parva (Aitong)	A[b]	7.0 (1)[c]	–	–	4	1	–
					B[b]	8.6 (5)	10.8 (5)	22.6 (5)	–	–	5
5	–	2	3	T. parva (Kiambu K1)	A	10.0 (4)	10.3 (3)	–	1	1	3
					B	8.2 (5)	10.6 (5)	16.8 (5)	–	–	5
5	–	4	1	T. parva (Kiambu K4)	A	8.5 (2)	–	–	3	2	–
					B	8.8 (5)	10.8 (5)	22.6 (5)	–	–	5
5	–	3	2	T. parva (Kiambu K5)	A	8.3 (3)	–	–	2	2	1
					B	9.6 (5)	11.3 (4)	18.0 (2)	–	1	4
5	–	5	–	T. lawrencei (Serengeti-transformed)	A	8.0 (4)	–	–	1	4	–
					B	7.2 (5)	9.8 (5)	15.8 (5)	–	–	5

(a) From Radley et al. 1975a.
(b) A = T. parva (Muguga) immunes. B = controls.
(c) Figure in parentheses = number of cattle used for estimation of mean.

Table 2

The Reactions of ECF-Susceptible Cattle During Immunization Against Various Theilerial Strains, Isologous Challenge, and Challenge With *Theileria parva* (Muguga)[a]

Number of Animals	Strain	Reactions During Immunization Severity			Reactions During Isologous Challenge Severity			Reactions During *T. parva* (M) Challenge Severity		
		No Reaction	Mild	Severe	No Reaction	Mild	Severe	No Reaction	Mild	Severe
5	*T. parva* (Aitong)	1	4	–	5	–	–	5	–	–
5	*T. parva* (Kiambu K1)	–	5	–	3[b]	1	–	4	–	–
5	*T. parva* (Kiambu K4)	–	4	–	4	1	–	5	–	–
5	*T. parva* (Kiambu K5)	1	4	–	5	–	–	5	–	–
5	*T. lawrencei* (Serengeti-transformed)	1	4	–	5	–	–	5	–	–
5	Susceptible controls							–	1	4[c]

(a) From Radley et al. 1975a.
(b) One animal died 9 days after isologous challenge. Its death was most probably due to haemonchiasis.
(c) All 4 died from ECF.

Table 3

The Reactions of ECF-Susceptible Cattle to the Inoculation of Various Theilerial Strains, With and Without Chemoprophylaxis, and to Subsequent Challenge With a Lethal Dose of *T. lawrencei* (KB5) Stabilate[a]

| Immunizing Strains | Number of Animals | Reactions to Immunization Severity | | | Reactions to Challenge with *T. lawrencei* KB5 | | | | | |
		No Reaction	Mild	Severe	Mean time (days) Prepatent Period	Febrile Response	Death	Severity No Reaction	Mild	Severe
T. parva (Muguga)	6	–	1	5	6.2 (6)[b]	13.0 (3)	16.0 (3)	–	–	6
T. parva (Kiambu 5)	4	–	2	2	6.5 (4)	–	28.0 (1)	–	–	4
T. lawrencei (Serengeti-transformed)	4	–	3	1	9.0 (3)	10.0 (1)	20.0 (1)	1	1	2
T. lawrencei (Solio)	6	2	4	–	10.0 (1)	–	–	5	1	–
Controls	5				5.6 (5)	9.5 (4)	14.7 (3)	–	–	5

(a) From Radley et al. 1975b.
(b) Figure in parentheses = number of cattle used for estimation of mean.

Table 4

The Reactions of Cattle Chemoprophylactically Immunized Against T. lawrencei (KB5) and of Susceptible Cattle to Challenge With Various Theilerial Strains[a]

Strain Used for Challenge	Group	Number of Animals	Mean Time (days)			Reactions to Various Challenge Strains Severity		
			Prepatent Period	Febrile Response	Death	No Reaction	Mild	Severe
T. parva Kiambu 1	T. lawrencei KB5 immunes	5	10.8 (5)[b]	17.0 (1)	—	—	2	3
	controls	5	7.2 (5)	12.3 (4)	19.2 (5)	—	—	5
T. lawrencei (Serengeti-transformed)	T. lawrencei KB5 immunes	5	9.5 (5)	14.0 (1)	21.0 (1)	1	3	1
	controls	5	6.8 (5)	11.8 (4)	18.0 (5)	—	—	5
T. lawrencei Solio KB1	T. lawrencei KB5 immunes	5	11.0 (1)	—	—	4	1	—
	controls	5	8.0 (5)	14.5 (4)	22.8 (4)	—	—	5

Table 4 *(Continued)*

Strain Used for Challenge	Group	Number of Animals	Mean Time (days)			Severity		
			Prepatent Period	Febrile Response	Death	No Reaction	Mild	Severe
T. lawrencei Solio KB2	*T. lawrencei* KB5 immunes	5	–	–	–	5	–	–
	controls	5	6.6 (5)	11.5 (2)	16.0 (1)	–	–	5
T. lawrencei KB5 Isologous	*T. lawrencei* KB5 immunes	5	7.3 (3)	–	–	2	3	–
	controls	5	6.8 (5)	13.5 (4)	19.2 (5)	–	–	5
T. lawrencei KB5 Homologous	*T. lawrencei* KB5 immunes	5	17.0 (2)	–	–	3	2	–
	controls	5	7.2 (5)	16.0 (1)	26.0 (1)	–	–	5

(a) From Radley et al. 1975b.
(b) Figure in parentheses = number of cattle used for estimation of mean.

Table 5

Reactions of Cattle Immunized Against Various Strains of *Theileria* to Challenge With a Lethal Dose of *T. parva* (Kiambu 1)[a]

Strains Used in Immunization	Number of Animals	Reactions to Challenge					
		Mean Time (days)			Severity		
		Prepatent Period	Febrile Response	Death	No Reaction	Mild	Severe
T. parva (Muguga) + *T. parva* (Kiambu 5) + *T. lawrencei* (Serengeti-transformed)	5	11.5 (2)[b]	—	—	3	2	—
T. parva (Muguga) + *T. parva* (Kiambu 5)	5	12.3 (4)	13.0 (2)	23.0 (1)	1	1	3
T. parva (Muguga) + *T. lawrencei* (Serengeti-transformed)	4	8.7 (3)	14.0 (3)	—	1	—	3

(a) From Radley et al. 1975c.
(b) Figure in parentheses = number of cattle used for estimation of mean.

Table 5 *(Continued)*

Strains Used in Immunization	Number of Animals	Mean Time (days)		Reactions to Challenge	Severity		
		Prepatent Period	Febrile Response	Death Due to ECF	No Reaction	Mild	Severe
T. parva (Muguga)	5	12.3 (4)	16.0 (2)	24.0 (1)	1	1	3
T. lawrencei (Serengeti-transformed)	5	9.8 (5)	14.0 (1)	21.0 (4)	—	—	4
Challenge controls	5	7.4 (5)	11.5 (4)	16.8 (5)	—	—	5

Table 6

Reactions of Cattle Immunized Against a Combination of Strains of *Theileria* to Challenge With *T. lawrencei* (Solio KB1)[a]

Strains Used for Immunization	Number of Animals	Reactions to Challenge					
		Mean Time (days)		Death Due to ECF	Severity		
		Prepatent Period	Febrile Response		No Reaction	Mild	Severe
T. parva (Muguga) + *T. parva* (Kiambu 5) + *T. lawrencei* (Serengeti-transformed)	5	17.0 (3)[b]	–	–	2	3	–
Challenge controls	5	8.4 (5)	–	–	–	–	5

(a) From Radley et al. 1975c.
(b) Figure in parentheses = number of cattle used for estimation of mean.

Table 7

Reactions of Cattle Immunized Against a Combination of Strains of *Theileria* Challenged With Recently Isolated Field Strains[a]

Strains Used for Challenge	Group	Number of Animals	Reactions to Various Challenges					
			Mean Time (days)			Severity		
			Prepatent Period	Febrile Response	Death Due to ECF	No Reaction	Mild	Severe
T. parva Entebbe 1	A[b]	6	15.0 (6)[c]	15.0 (1)	–	–	6	–
	B[d]	5	11.2 (5)	17.0 (4)	32.3 (3)	–	–	5
T. parva Entebbe 2	A	6	10.4 (5)	–	–	1	5	–
	B	5	6.6 (5)	13.5 (2)	18.0 (5)	–	–	5
T. parva Ukunda	A	5	11.25 (4)	–	–	1	4	–
	B	5	8.4 (5)	13.5 (4)	17.2 (5)	–	–	5

(a) From Radley et al. 1975c.
(b) Group A Immunized with *T. parva* (Muguga), *T. parva* (Kiambu 5), and *T. lawrencei* (Serengeti-transformed).
(c) Figures in brackets = number of cattle used for estimation of mean.
(d) Group B = susceptible controls.

In the second trial three groups of cattle were exposed on a farm near Mount Kenya (Cunningham et al. 1974b): (1) susceptible cattle; (2) cattle immunized against *Theileria parva* (Muguga); and (3) cattle immunized against *Theileria parva* (Muguga) and also against *Theileria lawrencei*. Eighty percent of cattle in groups 1 and 2 died, all cattle in group 3 survived.

Two trials have been carried out in tick-infested paddocks at EAVRO as follows:

1. Four cattle immunized against *Theileria parva* (Muguga) by simultaneous inoculation of stabilate and a single dose of long-acting oxytetracycline have been exposed for 60 days to unlimited tick challenge in a paddock infested with *R. appendiculatus* infected with *Theileria parva* (Muguga) (Radley et al. 1975d). All of the immune cattle withstood this challenge with minimal reactions and improved in condition during the period of exposure.

   Three groups of four susceptible cattle were introduced into the paddock with the immune cattle on days 0, 20, and 40. All of the susceptible cattle died of ECF between 14 and 21 days after exposure in the paddock, indicating that the immune cattle had withstood a continuous high challenge with *Theileria parva* (Muguga).

2. Two groups of four cattle were immunized against *Theileria lawrencei* stabilate 48 and *Theileria lawrencei* stabilate 58, respectively, by simultaneous inoculation of the stabilates and a single dose of long-acting oxytetracycline. Both groups of immune cattle were exposed for 77 days in a tick-infested *(R. appendiculatus)* paddock in which two adult buffaloes were maintained. These buffaloes were carriers of *Theileria lawrencei*. Stabilate 48 was isolated directly from one of them using a single batch of ticks. Stabilate 58 was obtained from successive batches of ticks fed on the same buffalo at a later date. Seven of the eight immunized cattle withstood this challenge with minimal reactions and improved in condition during the period of exposure.

Three groups of four susceptible cattle were introduced into the paddock with the immune cattle and the buffaloes on days 0, 21, and 43. All of the susceptible cattle died of *Theileria lawrencei* infection between 14 and 25 days after exposure in the paddock, indicating that the immunized cattle had withstood a continuous high challenge with *Theileria lawrencei* probably derived from both buffalo (Young et al., in preparation).

CONCLUSIONS

Assuming that there is a limit to the number of immunogenic types of theil-erial parasites involved in the ECF syndrome, and assuming that they can be identified and isolated, it is anticipated that chemoprophylactic vaccination can be used in the control of the disease.

The use of tissue culture material to immunize cattle requires further develop-ment and cannot yet be considered to be a practical method of vaccination.

BIBLIOGRAPHY

Barnett, S.F. 1957. Theileriosis control. *Bull. Epizoot. Dis. Afr.* 5: 343-357.

Barnett, S.F. & Brocklesby, D.W. 1966. The passage of *"Theileria lawrencei* (Kenya)"* through cattle. *Brit. Vet. J.* 122: 396-409.

Brocklesby, D.W. & Bailey, K.P. 1965. The immunization of cattle against East Coast fever (*Theileria parva* infection) using tetracyclines: a review of the literature and a reappraisal of the method. *Bull. Epizoot. Dis. Afr.* 13: 161-168.

Brown, C.G.D., Malmquist, W.A., Cunningham, M.P., Radley, D.E. & Burridge, M.J. 1971. Immunization against East Coast fever. Inoculation of cattle with *Theileria parva* schizonts grown in cell culture. *J. Parasitol.* 57: 59-60.

Brown, C.G.D., Stagg, D.A., Purnell, R.E., Kanhai, G.K. & Payne, R.C. 1973. Letter: infection and transformation of bovine lymphoid cells *in vitro* by infective particles of *Theileria parva. Nature* (Lond.) 245: 101-103.

Burridge, M.J., Morzaria, S.P., Cunningham, M.P. & Brown, C.G.D. 1972. Dura-tion of immunity to East Coast fever (*Theileria parva* infection of cattle). *Parasitology* 64: 511-515.

Cunningham, M.P., Brown, C.G.D., Burridge, M.J., Irvin, A.D., Kirimi, I.M., Purnell, R.E., Radley, D.E. & Wagner, G.G. 1974b. Theileriosis: the exposure of immunized cattle in a *Theileria lawrencei* enzootic area. *Trop. Anim. Health Prod.* 6: 39-43.

Cunningham, M.P., Brown, C.G.D., Burridge, M.J., Musoke, A.J., Purnell, R.E. & Dargie, J.D. 1973b. East Coast fever of cattle: 60 Co-irradiation of infective particles of *Theileria parva. J. Protozool.* 20: 298-300.

Cunningham, M.P., Brown, C.G.D., Burridge, M.J., Musoke, A.J., Purnell, R.E., Radley, D.E. & Sempebwa, C. 1974a. East Coast fever: titration in cattle of suspensions of *Theileria parva* derived from ticks. *Br. Vet. J.* 130: 336-345.

Cunningham, M.P., Brown, C.G.D., Burridge, M.J. & Purnell, R.E. 1973a. Cryo-preservation of infective particles of *Theileria parva. Int. J. Parasitol.* 3: 583-587.

Jarrett, W.F.H., Crighton, G.W. & Pirie, H.M. 1969a. *Theileria parva:* kinetics of replication. *Exp. Parasitol.* 24: 9-25.

Jarrett, W.F.H., Pirie, H.M. & Sharp, N.C.C. 1969b. Immunization against East Coast fever using tick infections and chlortetracycline. *Exp. Parasitol.* 24: 147-151.

Jezierski, A., Lambelin, G. & Lateur, L. 1959. Immunisation des bovinés contre l' "East Coast fever." (E.C.F.) (Theilériose à Theileria parva) *Bull. Inf. Inst. Agron. Congo Belge* 8: 1-21.

Lewis, E.A. 1950. Conditions affecting the East Coast fever parasite in ticks and in cattle, *E. Afr. Agric. J.* 16: 65-77.

Lowe, H.J., 1933. East Coast fever. *In* Annual Report of the Department of Veterinary Science and Animal Husbandry: 7. Dar es Salaam, Tanganyika Tertitory, 1932.

Malmquist, W.A., Nyindo, M.B.A. & Brown, C.G.D. 1970. East Coast fever: cultivation *in vitro* of bovine spleen cell lines infected and transformed by *Theileria parva. Trop. Anim. Health Prod.* 2: 139.

Neitz, W.O. 1953. Aureomycin in *Theileria parva* infection. *Nature* (Lond.) 171: 34-35.

Purnell, R.E. & Joyner, L.P. 1968. The development of *Theileria parva* in the salivary glands of the tick, *Rhipicephalus appendiculatus. Parasitology* 58: 725-732.

Radley, D.E. Chemoprophylactic immunization against East Coast fever. In preparation.

Radley, D.E., Brown, C.G.D., Burridge, M.J., Cunningham, M.P., Kirimi, I.M., Purnell, R.E. & Young, A.S. 1975a. East Coast fever: 1. Chemoprophylactic immunization of cattle against *Theileria parva* (Muguga) and five theilerial strains. *Vet. Parasitol.* 1: 35-41.

Radley, D.E., Brown, C.G.D., Cunningham, M.P., Kimber, C.D., Musisi, F.L., Purnell, R.E., Stagg, S.M. & Punyua, D.K. 1975d. East Coast fever: challenge of immunized cattle by prolonged exposure to infected ticks. *Vet. Rec.* 96: 525-527.

Radley, D.E., Brown, C.G.D., Cunningham, M.P., Kimber, C.D., Musisi, F.L., Payne, R.C., Purnell, R.E., Stagg, S.M. & Young, A.S. 1975c. East Coast fever: 3. Chemoprophylactic immunization of cattle using oxytetracycline and a combination of theilerial strains. *Vet. Parasitol.* 1: 51-60.

Radley, D.E., Young, A.S., Brown, C.G.D., Burridge, M.J., Cunningham, M.P., Musisi, F.L. & Purnell, R.E. 1975b. East Coast fever: 2. Cross-immunity trials with a Kenya strain of *Theileria lawrencei. Vet. Parasitol.* 1: 43-50.

Robson, J., Yeoman, G.H. & Ross, J.P.J. 1961. *Rhipicephalus appendiculatus* and East Coast fever in Tanganyika. *E. Afr. Med. J.* 38: 206-214.

Roe, J.E.R. 1962a. Tanganyika. Annual Report of the Department of Veterinary Services, Dar es Salaam, Government Printer, 1960, 60 pp.

Roe, J.E.R. 1962b. Tanganyika. Annual Report of the Department of Veterinary Services, Dar es Salaam, Government Printer, 1961.

Snodgrass, D.R., Trees, A.J., Bowyer, W.A., Bergman, J.R., Daft, J. & Wall, A.E. 1972. East Coast fever: field challenge of cattle immunized against *Theileria parva* (Muguga). *Trop. Anim. Health Prod.* 4: 142-151.

Spreull, J. 1914. East Coast fever inoculation in the Transkeian Territories, South Africa. *J. Comp. Pathol. Ther.* 27: 299-304.

Stobbs, T.H. 1964. Progress Report on the Serere Boran Experiment. Report 12/7 to the Commissioner for Agriculture, Entebbe. March 12, 1964.

Theiler, A. 1912. The immunization of cattle against East Coast fever. *In* 2nd Report, Director of Veterinary Research: 216-314. Union of South Africa, Pretoria.

Uilenberg, G. 1976. Tick-borne livestock diseases and their vectors: 2. Epizootiology of tick-borne diseases. *World Anim. Rev.* 17: 8-15.

Walker, J. & Whitworth, S.H. 1930. Artificial immunization and immunity in their relation to the control of East Coast fever. *In* Proceedings of the Pan-African Agricultural and Veterinary Conference, 1929. Pretoria, South Africa: 158.

Wilde, J.K.H., Brown, C.G.D., Hulliger, L., Gall, D. & McLeod, W.G. 1968. East Coast fever: experiments with the tissues of infected ticks. *Br. Vet. J.* 124: 196-208.

Wilson, S.G. 1950a. An experimental study of East Coast fever in Uganda. I. A study of the type of East Coast fever reactions produced when the number of infected ticks is controlled. *Parasitology* 40: 195-209.

Wilson, S.G., 1950b. An experimental study of East Coast fever in Uganda. II. The durability of immunity in East Coast fever. *Parasitology* 40: 210-214.

Wilson, S.G. 1951. An experimental study of East Coast fever in Uganda. III. A study of the East Coast fever reactions produced when infected ticks 31 days old are fed on susceptible calves in limited numbers over a period of 3 weeks. *Parasitology* 41: 23-35.

Young, A.S. & Purnell, R.E. 1973. Transmission of *Theileria lawrencei* (Serengeti) by the ixodid tick, *Rhipicephalus appendiculatus*. *Trop. Anim. Health Prod.* 5: 146-152.

Young, A.S., Radley, D.E., Brown, C.G.D., Cunningham, M.P., Kimber, C.D., Musisi, F., Payne, R.C. & Purnell, R.E. The exposure of cattle immunized by chemoprophylaxis to a prolonged natural challenge of *Theileria lawrencei* derived from African buffalo (*Syncerus caffer*). In preparation.

11

IMMUNOPROPHYLAXIS AGAINST AFRICAN TRYPANOSOMIASIS

Max Murray
International Laboratory for Research on Animal Diseases
Nairobi, Kenya

G.M. Urquhart
Glasgow University Veterinary School
Glasgow, Scotland

INTRODUCTION

To put the subject matter of this chapter in its proper perspective, it should first be made clear that the development of a vaccine against trypanosomiasis of cattle and sheep is perhaps the last practical possibility which would occur to most people whose daily business is concerned with the control of trypanosomiasis in the field in Africa today. The simple fact is that no one has yet evolved a technique of immunization which has been clearly shown to confer a significant degree of protection to domestic animals grazing in endemic areas.

In contrast, some considerable success has attended both the eradication of the tsetse fly vector by insecticides or bush clearing and the use of drugs with curative and prophylactic properties. Before embarking on an intensive study of immunoprophylaxis, it therefore seems desirable to consider briefly the merits and demerits of these techniques that are currently not only more efficacious but have the benefit of being immediately applicable.

The destruction of the tsetse fly by bush clearing and the use of ground or aerial insecticides has been practiced for many years with an increasing degree of sophistication. There is little doubt that tsetse flies may now be almost completely eradicated in many areas by these techniques, particularly by the use of insecticides. Unfortunately, very few areas of tsetse infestation have circumscribed boundaries, and unless cleared areas are vigorously and permanently settled, reinvasion of tsetse inevitably occurs. For a variety of reasons in the past, such settlement has not usually occurred. Perhaps the problem, i.e., the geographical and strategic use of insecticides, requires a degree of inter-African cooperation, sponsored by the United Nations, such as has led to the virtual eradication of rinderpest in the last few years. The second control technique, chemotherapy or chemoprophylaxis with trypanocidal drugs, has been of inestimable benefit in the control of trypanosomiasis, particularly in areas on the periphery of the tsetse belts. In areas of high tsetse challenge, however, two problems arise. First, the frequency of the treatment has to be stepped up, often to economically unacceptable levels. Secondly, one is frequently faced with the eventual emergence of drug-resistant strains, and unfortunately there are relatively few trypanocidal drugs available. Possibly both of these problems could be overcome by the sophisticated administration of a program incorporating a system of monitoring the duration of prophylaxis between chemotherapy, but areas of endemic trypanosomiasis, because of the very presence of the disease, are usually undeveloped and lacking in trained personnel and laboratory facilities.

It seems to us, therefore, that neither of these techniques, as used at present, offers an ideal answer to the control of trypanosomiasis, and that there is every justification for examining the prospects of immunization. Incidentally, our remarks are confined to trypanosomiasis of domestic animals and laboratory animal model systems, although the development and exploitation of a practical vaccine for bovine and ovine trypanosomiasis would perhaps increase the incidence of disease in man in at least some areas. This potential problem, however, might be countered in the future by development of a vaccine against human trypanosomiasis.

Unfortunately, we immediately run into the problem of antigenic variation. It now seems well established (see review by Gray 1967; Goedbloed et al. 1973; Wilson et al. 1973; Dar et al. 1973) that the numbers of antigenic variants of *T. brucei, T. vivax,* and *T. congolense* circulating as metacyclic (infective) trypanosomes in wild tsetse are very large indeed. Moreover, one fly may inoculate a mixture of antigenic variants on a single occasion (Dar et al. 1973). There is, it is true, considerable evidence to show that these variant antigens are responsible for the production of a very effective protective immunity, but this is directed solely against the particular variant inoculated and apparently confers no protection against other variants. On these grounds most workers have conceded that the possibility of vaccination is remote. Perhaps one should mention that this situation is also bedevilled by the fact that the detection, isolation, and serological typing of these isolates as currently practiced is laborious, inefficient, and expensive, particularly in the case of *T. vivax,* which will not readily infect laboratory animals.

CATTLE AND SHEEP

In these circumstances it is perhaps worthwhile to first examine those few reports which described the production of a significant degree of immunity in cattle and sheep under conditions of natural challenge.

Bevan (1928, 1936) in Southern Rhodesia was perhaps the first worker to note that clinical cases of bovine trypanosomiasis which recovered after treatment frequently remained in good health despite reinfection, as shown by positive blood smears. This type of immunity, characterized by a healthy state despite evidence of parasitemia, was described by Bevan as "tolerance."

Whiteside (1962) introduced three groups of Zebu cattle at different times into a trypanosome area near Lake Victoria in Kenya. Each group contracted trypanosomiasis within 4 weeks as shown by blood parasitemia and this was treated with the curative drug Berenil (Farbwerke Hoechst A.G., Frankfurt, West Germany), which is rapidly excreted and has little prophylactic effect. Subsequent reinfection of these groups, which always occurred about 4 weeks after treatment, was also treated with Berenil. After four such infections the intervals between parasitemia in the cattle of all the groups lengthened to 8 weeks. This extended interval between infections was considered by Whiteside to be due to the development of a degree of immunity. However, when the infection rate became very high, i.e., trypanosomiasis 2 weeks after the introduction of new cattle, the interval between parasitemia even after repeated drug treatments decreased to only 3½ weeks.

Incidentally, Whiteside also noted that the calves of cows newly introduced into an endemic area developed trypanosomiasis within 5 weeks of birth. Those born 8 months later took an average time of 14 weeks, and calves born 12 months later did not become infected until 30 weeks of age. Since the cows received trypanocidal drugs intermittently it is, we think, debatable whether this is evidence of a genuine maternally derived immunity or merely drug residues in fetal tissue or milk. However, a similar view, i.e., that calves born of dams with experience of trypanosomiasis resulting from light exposure to tsetse resist or tolerate infection with pathogenic trypanosomes, is stated with conviction and supported with field observations by Fiennes (1970) who worked in Kenya for many years.

Further evidence that cattle develop an immunity or at least a tolerant state to trypanosomiasis is given by Cunningham's description (1966) of how thousands of Zebu cattle survive around the northeast shore of Lake Victoria despite the fact that they are continuously exposed to trypanosome challenge. One interesting aside on this observation was that the incidence of infection as measured by blood parasitemia and the presence of neutralizing antibodies was 30%

and 90%, respectively. This was in fact similar to that encountered in game animals such as bushbuck and waterbuck, generally considered to be resistant to trypanosomiasis.

More recently, Wilson and his colleagues (1974, 1975a, 1975b, 1976) working in East Africa attempted to find if the strategic use of drugs over a period of 2 to 3 years would eventually enable young cattle to develop a degree of immunity. Immunity was assessed on trypanocidal drug requirement, development of parasitemia, ability to maintain normal blood values, growth rate (in the beef cattle), and the response to challenge after withdrawal of drugs. In one experiment with a breeding herd in a high tsetse challenge area, the frequency of drug treatment (Berenil) was based on the appearance of clinical signs and packed cell volume values below 20% (Wilson et al. 1975a). They found that immunity did not develop during 2 years of continuous exposure to the disease. However, during the second year the number of abortions and the calf mortality decreased. In addition, they maintained a beef herd under three different trypanocidal drug regimes in an area of medium tsetse challenge (Wilson et al. 1975b, 1976). In one group in which cattle were treated with Berenil upon development of clinical disease (or PCV 20%), it was concluded that a partial immunity to trypanosomiasis had developed after 2 years. On the other hand, cattle treated as a group with Berenil on the development of a patent parasitemia in any one animal of the group did not develop immunity, although they did have a better growth rate than the first group. Cattle treated as a group with Samorin (May and Baker, Ltd., Dagenham, Essex, England), using the same criterion for treatment, developed a degree of immunity and it was concluded that this regime was the most suitable of the three tried for the maintenance of beef cattle in a tsetse-infested area. In these studies no drug resistance was detected.

Tentative evidence of the development of a sterile immunity in two small groups of Zebu cattle on the Kenya coast was described by Soltys (1955). The first group comprising three cattle received the prophylactic drug Antrycide every 2 months for 28 months. Despite no further treatment they subsequently survived for 18 months with no evidence of infection. The second group of four cattle subjected to the same prophylactic regime was removed to a tsetse-free area for 10 months and then returned to the endemic area. All remained free of infection for the observation period of 8 months. Five control cattle introduced at the same time all contracted severe *T. congolense* infections within 3 weeks. Unfortunately, an experimental attempt to confirm this work by Smith (1958) indicated that repeated doses of Antrycide may leave tissue residues sufficient to confer prophylaxis for many months afterwards, and the validity of the "sterile immunity" described by Soltys still awaits confirmation.

Turning now to attempts to induce immunity by the deliberate use of trypano-some antigen, it is apparent that three techniques have been used: infection followed by treatment, the inoculation of trypanosome extracts, and infection with irradiated trypanosomes.

Koch (1901) was probably the earliest worker to attempt to immunize by the inoculation of living trypanosomes passaged through other host species. However, this was soon abandoned and Bevan (1928) was apparently the first to suggest that "vaccination" or "tolerance" might be achieved if cattle were given a try-panocidal drug after the deliberate inoculation of a laboratory-passaged strain of *T. congolense.* However, he subsequently reported in 1936 that the tolerance of his vaccinated cattle broke down when subjected to adverse conditions such as *T. vivax* infection, piroplasmosis, and malnutrition.

Around the same period Schilling (1935) in Tanganyika claimed to have achieved "full immunity" in cattle by vaccination with dead *T. brucei, T. congo-lense,* and *T. vivax* or by "mininal infection." However, Hornby (1941) who took over his observations considered his conclusions premature and invalid.

Soltys (1964) reported the successful immunization of two sheep given 10 inoculations of formalized *T. brucei* every two days in that 2 and 6 weeks later the sheep, when challenged with 200 *T. brucei* organisms (apparently the same variant), showed no evidence of infection for 6 months. Unfortunately, no con-trol sheep were apparently infected at the same time. In a second experiment, eight sheep given two inoculations of formalized trypanosomes in Freund's adju-vant all became infected on challenge.

Stephen (1966) in Nigeria infected six calves with wild-caught tsetse at monthly intervals for over 2 years (treating on only one or two occasions) and showed that despite intermittent parasitemias of *T. vivax* and *T. congolense* the calves sur-vived, although in poor condition. Untreated cattle in this area generally died within 3 months of infection.

In 1968, Cunningham reported the result of a small experiment in which six cattle were inoculated with a *T. brucei* stabilate and treated with Berenil 14 days later; six controls were treated with Berenil at the same time. Two animals from each group were challenged 1, 2, and 3 months later with the same stabilate. Of the cattle challenged one month after treatment one of the control animals was parasitemic on one occasion and subsequently remained negative. None of the remaining three cattle became infected. This result was attributed to the residual effect of Berenil. Of the cattle challenged 2 or 3 months later only one of the four vaccinates became parasitemic, whereas all four controls became infected. The four animals which were challenged one month after treatment were challenged again 8 months later. Both controls were parasitemic within 7 days, while both vaccinates successfully resisted challenge.

In two experiments of a similar type in Uganda, Wilson (1971) infected five cattle with two doses of a stabilate of *T. congolense* at an interval of 11 weeks. Berenil treatment was given 21 days after each infection. All of the cattle resisted challenge with the same stabilate 22 weeks after the first immunizing infection, although on subsequent challenge over the next few months three of the five became infected. In the second experiment, 10 cattle received five doses of metacyclic trypanosomes obtained from wild-caught tsetse over a period of 320 days, receiving Berenil after each inoculation 21 days later. On the sixth challenge all became parasitemic. Of these, six required a further treatment with Berenil to keep them alive, while four remained clinically unaffected for at least 50 days thereafter. Wilson considered that the latter group developed a "nonsterile immunity," i.e., the "tolerant" state of Bevan.

Using tsetse-transmitted *T. congolense* to immunize sheep, Uilenberg (1974) concluded that a cyclical infection—eliminated by treatment—may protect against subsequent cyclical infections with the same strain but not other strains of *T. congolense*. This finding suggests the emergence of "basic strain antigen" following cyclical transmission (see review by Gray 1967; Uilenberg 1974; Doyle 1975).

The third technique of immunization, gamma-irradiated trypanosomes, has been studied in *T. congolense* infection in cattle in Kenya by Duxbury, Sadun, and their colleagues (1972a). In contrast to the relatively successful results obtained in mice, four to seven weekly inoculations of 1×10^8 to 1×10^9 *T. congolense* conferred little or no protection in cattle to the challenge infection of 1×10^4 to 1×10^5 organisms. The only evidence of protection was a delay in the appearance of parasitemia from a normal period of 6 days to around 9 days. In discussing their results, the authors point out the possibility of antigenic variation having occurred in their immunizing and challenging inocula.

Immunization with irradiated *T. rhodesiense* induced strong and lasting resistance to homologous but not heterologous strain challenge in cattle (Wellde et al. 1973). Immunity lasted at least 8 months but was waning by 14 months. The outcome was dependent on the amount of trypanosome antigen used for immunization. For example, of three cattle immunized intravenously with 1×10^9 at 3 weekly intervals only one was completely resistant to challenge, whereas the five cattle given 6 weekly intravenous inoculations of amounts ranging from 4.4 to 22.9 $\times 10^9$ trypanosomes were completely resistant to challenge one week and 8 months later. Cattle used as infectivity controls in this study underwent spontaneous cure and were also found to be resistant to homologous strain challenge.

In a small experiment three cattle were immunized with irradiated *T. brucei* three times at weekly intervals and then, one week later, they were challenged along with infectivity controls. The prepatent period to parasitemia was 5 days in the controls and 8, 9, and 13 days in the vaccinates, possibly indicating the development of some immunity (Duxbury et al. 1973).

LABORATORY ANIMALS

As with domestic animals, in many of the vaccination studies carried out in laboratory animals the number of animals employed was frequently small, the experiments poorly controlled, and the results difficult to interpret. This was mainly because many of the experiments were done with organisms maintained by serial passage and the exact nature of the vaccinate and challenge antigens was not known. Nevertheless, it has been clearly shown that protection is readily achieved using a range of trypanosome preparations, although the evidence available points to the fact that successful protection only occurred when the host was challenged with the homologous antigenic variant. Most studies into immunoprophylaxis in laboratory animals have been carried out with the *T. brucei* subgroup (*T. rhodesiense, T. gambiense,* and *T. brucei*). With regard to the major trypanosomes of cattle, *T. congolense* and *T. vivax,* only a few investigations have been done on *T. congolense* and, as far as we are aware, none at all with *T. vivax,* no doubt because of the difficulty of establishing *T. vivax* in laboratory animals.

Trypanosoma rhodesiense

It has been possible to achieve considerable levels of protection against *T. rhodesiense* in mice, rats, and monkeys. These results were produced using exoantigen found in sera of infected rats (Seed & Weinman 1963; Seed 1963), trypanosome antigen and metabolic products (Seed 1963; Duxbury et al. 1974), and trypanosomes attenuated by x-irradiation (Duxbury & Sadun 1969; Duxbury et al. 1972b; Wellde et al. 1975).

It was found that the irradiation dose required to suppress normal division and infectivity was only a fraction of that required to kill the trypanosome and that trypanosomes remain immunogenic over a considerable range of irradiation from 20 kR to 1000 kR, losing their motility at about 640 kR (Duxbury & Sadun 1969). The protection achieved in mice, rats, and monkeys using x-irradiated trypanosomes (60 to 70 kR) was considerable, and in many experiments survival was 100% with none of the challenge trypanosomes becoming established as determined by blood smears and subinoculation. It was shown in rats that the level of protection to a 1 X 10^4 trypanosome challenge was dose-dependent: 57% survival with one dose of 4 X 10^6, 85% with two such immunizing inoculations, and 97% with three doses. In addition, the immunity achieved lasted for several months, starting to wane only after 5 months (Duxbury & Sadun 1969). In these studies the mice and rats were challenged with a homologous strain collected from the first wave of parasitemia; it was assumed that antigenic variation had not occurred (Duxbury & Sadun 1969; Duxbury et al. 1972b), although this was not definitely established. On the other hand, in immunized monkeys where protection was also achieved (five out of six monkeys were completely immune), the challenge dose of trypanosomes was from a relapsing parasitemia with the likelihood of different variants. However, the antigenic specificity was not determined (Duxbury et al. 1972b). The most probable explanation for this result was that the trypanosomes of the challenging infection were, by chance, of the same antigenic specificity as that of at least one of the six prior immunizing inoculations. More speculatively, it might reflect the existence in *T. rhodesiense* of some common antigen that is involved in the development of protective immunity. Thus, Wellde et al. (1975) demonstrated some such possible cross-protective effect in rats immunized with irradiated *T. rhodesiense*. When challenged with a serologically distinct relapsing variant they all succumbed, but some survived significantly longer than the infectivity controls.

One hundred percent protection, as judged by survival at day 30 and absence of parasitemia to homologous strain challenge, was achieved in mice using trypanosome excretion-secretion products collected *in vitro* from living trypanosomes (Duxbury et al. 1974). With lyophilized whole trypanosomes the levels of protection obtained were only slightly less (95%). These results were obtained whether or not the adjuvant aluminum hydroxide was used. When challenged with a different strain of *T. rhodesiense* all immunized mice died, but perhaps significantly their survival time increased to 20.6 days as compared with 15.3 days in the infectivity controls (Duxbury et al. 1974). In another study, the presence of a soluble exoantigen with protective qualities in the serum of infective animals was demonstrated when sera from infected rats were successfully used to immunize mice against a homologous strain challenge (Seed & Weinman 1963; Seed 1963). This was assessed by a significant increase in survival time.

Trypanosoma gambiense

Successful immunization against *T. gambiense* has been achieved in laboratory animals with a range of immunogens, including plasma from infected animals, trypanosome homogenates or extracts, and live trypanosomes.

Serum from infected mice and rats produced significant levels of protection to homologous strain challenge when used to immunize guinea pigs, rats, and mice (Dodin & Fromentin 1962; Dodin et al. 1962; Seed & Gam 1966a, 1966b; Fromentin 1974). This was judged by increased survival times and in some cases by complete survival (Dodin & Fromentin 1962; Fromentin 1974). Dodin & Fromentin (1962) found considerable cross-protection between two different strains of *T. gambiense;* however, detailed investigations into the antigenic nature of these were not carried out.

Dead trypanosome preparations also produced marked levels of protection. Lapierre & Rousset (1961) achieved protection to homologous strain challenge in mice using trypanosomes killed by Formalin or acetic acid. In a high proportion of mice there was complete protection: 8 out of 10 with the formalized vaccine and 14 out of 19 with trypanosomes treated with acetic acid. With the formalized vaccine, immunity developed later but lasted longer. Immunizing with three subcutaneous inoculations of 1.5 mg frozen and thawed trypanosome protein at 3-day intervals, Fromentin (1974) induced protection in mice to homologous strain challenge which lasted as long as 6 weeks. Kligler & Berman (1935) immunized rats with 8×10^5 killed *T. gambiense* on 5 successive days and challenged 3 to 5 days later with homologous strain. In this way survival time was increased significantly from 6.4 to 15.8 days. When challenged with *Trypanosoma evansi* or *Trypanosoma equi* there was no evidence of cross-reactivity as judged by increased survival time.

With a trypanosome extract obtained by DEAE-Sepharose fractionation, Seed (1972) achieved as much as 80% protection in mice based on survival at day 17. Infectivity controls lived only 5 days. Fromentin (1974), immunizing mice with a Sephadex-G 200-extracted fraction of the parasite, increased survival time from 5 to 20 days after a homologous strain challenge.

Perhaps the most intriguing result was produced by Petithory et al. (1971) who implanted diffusion chambers with millipore filters of pore size 0.45 μ into the peritoneal cavity of mice. In these chambers were 10^4 *T. gambiense.* The chambers were left for 45 days and then the mice were challenged with a homologous or heterologous strain of *T. gambiense.* Cross-protection ranging from 37% to 63% complete survival was achieved on heterologous strain challenge; similar results were obtained with homologous challenge.

Trypanosoma brucei

Similar results were achieved in mice, rats, and rabbits with *T. brucei*.Thus, killed trypanosomes (Soltys, 1964, 1967; Herbert & Lumsden 1968), trypanosome extracts (Lanham & Taylor 1972; Cross 1975), and soluble exoantigen in plasma of infected animals (Weitz 1960; Dodin & Fromentin 1962; Miller 1965; Soltys 1967; Herbert & Lumsden 1968; Lanham & Taylor 1972), produced protection to challenge with homologous variant or strain. It has been found that plasmanemes (filopodia) of *T. brucei* become readily detached from the organism and can be recovered from infected serum by centrifugation. It was suggested that they represent the released exoantigen of the trypanosome (Macadam & Herbert 1970a, 1970b). It was found that infected sera or filopodia-containing pellets centrifuged from infected sera gave better protection (8 of 10 surviving challenge) than infected sera free of filopodia (4 out of 10) (Herbert & Macadam 1971). The immunizing procedure involved the use of equivalent amounts of immunogen prepared in water-in-oil emulsion. The animals were challenged 8 weeks later with the same antigenic type. The above result was taken as evidence that a protective antigen is present in a fully soluble form in infected sera as well as in association with the filopodia. In addition, Herbert & Lumsden (1968) showed that infected formalized whole blood conferred protection. They were able to achieve simultaneous protection against four different variants of *T. brucei*; no cross-reactivity could be demonstrated when mice were immunized with single variants and cross-challenged. The ability of soluble protective antigen to absorb to red blood cells was demonstrated when Herbert & Inglis (1973) successfully immunized mice against *T. brucei* of the same antigenic type. The immunogen used was syngeneic red blood cells exposed to plasma from infected mice. It was repeatedly washed and administered intravenously. No further details have become available.

X-irradiation of *T. brucei* was carried out by James et al. (1973) who found that rats immunized by attenuated trypanosomes were protected to some extent against challenge with a homologous variant. A few were completely protected (2 of 13), while the remainder showed an increased survival time.

It was found that a number of factors influenced the level of protection and its rate of development. Firstly, the way in which trypanosomes were inactivated; β-propiolactone and 0.5% Formalin were superior to freezing and thawing, which in turn was better than phenol, heating at 56 C for 30 minutes, or lysis in distilled water (Soltys 1964, 1967). Secondly, it was demonstrated that some strains were more immunogenic than others when used in vaccination studies (Soltys 1964). Thirdly, apparently the number of doses employed to immunize was important. Soltys (1964) considered that multiple doses closely spaced (every 2 days) gave better results than doses 2 weeks apart, although the same total quantity of antigen was used. Fourthly, the route of administration of the immunizing dose was also found to influence the outcome of an intraperitoneal challenge; when the antigen was administered intravenously it gave significantly better protection than when given subcutaneously (Herbert & Lumsden 1968). Fifthly, it has been shown that the outcome of immunization was affected by the time of challenge. Using trypanosomes inactivated by 0.1% β-propiolactone as immunogen, Soltys (1967) found that 6 out of 10 immunized mice resisted challenge on day 7, 10 out of 10 on day 21, and 8 out of 10 on day 42. In this respect, preliminary observations indicated that the rate of development of immunity to a protective level might also be influenced by the method of antigen preparation (see *T. gambiense,* Lapierre & Rousset 1961), route of administration used and, possibly, the use of adjuvants. Thus, with plasma absorbed to aluminum hydroxide, formalized plasma, or whole blood from infected mice, Herbert & Lumsden (1968) found that when given intravenously 100% protection—based on survival at 14 days—was achieved by 7 to 14 days after immunization. However, by 159 days protection was falling off. With water-in-oil emulsion adjuvants, where much smaller amounts of antigen were used and administered subcutaneously, immunity took several weeks to rise to a protective level but lasted considerably longer.

In the studies involving killed *T. brucei* antigen given subcutaneously (Soltys 1964; Herbert & Lumsden 1968), the antigen was always used in water-in-oil emulsion and the effects of the adjuvant could not be evaluated.

Trypanosoma congolense

The data on *T. congolense* are more limited, although results similar to those with *T. rhodesiense, T. gambiense,* and *T. brucei* have been obtained. Protection has been achieved against challenge with a homologous strain using killed trypanosomes (Johnson et al. 1963), plasma from infected mice (Dodin & Fromentin 1962; Johnson et al. 1963), and x-irradiated trypanosomes (Duxbury et al. 1972a).

Johnson et al. (1963) used *T. congolense* killed by freezing and thawing with and without various adjuvants. It was found that antigen alone was not effective, but antigen with saponin increased the prepatent period and the number of survivors (five out of six). Similar results were obtained with plasma antigen. *N*-hexadecylamine was not as effective, whereas other adjuvants including Arquad 2HT, Freund's complete or incomplete, and potash alum were not effective at all. A potentially significant finding was that 19 weeks later the five surviving mice were challenged with a different strain of *T. congolense* and two survived, possibly indicating cross-protection.

In this preliminary study, other flagellates related to *Trypanosoma* were examined for protective properties when prepared as above and mixed with adjuvant. The flagellates were *Crithridia fasiculata, Leptomonas collosoma, T. melophagium,* and *T. mega.* The first two protected against *T. cruzi* challenge, but there was no cross-protection against *T. congolense.*

Trypanosoma congolense attenuated by x-irradiation produced protection as judged by the lengthening of the prepatent period and increased survival percentage (in certain experiments 100% survival) when mice were challenged with the homologous strain (Duxbury et al. 1972a). In dogs and in cattle immunized with irradiated *T. congolense,* little effect was achieved other than lengthening of the prepatent period.

CHEMOTHERAPEUTIC AGENTS AND IMMUNITY

As with cattle, mice infected with trypanosomes and then treated with a trypanocidal drug develop immunity to subsequent challenge with a homologous strain or variant. In some cases the mice remained resistant for as long as one year. Such studies have been done with *T. rhodesiense* (Lourie & O'Connor 1937; Fulton & Lourie 1946), *T. brucei* (Browning & Gulbransen 1936, who also reviewed the situation; Lourie & O'Connor 1937; Herbert & Lumsden 1968), and *T. congolense* (Browning & Calver 1943; Fulton & Lourie 1946). Browning & Gulbransen (1936) also showed that rabbits infected with *T. brucei* and then treated possess a high degree of resistance to reinoculation with homologous strain and that this resistance persists for long periods.

James (1976) employed trypanocidal drugs in an attempt to attenuate suspensions of rodent-adapted strains of *T. brucei* and *T. congolense.* This was done briefly, exposing the trypanosomes *in vitro* to low concentrations of one or another of two trypanocidal drugs: Samorin and Berenil. The concentration of drug employed was too low to have any prophylactic effect when inoculated into animals. Trypanosomes treated in this way were detected after intravenous inoculation 30 minutes, 3 hours, and 24 hours later but not at 48 or 72 hours. Single or multiple immunizing inocula of from 10^6 or 10^7 treated parasites gave complete protection to challenge with 10^4 organisms and almost complete protection with 10^5 (*T. brucei* in rats and *T. congolense* in mice). Also, attenuation with Samorin gave better protective results than attenuation with Berenil. However, as with other vaccination procedures, protection was achieved only following homologous strain challenge.

THE NATURE OF THE PROTECTIVE ANTIGEN

This has been reviewed by Seed (1974) and also by Doyle (1975). The most notable advance in this area has come from Cross (1975) studying a *T. brucei* clone. He found that a characteristic and predominant glycoprotein could be isolated from each clone and that this molecule was the major constituent of the parasite surface coat. Each glycoprotein had a molecular weight of approximately 65,000 and consisted of about 600 amino acid residues and 20 monosaccharide residues. Although these clone-specific glycoproteins had a similar molecular weight, they differed in their isoelectric points (pI 8.19 to 6.46) and preliminary structural studies indicated that there were large differences in the amino acid sequences dispersed over more than one half of the polypeptide chain. Immunization with purified clone-specific glycoproteins gave complete protection against challenge with the homologous but not heterologous clones and resulted in the formation of both precipitating and agglutinating antibodies.

So far no antigen with protective qualities and common to a trypanosome species has been demonstrated. This would appear to be an area worthy of further investigation and no doubt the situation will be made clearer by further work along the lines of Cross (1975).

EFFECTOR MECHANISMS IN PROTECTION

It is likely that the most effective effector mechanism in dealing with the African trypanosomes, at least the intravascular ones, is antibody, and this has been confirmed both *in vivo* and *in vitro*. Thus, it has been shown that homologous antibody passively transferred is protective. This has been done with *T. gambiense* in mice and rabbits (Dodin & Fromentin 1962; Seed & Gam 1966a 1966b; Takayanagi 1971; Seed 1972; Takayanagi et al. 1973), *T. brucei* in mice (Watkins 1964), and *T. rhodesiense* in mice (Seed 1963). It was found that antibody was most effective when administered at the same time as the challenge infection (Seed & Gam 1966b) and that the outcome depended on the quantity of antiserum used (Dodin & Fromentin 1962; Watkin 1964; Seed & Gam 1966b). Protective antibody, successfully used for passive transfer, was detectable as early as 2 days after infection (Takayanagi et al. 1973). While both specific IgG and IgM are protective (Seed 1972; Takayanagi et al. 1973; Zahalsky & Weinberg 1976), IgM was found to be more effective than IgG at neutralizing *T. gambiense* in that much smaller quantities of IgM were required to neutralize a given number of trypanosomes (Takayanagi & Enriquez 1973). On the other hand, Zahalsky & Weinberg (1976) studying *T. brucei* in rats presented preliminary data that suggested that IgG was more effective than IgM in producing protection: mice given IgM-treated trypanosomes lived 2 or 3 days longer than controls, whereas mice receiving IgG-treated trypanosomes survived for at least 4 days longer than controls. Further work is required to establish the major protective immunoglobulin class or classes in trypanosomiasis.

In vitro studies have shown that homologous antibody is capable of lysing trypanosomes with or without complement. In the presence of complement, however, lysis occurred more rapidly (Lourie & O'Connor 1936). The trypanosomes involved were mouse-adapted *T. brucei* and *T. rhodesiense* as well as *T. equiperdum*. Diggs et al. (1976) demonstrated the cytotoxicity of serum from rats immunized with irradiated *T. rhodesiense*. This was assessed by the uptake of radiolabeled leucine. Incorporation was completely prevented if the organisms were treated with fresh serum from immunized animals. This reaction was abrogated by heat inactivation but fully restored by adding fresh rat or guinea pig serum to the heated immune serum, suggesting the involvement of complement in the cytotoxic events. The immunoglobulin class or classes involved were not investigated.

Passive protection has also been achieved in syngeneic mice by the transfer of sensitized cells (Luckins 1972; Takayanagi et al. 1969, 1973; Takayanagi & Nakatake 1975; Dodin et al. 1962). In the first four studies, cells were obtained from mice infected with trypanosomes and then treated with a trypanocidal drug, while in the fifth investigation the cells were recovered from the mice immunized with plasma from *T. gambiense*-infected animals. Luckins (1972) induced immunity to *T. brucei* in mice by transfer of spleen, lymph node, and bone marrow cells. The initial parasitemia was depressed and survival time increased from 4 to 9.6 days. Takayanagi et al. (1969, 1973) found that the outcome of their spleen cell transfer experiments depended on the number of cells transferred, there being a direct relationship between number of cells used and the level of protection achieved, and the degree of sensitization of the cells. Moreover, cells collected during the first 10 days of an infection were much more effective than cells collected after that. Following passage of spleen cells from immunized animals through columns of glass beads, it was found that the adherent cells, likely to be the antibody-producing cells, were more protective than the cells which appeared in the filtrate (Takayanagi & Nakatake 1975). When cortisone or antithymocyte serum was given prior to immunization, protective responses were depressed. These results suggested that antibody-producing cells were important in the effector aspect of the immune protective response but that thymus-dependent cells played a major role in the induction of the response. Following this Takayanagi & Nakatake (1976) demonstrated that thymic cells from immune animals when transferred to adult thymectomized irradiated (800 R) mice conveyed protection to homologous strain challenges 5 days later, providing the mice were immunized with a 1% parasite antigen solution (homologous strain) just after cell transfer. Agglutinating antibody was also induced. Neither immune thymic cells without parasitic antigen solution nor normal thymic cells with parasite antigen solution produced protection or agglutinins. Takayanagi & Nakatake (1976) concluded that immune thymic cells were responsible for protection and agglutinin production. An alternative explanation is that the adult thymectomized irradiated mice still had a population of B cells present. Thus, protection and production of agglutinins only occurred when both immune thymic cells were transferred and when B cells in the recipient were sensitized by inoculation with parasite antigen solution. In all the above studies, successful protection was achieved only when the animals were challenged with a homologous strain.

There is evidence that cells may have an effector role in the protective mechanisms in trypanosomiasis. Macrophages are capable of phagocytosing trypanosomes and possibly destroying them (Goodwin 1970). Phagocytosed *T. congolense* have been found in circulating macrophages of the African buffalo (Young et al. 1975). Preliminary observations with mouse peritoneal macrophages (Lumsden & Herbert 1967) indicated that bloodstream forms of *T. brucei* are rarely phagocytosed in the presence of normal mouse serum but are actively ingested in the presence of homologous variant antiserum. Trypanosome antibody, cytophilic for macrophages, has been demonstrated in *T. brucei* infections in rabbits (Tizard & Soltys 1971a). This antibody appeared to be of the IgG class and was not complement-dependent; the reaction was not inhibited by heating for 30 minutes at 56 C. Similarly, the presence of specific antiserum to a particular variant of *T. gambiense* was found to be a prerequisite for the attachment and ingestion of trypanosomes by rat macrophages (Takayanagi et al. 1974; Takayanagi & Nakatake 1976). This antibody was thought to be related to agglutinating antibody: the reaction was heat-stable and not complement-dependent. Macrophages from normal, immune, and irradiated donors were equally effective.

Another possible effector mechanism might be antibody-mediated cellular cytotoxicity. Mkwananzi et al. (1976) have demonstrated that normal human lymphoid cells in the presence of specific antibody can cause isotope leakage reflecting death of culture forms of *Trypanosoma dionisii*, a parasite related to *Trypanosoma cruzi*. While such an effector mechanism might appear unlikely with the intravascular forms of the African trypanosome, it might be operative against the tissue forms of the *T. brucei* subgroup where a whole range of potential effector cell types are present in the tissues including lymphoid cells and macrophages (Murray et al. 1974).

The role of cell-mediated immunity in protective mechanisms in African trypanosomiasis awaits evaluation. Only in rabbits infected either with *T. brucei, T. rhodesiense,* or *T. congolense* have studies been made. It was found in rabbits with *T. brucei* or *T. rhodesiense* (trypanosomes which are located both intravascularly and extravascularly) that both immediate and delayed-type hypersensitivity reactions developed. This was judged by skin reactions and histology as well as by the demonstration that the delayed hypersensitivity reaction could be passively transferred by living spleen cells from an infected rabbit (Tizard & Soltys 1971b). On the other hand, rabbits infected with *T. congolense* (a trypanosome apparently confined to the circulation) developed an immediate hypersensitivity reaction but not a delayed one (Mansfield & Kreier 1972).

MANIPULATION OF HOST RESISTANCE

It has been demonstrated in laboratory animals that host resistance to African trypanosomes can be increased in a number of ways. For example, it has been found that mice pretreated intraperitoneally with endotoxin (*E. coli* lipopolysaccharide) were rendered more resistant to infection with *T. congolense, T. rhodesiense,* and *T. musculi* as judged by prolonged survival time and delay in onset of peak parasitemia (Singer et al. 1964). If the endotoxin was given on the day of challenge with trypanosomes or subsequent to challenge no such effect was achieved. Indeed, when endotoxin was given subsequent to trypanosome infection, survival time of infected mice was significantly shortened. Why endotoxin should have this effect is not known, and it is difficult to speculate as endotoxins have such wide-ranging immunologic and pharmacological activities (reviewed by Cluff 1970). It might be its effect in stimulating the mononuclear phagocytic system, its adjuvant activity, its effect on complement or in stimulating the alternate pathway, or its role as an interferon stimulator that causes this sequela.

Intravenous infection of the synthetic polyribonucleotide, polyinosinic acid-polycytidylic acid (Poly I : Poly C) increased resistance of mice to *T. congolense* as judged by increased survival time and reduced parasitemias (Herman & Baron 1971). This effect was dose-dependent and best protection was obtained when the injection was given around the time of infection. In this study it was concluded that the protective effect achieved was probably due to the immunologic enhancing capacity of Poly I : Poly C and not to its ability to stimulate interferon production. This was based on the fact that viral interferon inducers, Newcastle disease virus and Semliki Forest virus, had no effect on protection against *T. congolense,* whereas cyclophosphamide reversed the protective effect. On the other hand, Van Dijick et al. (1970) found that prior administration of the polyanion polyacrylic acid did not protect mice against subsequent challenge with *T. congolense.*

In preliminary studies, we have been able to increase host resistance in mice by administration of Bacillus Calmette-Guerin (BCG) prior to challenge with *T. brucei* or *T. congolense.* The rationale behind this experiment is discussed later.

It is worth noting that several agents have been used to alter host reactivity to other protozoal diseases including murine malaria, *Trypanosoma cruzi,* and *Toxoplasma gondii.*

The administration of Newcastle disease virus, statolon, the complex of Poly I : Poly C, or polyacrylic acid to mice, a few hours before or after *Plasmodium berghei* challenge resulted in complete protection or an increase in survival time (Jahiel et al. 1968a, 1968b; Schultz et al. 1968; Jahiel et al. 1969; Van Dijick et al. 1970; Jahiel et al. 1970). These agents are all recognized for their ability to stimulate interferon production. Further evidence that interferon might be involved was obtained when mouse blood infected with *P. berghei* was incubated in serum containing a high concentration of interferon (Schultz et al. 1968). When subsequently inoculated into susceptible mice it was found that there was a significant increase in survival time (some mice survived completely) as compared with infected blood incubated in normal serum. There is evidence, however, that interferon is more effective against sporozite-induced infections than against blood-form-induced infections. It was demonstrated that mouse serum with high levels of interferon exerted a significant protective effect against sporozite-induced *P. berghei* when it was injected during the pre-erythrocytic phase of development (which ends about 42 to 48 hours after sporozoite inoculation). The failure to demonstrate protection when serum with interferon was injected 45 hours after sporozoite inoculation suggested that interferon was not as effective on the erythrocytic phase of the infection (Jahiel et al. 1970).

Clark et al. (1976) found that intravenous inoculation of 2×10^7 BCG protected mice against *Plasmodium* sp. and *Babesia* sp. challenge one month later. Inoculation of BCG subcutaneously had no effect. They provided tentative evidence that neither antibody specific for surface antigens of the parasite nor increased phagocytic capacity was responsible for this protection, but the protective factor was a nonantibody-soluble mediator. *Corynebacterium parvum* was used in the same way. Nussenzweig (1967) found that intravenous treatment with heat-inactivated *C. parvum* resulted in complete protection or a significantly increased survival in mice challenged with sporozoites of *P. berghei* 1 to 3 weeks later. Comparable results were achieved with Freund's adjuvant. It was suggested that the mechanism of this type of protection was unknown, but protection occurred under conditions in which phagocytosis was increased as judged by a seven-to ninefold increase in carbon clearance (Halpern et al. 1963).

Similar studies were made with the model system of *T. cruzi* in the mouse. *Escherichia coli* endotoxin, whether given before, simultaneous with, or after inoculation with *T. cruzi,* did not increase host resistance (Kierszenbaum & Saavedra 1972). On the other hand, intravenous injection of *C. parvum* before or after intraperitoneal infection with a highly reticulotropic strain of *T. cruzi* produced enhanced resistance against the infection in mice (Kierszenbaum 1975). No such effect was achieved by intraperitoneal infection of *C. parvum.* It was thought that *C. parvum's* potent stimulant effect on the mononuclear phagocytic system might be responsible for this result. This proposal is supported by the fact that manipulation of the mononuclear phagocytic system can affect the course of experimental Chagas' disease. Kierszenbaum et al. (1974) found that stimulation of the mononuclear phagocytic system by diethylstilbestrol resulted in greater longevity, reduced mortality, and decreased parasitemia in *T. cruzi*-infected mice. They also confirmed the work of Goble & Boyd (1962) showing that depression of the mononuclear phagocytic system resulted in increased severity of the disease.

Studies employing BCG to increase host resistance have been equivocal. Kuhn et al. (1975) found that intravenous inoculation of BCG 21 days before challenge with *T. cruzi* did not alter the course of the disease in mice. Hoff (1975) also failed to increase host resistance to *T. cruzi.* He used 4×10^5 to 9×10^5 organisms given intraperitoneally 18 and 3 days before challenge. On the other hand, Ortiz-Ortiz et al. (1975) gave 4×10^6 organisms intravenously 11 days and 1 day before challenge and significantly increased survival time; some mice made a complete recovery. This success was attributed to macrophages being activated by BCG to kill ingested parasites, a mechanism established by Kress et al. (1975) and Hoff (1975). Furthermore, it was shown that the uptake of *T. cruzi* by BCG-activated macrophages was facilitated by the presence of cytophilic antibody (Hoff 1975). It is of interest that whereas Hoff (1975) found that BCG-activated macrophages were capable of killing *T. cruzi in vitro,* with *in vivo* studies he failed to produce protection by prior inoculation with BCG. This result might be attributed to the route of administration of BCG he employed, intraperitoneal as opposed to intravenous.

Tabbara et al. (1975) found that prior intravenous inoculation of BCG (8×10^6) produced significant protection against *Toxoplasma gondii* injected into the suprachoroidal space 14 days later; the onset of the retinochoroiditis was delayed and the severity of the disease reduced. Inoculation of BCG locally by the retrobulbar route produced little or no effect, confirming observations of the other workers on the importance of the route of administration.

It would appear that several factors influence the outcome of the use of BCG. These include the strains and preparations employed (Mackaness et al. 1973), the dose (Mackaness et al. 1974a), the timing (Mathe et al. 1973; Mackaness et al. 1974a; Zatz 1976), and the route of administration (Mathe et al. 1973; Tabbara et al. 1975; Clark et al. 1976; Zatz 1976).

DISCUSSION

In attempting to draw some general conclusions, it is difficult to make a critical evaluation of many of the observations and experiments described for a variety of reasons. The small number of animals used, the antigenic diversity of challenge, the possibility of extended drug prophylaxis being confused with immunity, the difficulty in distinguishing reinfection, and the physical difficulties which attend field observations in areas of endemic trypanosomiasis in Africa all make critical evaluation difficult.

Nevertheless, certain general conclusions may be drawn. First, cattle exposed for a prolonged period to tsetse often appear to develop a degree of immunity to field challenge usually with the aid of intermittent chemotherapy. Sometimes this may be sterile but more frequently is associated with intermittent parasitemia and a variable degree of clinical illness. Second, in domestic animals the use of single stabilates for experimental immunization and challenge frequently produces sterile immunity, although this appears to be of somewhat limited duration in terms of potential practical value.

In laboratory animals similar results have been obtained, although the relative duration of immunity was generally longer. The nature of the immunogen used appeared to matter little. Successful immunization was produced with bloodstream trypanosomes, living or irradiated; whole trypanosome homogenates produced in a variety of ways; and also using metabolic or biochemical fractions.

The degree of protection demonstrated against heterologous variants of the same strain or against heterologous strains of the same species was rarely significant, and when achieved the exact antigenic nature of the trypanosomes used for immunization and challenge was rarely investigated. However, it is perhaps worth considering the circumstances under which apparent cross-protection was achieved. It was produced in monkeys immunized intravenously with six repeated doses of 1×10^8 or 1×10^9 irradiated trypanosomes (Duxbury et al. 1972b). Five of the monkeys survived subsequent challenge with what might be presumed to be a relapsing variant of the same strain. This was not checked immunologically. Increased survival time occurred in mice, 15.3 to 20.6 days immunized with the secretion-excretion products of one strain of *T. rhodesiense* and challenged with a separate isolate of *T. rhodesiense* (Duxbury et al. 1974). Again the antigenic relationship was not determined. However, in 2 of 10 rats immunized with irradiated *T. rhodesiense* and challenged with a serologically heterologous variant there was a significant increase in survival time (Wellde et al. 1975).

Cross-protection has been reported with *T. gambiense* in mice. Dodin & Fromentin (1962) recorded considerable cross-protection between two different strains of *T. gambiense*. Petithory et al. (1971), following implantation of diffusion chambers containing live trypanosomes into the peritoneal cavity of mice, reported significant cross-protection; however, the antigenic relationship of the different strains was not studied immunologically.

Cross-protection has also been reported in mice immunized with *T. congolense* (Johnson et al. 1963). The immunogen used was trypanosomes killed by rapid freeze thawing and administered with saponin as adjuvant. Two of five mice survived challenge with a different strain of *T. congolense*, although again its antigenic nature was not established.

Such results are difficult to analyze because of lack of data on the antigenic nature of the immunogen and of the challenge infection. They might indicate that a common or basic antigen involved in protection does exist. This might act as a priming or carrier antigen and allow quicker or secondary responses to subsequent variant (or hapten) antigens as suggested by Brown (1971) in malaria. Alternatively, and more likely, these results might reflect the antigenic diversity of the trypanosomes present in the strains or isolates used for immunization. The possible cross-reactivity result achieved using the adjuvant saponin with the immunogen (Johnson et al. 1963) might have depended on some intrinsic ability of the adjuvant to stimulate a broad-spectrum antibody response or "scatter" effect to the immunogen, thereby allowing the host to cope with different variants of the same trypanosome species.

When considering the feasibility of the production of a vaccine against trypanosomiasis it is worth remembering that there is evidence from field studies, as stated earlier, that cattle do develop at least some degree of immunity to trypanosome challenge. Several possible explanations exist.

It might be related to environmental factors, e.g., the chance that cattle have been fortunate not to have encountered highly pathogenic strains of trypanosomes while unprotected by drugs. Such strains also might deter the reactivity of the host to subsequent reinfection (see below). The age when infection was first experienced might influence the course of disease and this might be related to the system of husbandry and/or colostral intake of antibody.

Alternatively, it might be that survivors possess some genetic advantage which enables them to acquire a high degree of resistance. There is some evidence that N'dama cattle of West Africa are relatively resistant to trypanosomiasis as compared with Zebu. In Gambia, for instance, many N'dama survive without the aid of drugs, insecticides, or bush clearing in areas continuously infested by tsetse. However, this immunity is not absolute by any means and we have found in Gambia that considerable numbers of cattle become infected and a significant percentage die. Thus, one might conclude that just as N'dama are not all resistant, so Zebu cattle are not all wholly susceptible as Cunningham's (1966) observation would confirm. However, on present evidence it would be reasonable to conclude that the two breeds occupy different positions on the spectrum of resistance. As part of future research it is essential that the immunologic secrets of cattle, both N'dama and Zebu, that survive in enzootic areas should be unraveled. Are these secrets environmental or are factors under genetic control important, such as complement, properdin, and conglutinin levels, the ability to mount, and the quality of humoral and cell-mediated responses?

There are a number of possible explanations for survival based on immunologic phenomena. It might be that although the immune response to a succession of variant antigens is predominantly specific, it conditions the host in some way for a brisk response of a secondary type against new variants. It may be that there develops a carrier-hapten situation with the somatic antigen acting as common carrier and allowing secondary responses to a series of hapten variants from the trypanosome exoantigen as has been proposed by Brown (1971) in malaria. Conceivably cross-reacting antibody might be produced. Alternatively, provided cattle survive the initial stages of infection there may be the gradual development of a primed mononuclear phagocytic system which can rapidly cope, at least to some extent, with new variants. It is well recognized that an expanded mononuclear phagocytic system is one of the most prominent findings in bovine and ovine trypanosomiasis (Murray 1974; Mackenzie et al. 1973).

On the other hand, it may be that the number of potential variants is limited or that some variants are more common than others and certain cattle are fortunate enough to meet the same variant twice and survive. Wilson & Cunningham (1972) recorded the reappearance of an antigenic variant similar to the infecting one in a bovine with *T. congolense*. This immediately preceded the disappearance of detectable trypanosomes and the animal's recovery. Further possible evidence has been the demonstration of the same antigenic type in two series of variant populations derived in laboratory animals from two strains of *T. brucei* isolated 6 years apart in the same district of Uganda (Van Meirvenne et al. 1975a). Whether the number of variants is limited or not remains a vital question to be answered. So far the largest number recorded has been 24 with *T. gambiense* in mice, the original and 23 relapsed variants (Osaki 1959).

Another possibility is that repeated exposure alters the immunologic reactivity of the host. For example, it has recently been shown that laboratory animals (Allt et al. 1971; Goodwin et al. 1972; Murray et al. 1974a, 1974b; Mansfield & Wallace 1974), cattle (Holmes et al. 1974), and sheep (Mackenzie et al. 1975) infected with trypanosomes develop a degree of immunosuppression to a number of antigens. Perhaps cattle subjected to repeated infection develop a persistent immunosuppressed state. It is known that in chronically infected cattle the immunologic apparatus, particularly the lymph nodes, become atrophied and are small and depleted of lymphocytes (Murray 1974). If, as suggested, the most significant pathogenic lesions of trypanosomiasis, namely anemia and myocarditis (Murray 1974; Lambert & Houba 1974), are immunologically mediated, it might be that these immunosuppressed cattle are less likely to develop such lesions and, although parasitemic, have a greater chance of survival.

In considering the prospects of vaccination, it is obvious that the major stumbling block is the fact that it is the variant antigens that appear to be largely responsible for the production of protective antibody. Thus, one would like to see the problem of antigenic variation unraveled, particularly with regard to the relationship, if any, of various antigenic variants to each other, not only in terms of serologic specificity but also in relation to cross-protection. The demonstration of the existence of basic strain antigens following cyclical transmission and of predominant variant antigens (Osaki 1959; Gray 1967; Uilenberg 1974; Van Meirvenne et al. 1975b; Gray 1975; Doyle 1975; Paris et al. 1976) is fundamental to the question of immunoprophylaxis in trypanosomiasis and deserves further investigation. As stated by Van Meirvenne et al. (1975a), "of major importance would be a better knowledge of the number of serological types circulating as metacyclic forms in tsetse flies." While it seems likely that antigenicities of strains of trypanosomes do not always revert to basic types on passage through a tsetse, it may be that there are key variants which are relatively common and therefore important in the selection of antigenic types for vaccination. If the existence of key variants is confirmed, it might be that "cocktail" vaccines using a mixture of metacyclic forms isolated in a particular area might prove successful.

In planning a strategy of immunization or increasing host resistance nonspecifically, the basic mechanisms of the disease process and of how trypanosomes are killed must be more precisely understood. For example, a major feature of both human and animal trypanosomiasis is markedly elevated levels of immunoglobulin, especially IgM (Mattern et al. 1961; Luckins 1972), a large proportion of which would appear to be nonspecific (Freeman et al. 1970). At the same time the host develops a reversible immunosuppressive effect to a number of antigens (Allt et al. 1971; Goodwin 1970; Goodwin et al. 1972; Greenwood et al. 1973; Murray et al. 1974a, 1974b; Holmes et al. 1975; Mackenzie et al. 1975). It is interesting to speculate whether the host's response to the trypanosome might also be defective and that this might contribute to the survival of the parasites. It has been suggested that both of these phenomena, i.e., the elevated immunoglobulin levels and the immunosuppression, are largely the result of the trypanosome acting as a polyclonal B-cell mitogen (Urquhart et al. 1973; Greenwood 1974). Alternatively, immunosuppression might reflect some defect in lymphocyte function induced by blocking factors such as immune complexes which are demonstrable by elution, immunofluorescence, and electron microscopy studies (Lambert & Houba 1974; Murray 1974; Nagle et al. 1974). It might be that these complexes act as blocking factors on B cells (Diener & Feldmann 1972) and/or on T-lymphocyte surfaces and so depress a range of T-cell functions such as T-helper cell effects in immunoglobulin formation or cell-mediated immune responses. The blocking effect of immune complexes on T lymphocytes has been reviewed by Gorzynski et al. (1974). Another potential blocking factor is the presence of high levels of IgM which appear soon after infection. There is evidence to indicate that IgM may act as a suppressive factor in the host immune response. For example, in the immunologic unreactive state occurring in nonresponder mice after secondary antigen challenge, Ordal et al. (1976) presented data which indicated that IgM was responsible for this suppressed state.

Thus, it is unlikely that a magic potion of parasite extract will engender the quality of protection required. Instead one might perhaps initiate an immunologic engineering program involving the strategic use of adjuvants and immunogens, bearing in mind what is known of the basic mechanisms operative in the disease process. Thus, in trypanosomiasis one might attempt (1) the production of good quality, high-affinity antibody (this might involve a change of immunoglobulin class), (2) to help depress or remove immune complexes and obviate their potential blocking effect on the host's immune response, and (3) to allow full expression of or stimulate cell-mediated immunity.

In this respect the work of Mackaness et al. (1974a) has potential significance. They found in mice an inverse relationship between the dose of sheep red blood cells and delayed-type hypersensitivity reactions in the foot pad. They produced a good delayed-type hypersensitivity response with 10^5 but not with 10^8 sheep red blood cells. However, when BCG (10^7) was inoculated intravenously 12 days before sheep red blood cells, a good and long-lasting delayed-type hypersensitivity reaction with 10^8 sheep red blood cells was achieved. They were able to show that the blocking factor was in the serum and that it was the product of the interaction between antigen and antibody (Mackaness et al. 1974b). Why BCG achieved this was not precisely understood, but it was thought that it acted by expanding the mononuclear phagocytic system which removed immune complexes and allowed full expression of T-cell functions. In addition, it was likely that it directly increased the output of activated T cells.

In preliminary studies using the same regime, namely intravenous BCG (3×10^6) prior to challenge, we have found an increased prepatent period and survival time in C57 black mice challenged with *T. brucei* and an increased survival time in outbred mice challenged with *T. congolense*. While such regimes may not produce a sterile immunity, by altering the host's immune response they might produce a significant improvement that could be economically exploitable, especially in cattle, which unlike mice do not invariably die from a trypanosome infection.

BIBLIOGRAPHY

Allt, G., Evans, E.M.E., Evans, D.H.L. & Targett, G.A.T. 1971. Effect of infection with trypanosomes on the development of experimental allergic neuritis in rabbits. *Nature* (Lond.) 233: 197-199.

Bevan, L.E.W. 1928. Method of inoculating cattle against trypanosomiasis. *Trans. R. Soc. Trop. Med. Hyg.* 22: 147-156.

Bevan, L.E.W. 1936. Notes on immunity in trypanosomiasis. *Trans. R. Soc. Med. Hyg.* 30: 199-206.

Brown, K.N. 1971. Protective immunity to malaria parasites: A model for the survival of cells in an immunological hostile environment. *Nature* (Lond.) 230: 163-167.

Browning, C.H. & Calver, K.M. 1943. Effect of stage of infection on chemotherapeutic response of *T. congolense* and on immunity following cure. *J. Pathol. Bacteriol.* 55: 393-394.

Browning, C.H. & Gulbransen, R. 1936. Immunity following cure of experimental *Trypanosoma brucei* infection by chemotherapeutic agent. *J. Pathol. Bacteriol.* 43: 479-486.

Clark, I.A., Allison, A.C. & Cox, F.E. 1976. Protection of mice against Babesia and Plasmodium with BCG. *Nature* (Lond.) 259: 309-311.

Cluff, L.E. 1970. Effects of endotoxins on susceptibility to infections. *J. Infect. Dis.* 122: 205-215.

Cross, G.A.M. 1975. Identification, purification and properties of clone-specific glycoprotein antigens constituting the surface coat of *Trypanosoma brucei.* *Parasitology* 71: 393-417.

Cunningham, M.P. 1966. Immunity in bovine trypanosomiasis. *E. Afr. Med. J.* 43: 394-397.

Cunningham, M.P. 1968. Vaccination of cattle against trypanosomes by infection and treatment. *In* Isotopes and Radiation in Parasitology: 88-91. International Atomic Energy Agency. Vienna, Austria.

Dar, R.K., Paris, J. & Wilson, A.J. 1973. Serological studies on trypanosomiasis in East Africa. IV. Comparison of antigenic types of *Trypanosoma vivax* group organisms. *Ann. Trop. Med. Parasitol.* 67: 319-329.

Diener, E. & Feldmann, M. 1972. Relationship between antigen and antibody-induced suppression of immunity. *Transplant. Rev.* 8: 76-103.

Diggs, C., Flemmings, B., Dillon, J., Snodgrass, R., Campbell, G. & Esser, K. 1976. Immune serum-mediated cytotoxicity against *Trypanosoma rhodesiense. J. Immunol.* 116: 1005-1009.

Dodin, A. & Fromentin, H. 1962. Mise en évidence d'un antigéne vaccinant dans le plasma de souris expérimentalement infectées par *Trypanosoma gambiense* et par *Trypanosoma congolense. Bull. Soc. Pathol. Exot.* 55: 123-138.

Dodin, A., Fromentin, H. & Gleye, M. 1962. Mise en évidence d'un antigène vaccinant dans le plasma de souris expérimentalement inféctees par diverses espèces de trypanosomes. *Bull. Soc. Pathol. Exot.* 55: 291-299.

Doyle. 1975. Unpublished observation.

Duxbury, R.E., Anderson, J.S., Wellde, B.T., Sadun, E.H. & Muriithi, I.E. 1972a. *Trypanosoma congolense:* immunization of mice, dogs, and cattle with gamma-irradiated parasites. *Exp. Parasitol.* 32: 527-533.

Duxbury, R.E. & Sadun, E.H. 1969. Resistance produced in mice and rats by inoculation with irradiated *Trypanosoma rhodesiense. J. Parasitol.* 55: 859-865.

Duxbury, R.E., Sadun, E.H. & Anderson, J.S. 1972b. Experimental infections with African trypanosomes. II. Immunization of mice and monkeys with a gamma-irradiated, recently isolated human strain of *Trypanosoma rhodesiense. Am. J. Trop. Med. Hyg.* 21: 885-888.

Duxbury, R.E., Sadun, E.H., Anderson, J.S., Wellde, B.T., Muriithi, I.E. & Warui, G.M. 1973. Immunization of rodents, dogs, cattle, and monkeys against African trypanosomiasis by the use of irradiated trypanosomes. *In* Isotopes and Radiation in Parasitology III: 179-180. International Atomic Energy Agency. Vienna, Austria.

Duxbury, R.E., Sadun, E.H., Schoenbechler, M.J. & Stroupe, D.A. 1974. *Trypanosoma rhodesiense:* protection in mice by inoculations of homologous parasite products. *Exp. Parasitol.* 36: 70-76.

Fiennes, R.N. 1970. Pathogenesis and pathology of animal trypanosomiasis. *In* The African Trypanosomiasis. Mulligan H.W. & Potts, W.H., Eds.: 729-750. Allen and Unwin. London, England.

Freeman, T., Smithers, S.R., Targett, G.A. & Walker, P.J. 1970. Specificity of immunoglobulin G in rhesus monkeys infected with *Schistosoma mansoni, Plasmodium knowlesi,* and *Trypanosoma brucei. J. Infect. Dis.* 121: 401-406.

Fromentin, H. 1974. *Trypanosoma brucei gambiense.* Étude antigenique. I. Protection expérimentale de la souris. Résultats partiels. *Bull. Soc. Pathol. Exot.* 67: 277-280.

Fulton, J.D. & Lourie, E.M. 1946. Immunity of mice cured of trypanosome infections. *Ann. Trop. Med. Parasitol.* 40: 1-9.

Goble, F.C. & Boyd, J.L. 1962. Reticulo-endothelial blockade in experimental Chagas' disease. *J. Parasitol.* 48: 223-228.

Goedbloed, E., Ligthart, G.S., Minter, D.M., Wilson, A.J., Dar, F.K. & Paris, J. 1973. Serological studies of trypanosomiasis in East Africa. II. Comparisons of antigenic types of *Trypanosoma brucei* subgroup organisms isolated from wild tsetse flies. *Ann. Trop. Med. Parasitol.* 67: 31-43.

Goodwin, L.G. 1970. The pathology of African trypanosomiasis. *Trans. R. Soc. Trop. Med. Hyg.* 64: 797-817.

Goodwin, L.G., Green, D.G., Guy, M.W. & Voller, A. 1972. Immunosuppression during trypanosomiasis. *Brit. J. Exp. Pathol.* 53: 40-43.

Gorozynski, R., Kontiainen, S., Mitchison, N.A. & Tigelaar, R.E. 1974. Antigen-antibody complexes as blocking factors on the *T. lymphocyte* surface. *In* Cellular Selection and Regulation in the Immune Response. Edelman, G.M., Ed.: 143-154. Raven Press. New York, N.Y.

Gray, A.R. 1967. Some principles of the immunology of trypanosomiasis. *Bull. WHO* 37: 177-193.

Gray, A.R. 1975. A pattern in the development of agglutinogenic antigens of cyclically transmitted isolates of *Trypanosoma gambiense. Trans. R. Soc. Trop. Med. Hyg.* 69: 131-138.

Greenwood, B.M. 1974. Possible role of a B-cell mitogen in hypergamma-globulinaemia in malaria and trypanosomiasis. *Lancet* 1: 435-6.

Greenwood, B.M., Whittle, H.C. & Molyneux, D.H. 1973. Immunosuppression in Gambian trypanosomiasis. *Trans. R. Soc. Trop. Med. Hyg.* 67: 846-50.

Halpern, B.N., Prevot, A.R., Biozzi, G., Stiffel, C., Moulton, D., Morard, J.C., Bouthillier, Y. & Decreusefond, C. 1963. Stimulation de l'activité phagocytaire du système réticuloendothélial provoquée par *Corynebacterium parvum. J. Reticuloendothel. Soc.* 1: 77-96.

Herbert, W.J. & Inglis, M.D. 1973. Immunization of mice, against *T. brucei* infection, by the administration of released antigen adsorbed to erythrocytes. *Trans. R. Soc. Trop. Med. Hyg.* 67: 268.

Herbert, W.J. & Lumsden, W.H. 1968. Single-dose vaccination of mice against experimental infection with *Trypanosoma* (Trypanozoon) *brucei. J. Med. Microbiol.* 1: 23-32.

Herbert, W.J. & Macadam, R.F. 1971. The immunization of mice with *trypanosome plasmanemes* (filopodia). *Trans. R. Soc. Trop. Med. Hyg.* 65: 240.

Herman, R. & Baron, S. 1971. Immunologic-mediated protection of *Trypanosoma congolense*-infected mice by polyribonucleotides. *J. Protozool.* 18: 661-668.

Hoff, R. 1975. Killing *in vitro* of *Trypanosoma cruzi* by macrophages from mice immunized with *T. cruzi* or BCG, and absence of cross-immunity on challenge *in vivo. J. Exp. Med.* 142: 299-311.

Holmes, P.H., Mammo, C., Thomson, A., Knight, P.A., Lucken, R., Murray, P.K., Murray, M., Jennings, F.W. & Urquhart, G.M. 1974. Immunosuppression in bovine trypanosomiasis. *Vet. Rec.* 95: 86-87.

Hornby, H.E. 1941. Immunization against bovine trypanosomiasis. *Trans. R. Soc. Trop. Med. Hyg.* 35: 165-176.

Jahiel, R.I., Nussenzweig, R.S., Vanderberg, J. & Vilcek, J. 1968b. Antimalarial effect of interferon inducers at different stages of development of *Plasmodium berghei* in the mouse. *Nature* (Lond.) 220: 710-711.

Jahiel, R.I., Nussenzweig, R.S., Vilcek, J. & Vanderberg, J. 1969. Protective effect of interferon inducers on *Plasmodium berghei* malaria. *Am. J. Trop. Med. Hyg.* 18: 823-835.

Jahiel, R.I., Vilcek, J. & Nussenzweig, R.S. 1970. Exogenous interferon protects mice against *Plasmodium berghei* malaria. *Nature* (Lond.) 227: 1350-1351.

Jahiel, R.I., Vilcek, J., Nussenzweig, R.S. & Vanderberg, J. 1968a. Interferon inducers protect mice against *Plasmodium berghei* malaria. *Science* 161: 802-804.

James, D.M. 1976. Induction of immunity in rodents receiving living drug-treated trypanosomes. *Int. J. Parasitol.* 6: 179-182.

James, D.M., Fregene, A.O. & Salomon, K. 1973. The effect of irradiation on infectivity and immunogenicity of *Trypanosoma brucei. J. Parasitol.* 59: 489-492.

Johnson, P., Neal, R.A. & Gall, D. 1963. Protective effect of killed trypanosome vaccines with incorporated adjuvants. *Nature* (Lond.) 200: 83.

Kierszenbaum, F. 1975. Enhancement of resistance and suppression of immunization against exeprimental *Trypanosoma cruzi* infection by *Corynebacterium parvum*. *Infect. Immun.* 12: 1227-1229.

Kierszenbaum, F., Knecht, E., Budzko, D.B. & Pizzimenti, M.C. 1974. Phagocytosis: a defense mechanism against infection with *Trypanosoma cruzi*. *J. Immunol.* 112: 1839-1844.

Kierszenbaum, F. & Saavedra, L.E. 1972. The effects of bacterial endotoxin on the infection of mice with *Trypanosoma cruzi*. *J. Protozool.* 19: 655:657.

Kligler, I.J. & Berman, M. 1935. Susceptibility and resistance to trypanosome infection: specific character of immunity produced in rats by infection of suspensions of dead trypanosomes. *Ann. Trop. Med. Parasitol.* 29: 457-461.

Koch, R. 1901. Ein Versuch zur Immunisirung von Rindern gegen Tsetsekrankheit (Surra). *Dtsch Kolonialbl.* (Suppl.) 12(24): 4.

Kress, Y., Bloom, B.R., Wittner, M., Rowen, A. & Tanowitz, H. 1975. Resistance of *Trypanosoma cruzi* to killing by macrophages. *Nature* (Lond.) 257: 394-396.

Kuhn, R.E., Vaughn, R.T. & Herbst, G.A. 1975. The effect of BCG on the course of experimental Chagas' disease in mice. *Int. J. Parasitol.* 5: 557-560.

Lambert, P.H. & Houba, V. 1974. Immune complexes in parasitic diseases. *In* Progress in Immunology II. Brent, L. & Holborow, J., Eds. Vol. 5: 57. North Holland Publishing Company. Amsterdam, The Netherlands.

Lanham, S.M. & Taylor, A.E.R. 1972. Some properties of the immunogens (protective antigens) of a single variant of *Trypanosoma brucei*. *J. Gen. Microbiol.* 72: 101-116.

Lapierre, J. & Rousset, J.J. 1961. Étude de l'immunité dans les infections à *Trypanosoma gambiense* chez la souris blanche. Variations antigéniques au cours des crises trypanolytiques. *Bull. Soc. Path. Exot.* 54: 332-336.

Lourie, E.M. & O'Connor, R.J. 1936. Trypanolysis *in vitro* by mouse immune serum. *Ann. Trop. Med. Parasitol.* 30: 365-388.

Lourie, E.M. & O'Connor, R.J. 1937. Study of *Trypanosoma rhodesiense* relapse strains *in vitro*. *Ann. Trop. Med. Parasitol.* 31: 319-340.

Luckins, A.G. 1972a. Adoptive immunity in experimental trypanosomiasis. *Trans. R. Soc. Trop. Med. Hyg.* 66: 346-347.

Luckins, A.G. 1972b. Studies on bovine trypanosomiasis. Serum immunoglobulin levels in Zebu cattle exposed to natural infections in East Africa. *Brit. Vet. J.* 128: 523-528.

Lumsden, W.H.R. & Herbert, W.J. 1967. Phagocytosis of trypanosomes by mouse peritoneal macrophages. *Trans. R. Soc. Trop. Med. Hyg.* 61: 142.

Macadam, R.F. & Herbert, W.J. 1970a. Fine structural demonstration of cytoplasmic protrusions (filopodia) in Trypanosomes. *Exp. Parasitol.* 27: 1-8.

Macadam, R.F. & Herbert, W.J. 1970b. Studies of the filopodia of *T. brucei* and *T. rhodesiense. Trans. R. Soc. Trop. Med. Hyg.* 64: 181-182.

Mackaness, G.B., Auclair, D.J. & Lagrange, P.H. 1973. Immunopotentiation with BCG. I. Immune response to different strains and preparations. *J. Nat. Cancer Inst.* 51: 1655-1667.

Mackaness, G.B., Lagrange, P.H. & Ishibashi, T. 1974a. The modifying effect of BCG on the immunological induction of T cells. *J. Exp. Med.* 139: 1540-1542.

Mackaness, G.B., Lagrange, P.H., Miller, T.E. & Ishibashi, T. 1974b. Feedback inhibition of specifically sensitized lymphocytes. *J. Exp. Med.* 139: 543-549.

Mackenzie, P.K.I., Boyt, W.D., Emslie, V.W., Lander, K.P. & Swanepoel, R. 1975. Immunosuppression in ovine trypanosomiasis. *Vet. Rec.* 97: 452-453.

Mackenzie, P.K.I. & Cruickshank, J.G. 1973. Phagocytosis of erythrocytes and leucocytes in sheep infected with *Trypanosoma congolense* (Broden 1904). *Res. Vet. Sci.* 15: 256-262.

Mansfield, J.M. & Kreier, J.P. 1972. Tests for antibody- and cell-mediated hypersensitivity to trypanosome antigens in rabbits infected with *Trypanosoma congolense. Infect. Immun.* 6: 62-67.

Mansfield, J.M. & Wallace, J.H. 1974. Suppression of cell-mediated immunity in experimental African trypanosomiasis. *Infect. Immun.* 10: 335-339.

Mathé, G., Kamel, M., Dezfulian, M., Halle-Panenko, O. & Bourut, C. 1973. An experimental screening for "systematic adjuvants of immunity" applicable in cancer immunotherapy. *Cancer Res.* 33: 1987-1997.

Mattern, P., Masseyeff, R., Michel, R. & Peretti, P. 1961. Étude immuno-chemique de la B_2-macroglobuline des sérums de malades atteints de trypanosomiase africaine à T. gambiense. *Ann. Inst. Pasteur* (Paris) 101: 382-388.

Miller, J.K. 1965. Variation of the soluble antigens of *Trypanosoma brucei. Immunology* 9: 521-528.

Mkwananzi, J.B., Franks, D. & Baker, J.R. 1976. Cytotoxicity of antibody-coated trypanosomes by normal human lymphoid cells. *Nature* (Lond.) 259: 403-404.

Murray, M. 1974. The pathology of African trypanosomiasis. *In* Progress in Immunology II. Brent, L. & Holborow, J., Eds. Vol. 4: 181. North Holland Publishing Company. Amsterdam, The Netherlands.

Murray, M., Murray, P.K., Jennings, F.W., Fisher, E.W. & Urquhart, G.M. 1974. The pathology of *Trypanosoma brucei* infection in the rat. *Res. Vet. Sci.* 16: 77-84.

Murray, P.K., Jennings, F.W., Murray, M. & Urquhart, G.M. 1974a. The nature of immunosuppression in *Trypanosoma brucei* infections in mice. I. The role of the macrophage. *Immunology* 27: 815-824.

Murray, P.K., Jennings, F.W., Murray, M. & Urquhart, G.M. 1974b. The nature of immunosuppression in *Trypanosoma brucei* infections in mice. II. The role of the T and B lymphocytes. *Immunology* 27: 825-840.

Nagle, R.B., Ward, P.A., Lindsley, H.B., Sadun, E.H., Johnson, A.J., Berkaw, R.E. & Hildebrandt, P.K. 1974. Experimental infections with African Trypanosomes. VI. Glomerulonephritis. Involving the alternate pathway of complement activation. *Am. J. Trop. Med. Hyg.* 23: 15-26.

Nussenzweig, R.S. 1967. Increased nonspecific resistance to malaria produced by administration of killed *Corynebacterium parvum*. *Exp. Parasitol.* 21: 224-231.

Ordal, J., Smith, S., Ness, D., Gershon, R.K. & Grumet, F.C. 1976. IgM-mediated, T cell-independent suppression of humoral immunity. *J. Immunol.* 116: 1182-1187.

Ortiz-Ortiz, L., Gonzalez-Mendoza, A. & Lamoyi, E. 1975. A vaccination procedure against *Trypanosoma cruzi* infection in mice by nonspecific immunization. *J. Immunol.* 114: 1424-1425.

Osaki, H. 1959. Studies on the immunological variation in *Trypanosoma gambiense* (serotypes and the mode of relapse). *Biken J.* 2: 113-127.

Paris, J., Wilson, A.J. & Gray, A.R. 1976. A study of the antigenic relationships of isolates of *Trypanosoma brucei* from three areas in East Africa. *Ann. Trop. Med. Parasitol.* 70: 45-51.

Petithory, J., Rousset, J.J. & Liqoult, M.F. 1971. Immunisation de la souris contre une souche hétérologue par des trypanosomes virulents vivants en chambre de diffusion. *Bull. Soc. Path. Exot.* 64: 337-341.

Schilling, C. 1935. Immunization against trypanosomiasis. *J. Trop. Med. Hyg.* 38: 106-108.

Schultz, W.W., Huang, K.Y. & Gordon, F.B. 1968. Role of interferon in experimental mouse malaria. *Nature* (Lond.) 220: 709-710.

Seed, J.R. 1963. The characterization of antigens isolated from *Trypanosoma rhodesiense. J. Protozool.* 10: 380-389.

Seed, J.R. 1972. *Trypanosoma gambiense* and *T. equiperdum:* characterization of variant specific antigens. *Exp. Parasitol.* 31: 98-108.

Seed, J.R. 1974. Antigens and antigenic variability of the African trypanosomes. *J. Protozool.* 21: 639-646.

Seed, J.R. & Gam, A.A. 1966a. Passive immunity to experimental trypanosomiasis. *J. Parasitol.* 52: 1134-1140.

Seed, J.R. & Gam, A.A. 1966b. The properties of antigens from *Trypanosoma gambiense. J. Parasitol.* 52: 395-398.

Seed, J.R. & Weinman, D. 1963. Characterization of antigens isolated from *Trypanosoma rhodesiense. Nature* (Lond.) 198: 197-198.

Singer, I., Kimble, E.T., III & Ritts, R.E., Jr. 1964. Alterations of the host-parasite relationship by administration of endotoxin to mice with infections of trypanosomes. *J. Infect. Dis.* 114: 243-248.

Smith, I.M. 1958. The protection against trypanosomiasis conferred on cattle by repeated doses of antrycide, alone or with *Trypanosoma congolense. Ann. Trop. Med. Parasitol.* 52: 391-401.

Soltys, M.A. 1955. Studies on resistance to *Trypanosoma congolense* developed by Zebu cattle treated prophylactically with antrycide pro-salt in an enzoatic area of East Africa. *Ann. Trop. Med. Parasitol.* 49: 1-8.

Soltys, M.A. 1964. Immunity in trypanosomiasis. V. Immunization of animals with dead trypanosomes. *Parasitology* 54: 585-591.

Soltys, M.A. 1967. Comparative studies of immunogenic properties of *Trypanosoma brucei* inactivated with beta-propiolactone and with some other inactivating agents. *Can. J. Microbiol.* 13: 743-747.

Stephen, L.E. 1966. Observations on the resistance of West African N'dama and Zebu cattle to trypanosomiasis following challenge by wild *Glossina morsitans* from an early age. *Ann. Trop. Med. Parasitol.* 60: 230-246.

Tabbara, K.F., O'Connor, G.R. & Nozik, R.A. 1975. Effect of immunization with attenuated *Mycobacterium bovis* on experimental toxoplasmic retinochoroiditis. *Am. J. Ophthalmol.* 79: 641-47.

Takayanagi, T. 1971. Protection of mouse from Trypanosome infection. *Jap. J. Parasitol.* 20: 48.

Takayanagi, T. & Enriquez, G.L. 1973. Effects of the IgG and IgM immunoglobulins in *Trypanosoma gambiense* infections in mice. *J. Parasitol.* 59: 644-647.

Takayanagi, T., Kambara, H. & Enriquez, G.L. 1973. *Trypanosoma gambiense:* immunity with spleen cell and antiserum transfer in mice. *Exp. Parasitol.* 33: 429-432.

Takayanagi, T., Kambara, H. & Inoki, S. 1969. Studies of protection against infection of Trypanosoma gambiense. *Jap. J. Parasitol.* 18: 686-687.

Takayanagi, T. & Nakatake, Y. 1975. *Trypanosoma gambiense:* enhancement of agglutinin and protection in subpopulations by immune spleen cells. *Exp. Parasitol.* 38: 233-239.

Takayanagi, T. & Nakatake, Y. 1976. *Trypanosoma gambiense:* immunity with thymic cell transfer in mice. *Exp. Parasitol.* 39: 234-243.

Takayanagi, T., Nakatake, Y. & Enriquez, G.L. 1974. Attachment and ingestion of *Trypanosoma gambiense* to the rat macrophage by specific antiserum. *J. Parasitol.* 60: 336-339.

Tizard, I.R. & Soltys, M.A. 1971a. Macrophage cytophilic antibodies to *Trypanosoma brucei* in rabbits. *Trans. R. Soc. Trop. Med. Hyg.* 65: 407-408.

Tizard, I.R. & Soltys, M.A. 1971b. Cell-mediated hypersensitivity in rabbits infected with *Trypanosoma brucei* and *Trypanosoma rhodesiense*. *Infect. Immun.* 4: 674-677.

Uilenberg, G. 1974. Summary of studies on the immunology of *Trypanosoma congolense* infection carried out at Maisons-Alfort (I.E.M.V.T.) France, 1970-1972. *In* Control Programmes for Trypanosomes and Their Vectors. *Rev. Élevage Méd. Vét. Pays Trop.* (Suppl.): 207-208.

Urquhart, G.M., Murray, M., Murray, P.K., Jennings, F.W. & Bate, E. 1973. Immunosuppression in *Trypanosoma brucei* infections in rats and mice. *Trans. R. Soc. Trop. Med. Hyg.* 67: 528-535.

Van Dijck, P.J., Claesen, M. & De Somer, P. 1970. Effect of polyacrylic acid on experimental malaria and trypanosomiasis in mice. *Ann. Trop. Med. Parasitol.* 64: 5-9.

Van Meirvenne, N., Janssens, P.G. & Magnus, E. 1975b. Antigenic variation in syringe-passaged populations of *Trypanosoma* (Trypanozoon) *brucei*. I. Rationalization of the experimental approach. *Ann. Soc. Belge Méd. Trop.* 55: 1-23.

Van Meirvenne, N., Janssens, P.G., Magnus, E., Lumsden, W.H.R. & Herbert, W.J. 1975a. Antigenic variation in syringe-passaged populations of *Trypanosoma* (Trypanozoon) *brucei*. II. Comparative studies on two antigenic type collections. *Ann. Soc. Belge Méd. Trop.* 55: 25-30.

Watkins, J.F. 1964. Observations on antigenic variation in a strain of *Trypanosoma brucei* growing in mice. *J. Hyg.* 62: 69-80.

Weitz, B. 1960. The properties of some antigens of *Trypanosoma brucei*. *J. Gen. Microbiol.* 23: 589-600.

Wellde, B.T., Duxbury, R.T., Sadun, E.H., Langbehn, H.R., Lotzsch, R., Deindl, G. & Warui, G. 1973. Experimental infections with African trypanosomes. IV. Immunization of cattle with gamma-irradiated *Trypanosoma rhodesiense*. *Exp. Parasitol.* 34: 62-68.

Wellde, B.T., Schoenbechler, M.J., Diggs, C.L., Langbehn, H.R. & Sadun, E.H. 1975. *Trypanosoma rhodesiense:* variant specificity of immunity of immunity endured by irradiated parasites. *Exp. Parasitol.* 37: 125-129.

Whiteside, E.F. 1962. Interactions between drugs, trypanosomes and cattle in the field. *In* Drugs, Parasites and Hosts. Goodwin, L.G. & Nimmo-Smith, R.H., Eds.: 116-141. Churchill. London, England.

Wilson, A.J. 1971. Immunological aspects of bovine trypanosomiasis. III. Patterns in the development of immunity. *Trop. Anim. Health Prod.* 3: 14-22.

Wilson, A.J. 1974. Immune reaction in the vertebrate host. *In* Control Programmes for Trypanosomes and Their Vectors. *Rev. Élevage Méd. Vét. Pays. Trop.* (Suppl.): 211-213.

Wilson, A.J. & Cunningham, M.P. 1972. Immunological aspects of bovine trypanosomiasis. I. Immune response of cattle to infection with *Trypanosoma congolense* and the antigenic variation of the infecting organisms. *Exp. Parasitol.* 32: 165-173.

Wilson, A.J., Dar, F.K. & Paris, J. 1973. Serological studies on trypanosomiasis in East Africa. III. Comparison of antigenic types of *Trypanosoma congolense* organisms isolated from wild flies. *Ann. Trop. Med. Parasitol.* 67: 313-317.

Wilson, A.J., Le Roux, J.G., Paris, J., Davidson, C.R. & Gray, A.R. 1975b. Observations on a herd of beef cattle maintained in a tsetse [glossina] area. I. Assessment of chemotherapy as a method for the control of trypanosomiasis. *Trop. Anim. Health Prod.* 7: 187-199.

Wilson, A.J., Paris, J. & Dar, F.K. 1975a. Maintenance of a herd of breeding cattle in an area of high trypanosome challenge. *Trop. Anim. Health Prod.* 7: 63-71.

Wilson, A.J., Paris, J., Luckins, A.G., Dar, F.K. & Gray, A.R. 1976. Observations on a herd of beef cattle maintained in a tsetse [glossina] area. II. Assessment on the developments of immunity in association with trypanocidal drug treatment. *Trop. Anim. Health Prod.* 8: 1-11.

Young, A.S., Kanhai, G.K. & Stagg, D.A. 1975. Phagocytosis of *Trypanosoma* (Nannomonas) *congolense* by circulating macrophages in the African buffalo *(Syncerus caffer). Res. Vet. Sci.* 19: 108-110.

Zahalsky, A.C. & Weinberg, R.L. 1976. *Trypanosoma brucei:* humoral response. *J. Parasitol.* 62: 15-19.

Zatz, M. 1976. Effects of BCG on lymphocyte trapping. *J. Immunol.* 116: 1587-1591.

12

IMMUNOPROPHYLAXIS AGAINST CHAGAS' DISEASE

Antonio R.L. Teixeira

Faculdade de Ciencias da Suade da Universidade de Brasilia
Brasilia, Brazil

INTRODUCTION

Chagas' disease is caused by *Trypanosoma cruzi*, a flagellate protozoan transmitted by an hematophagus reduviid bug. This disease, identified by Dr. Carlos Chagas in 1909 (Chagas 1909, 1910), is a major public health problem in rural areas of Central and South America. Approximately 35 million people are estimated to be at risk of *Trypanosoma cruzi* infection, and at least 7 million have already been infected (Pan American Health Organization 1970). Human cases have been described from the southern United States to southern Argentina (Marsden 1971). Where Chagas' disease is endemic, chronic myocarditis is the leading cause of sudden death and heart failure (Laranja et al. 1956). Certain digestive disturbances are also common manifestations of chronic Chagas' disease (Vampré 1923; Prado 1945; Köberle & Nador 1955).

In addition to humans, *Trypanosoma cruzi* infects more than 100 species of domestic and wild mammals, including members of several orders (Chagas 1912; Pessoa 1958; Barretto 1967; Hoare 1972). These species maintain the parasite in the wild state, making it very difficult to eradicate.

LIFE CYCLE OF *TRYPANOSOMA CRUZI* IN THE VECTOR AND THE HOST

The Agent

Trypanosoma cruzi is one of those mammalian trypanosomes of the sub-genus *Schizotrypanum* (Chagas 1909), that are pathogenic to man and certain animals. The adult blood trypanosomes are relatively small, dimorphic forms represented by broad and slender types measuring 11.7 to 28 μm in length. A striking feature of these trypanosomes is the large round or oval kinetoplast situated near the short, pointed posterior end of the body. The nucleus is slightly anterior to the middle of the body. This trypanosome always has a free flagellum with two or three shallow convolutions (Hoare 1972). *Trypanosoma cruzi* can be readily cultured in the laboratory (Figure 1).

Different strains of *Trypanosoma cruzi* have been recognized on the basis of virulence (Brumpt 1913), tissue affinity and course of parasitemia (Villela 1925; Souza Campos 1927; Badinez 1945; von Brand et al. 1949), morphology (Brener & Chiari 1963), prepatent period (Brener 1965), aspects of early growth (Brener & Chiari 1965), drug susceptibility (Hauschka 1949; Goble 1961a), and antigenic   composition   (Moore   1957; Nussenzweig   et   al.   1962,   1963a; Nussenzweig & Goble 1966; Gonzalez-Cappa & Kagan 1969). Differences in strains might be responsible for the geographic variations in pathogenicity and manifestations of *Trypanosoma cruzi* infections.

Most criteria for differentiation of strains are difficult to standardize. However, the recent development of electrophoretic techniques for demonstrating enzyme variation in strains holds promise for the future (Kilgour & Godfrey 1973).

Trypanosomes closely resembling *Trypanosoma cruzi* have been described in monkeys and bats. They are distinguishable from *Trypanosoma cruzi* mainly on the basis of host-parasite relations. These *cruzi*-like trypanosomes are not pathogenic to man and laboratory animals (Hoare 1972).

The Vector

Blood-feeding reduviid bugs of the subfamily Triatominae are the intermediate hosts and natural vectors of *Trypanosoma cruzi*. The geographic range of these bugs is extensive, from about latitude $42° $ N in the United States to $43° $ S in Argentina. The most important transmitting species are *Triatoma infestans, Panstrongylus megistus,* and *Rhodnius prolixus.* These triatomids are nocturnal, hiding in the daytime and emerging at night when they attack the sleeping inhabitants. The bugs ingest *Trypanosoma cruzi* when feeding on infected vertebrate hosts (Hoare 1972).

The trypanosomes undergo development in their passage through the intestine of the bug. The ingested blood trypomastigotes are transformed into amastigotes in the foregut, into epimastigote forms in the midgut, and revert to metacyclic trypomastigotes in the hindgut of the bug. The trypomastigotes are the infective forms of *Trypanosoma cruzi.* They are discharged with the feces as the bug feeds on healthy individuals, and contaminate either the bite wound or the conjunctiva.

Chagas' disease can also be transmitted congenitally through the placenta (Howard & Rubio 1968; Bittencourt 1969), by blood transfusion (Dias 1949; Amato Neto 1968), and by accidental infection in the laboratory.

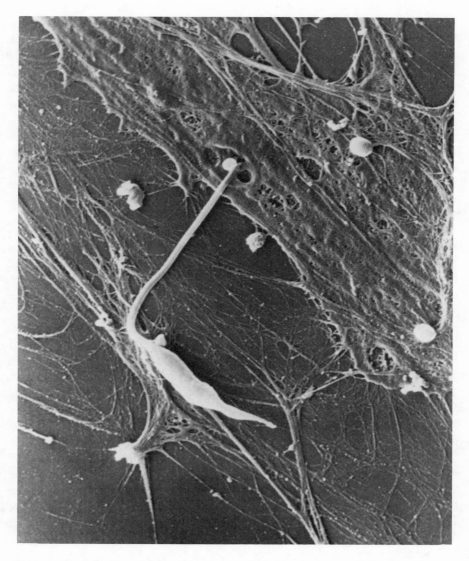

Figure 1. Trypomastigote of *Trypanosoma cruzi* infecting a culture cell. Scanning electron microscope (Teixeira & Santos-Buch 1974) X 6,300.

Host-Parasite Relations

Trypanosoma cruzi does not multiply in the peripheral blood of its verte-brate hosts (Chagas 1909; Vianna 1911; Dias 1934; Hoare 1972). The infective trypomastigotes that enter the body parasitize macrophages and other local tissue cells at the point of inoculation (Figure 2). Within the host cell the trypomastigotes change into round amastigotes, which multiply every 12 hours by binary fission. After 4 to 5 days the cytoplasm of the host cell is filled with parasites, forming a pseudocyst (Pizzi & Prager 1952; Pizzi et al. 1954). The amastigotes of heavily parasitized cells elongate their bodies and (probably passing through an epimastigote stage) become trypomastigotes, which are released to the external milieu and the bloodstream. Circulating trypomastigotes and intracellular amastigotes are abundant in the acute phase of infection. Any tissue or cell type can be parasitized, but cysts containing amastigotes are most often found in cardiac muscle, smooth muscle, skeletal muscle, and glial cells (Vianna 1911; Crowell 1923; Teixeira et al. 1970).

The course of *Trypanosoma cruzi* infection in the host is unpredictable. The degrees of infection in various animals range from low, transient parasitemia with rare tissue parasites to high parasitemia with abundant intracellular stages and extensive tissue damage. Whatever the outcome of the infection, no spontaneous cure with eradiction of parasites from the host has been reported. Host species vary in their susceptibility to the disease. Some strains of mice and rats are very susceptible to *Trypanosoma cruzi* and die early in the acute phase, when para-sitemia is high (Hauschka 1949; Hauschka et al. 1950; Pizzi et al. 1954). Other vertebrates such as rabbits, cebus monkeys, and humans are less susceptible and seldom die of acute Chagas' disease. Under experimental conditions, rabbits, cats, dogs, and monkeys survive the acute phase, but may later develop chronic Chagas' disease and die even when parasites are not found in the blood or in tissue cells (Chagas 1910; Torres 1930; Torres & Tavares 1958; Dias 1956; Goble 1961b; Guimarães & Miranda 1959; Teixeira et al. 1975).

The factors that modulate the host-parasite relationship are only partially understood. The strain of the parasite is definitely a major factor determining the course of the infection. The virulent strains produce fatal disease both in nature and under experimental conditions (Chagas 1909; Brumpt 1913; Hauschka 1949; Rubio 1954; Brener 1965; Brener et al. 1974). The size of the inoculum does not always correlate with the severity of the infection. Reducing the number of parasites in the inoculum may delay but not prevent the death of the infected animal (Phillips 1960). Age is an important factor. The most severe infections are usually seen in neonates and young hosts (Chagas 1916; Pizzi et al. 1954). The genetic background of the host is another important factor. Hauschka

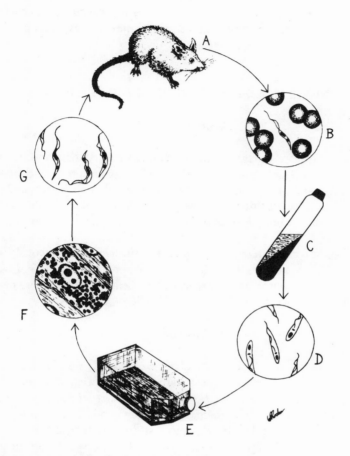

Figure 2. Maintenance of *Trypanosoma cruzi* in the laboratory. Mouse with *Trypanosoma cruzi* infection (A) shows parasite in the blood (B) which can be cultured in blood-agar diphasic medium (C). Epimastigote forms grown in culture (D) can be passaged to tissue culture (E) where they enter the cells and transform into intracellular amastigote states (F) which later transform into trypomastigotes (G). These are harvested from the culture medium and can be used to infect mouse.

et al. (1950) and Pizzi et al. (1954) observed variations in the susceptibility of in-bred strains of mice to *Trypanosoma cruzi* infection. The genetically controlled immune response plays a role in acquired resistance to *Trypanosoma cruzi* (Pizzi 1961). The role of humoral and cell-mediated immune response in Chagas' disease will be discussed later in this chapter.

CLINICAL MANIFESTATIONS OF CHAGAS' DISEASE

Acute Phase

Acute Chagas' disease usually occurs in children and is characterized by the presence of trypomastigotes in the peripheral blood. Its symptoms include fever, muscular pains, general malaise, and vomiting. The lymph nodes, liver, and spleen become enlarged. In 50% of the cases, the parasite leaves evidence of its route of entry, either a unilateral bipalpebral edema (Romana sign) or an indurated skin lesion (Chagoma).

In about 90% of cases in man, the infection subsides spontaneously within 2 to 3 months (Laranja et al. 1956; Mott 1967). Approximately 10% of patients with acute Chagas' disease die of myocarditis, meningoencephalitis, or inter-current infections (Chagas 1916; Laranja et al. 1956; Prath 1968).

Latent Phase

Individuals who recover from acute Chagas' disease, as well as many people who give no history of acute disease, can harbor *Trypanosoma cruzi* in the body for life. These carriers have antibodies to *Trypanosoma cruzi* that can be demon-strated by complement fixation, hemagglutination, and other serologic tests (Laranja et al. 1956; Prath 1968). The most striking case of a carrier was the woman who in 1909, at the age of 2 years, was the first case of American trypan-osomiasis described by Chagas. Salgado et al. (1962) examined this patient and found that she was still harboring *Trypanosoma cruzi,* although she showed no signs of Chagas' disease.

Chronic Phase

In asymptomatic patients diagnosed as having Chagas' disease by serologic tests, the onset of recurrent palpitations, electrocardiographic abnormalities, or heart failure are ominous signs (Laranja et al. 1956; Mott 1972). When these patients die of chronic Chagas' disease their hearts are enlarged. Microscopic examination of the myocardium reveals striking myocarditis, but parasites are not seen in the cardiac fibers (Torres 1930; Andrade 1958). Other common manifestations of chronic Chagas' disease are the mega conditions (Köberle 1957). Segments of the esophagus and colon are dilated and hypertrophied, conditions related to the destruction of ganglionic cells in the parasympathetic myenteric plexus (Köberle 1959, 1968).

MECHANISMS OF RESISTANCE AGAINST *TRYPANOSOMA CRUZI*

Natural Immunity

Birds and cold-blooded animals (Dias 1933, 1944; Rubio 1956) are generally refractory to *Trypanosoma cruzi*. Dias (1933) failed to infect reptiles (*Tropidurus torquatus, Ameiva surinamensis*) or amphibians (*Leptodactylus ocellatus, Bufo crucifer*) with blood trypanosomes derived from an infected guinea pig. Within 3 hours all trypanosomes had disappeared from the site of inoculation and could not be found alive in the blood. Further, the animals killed 7 days later did not show amastigote forms encysted in the tissues. Rubio (1956) showed that sera from fowl, frogs, and toads have a lytic effect on metacyclic (i.e., trypomastigote) trypanosomes.

Trypanosoma cruzi does not enter the blood of avians because the parasites are destroyed at the site of inoculation in the skin. The resistance of chickens to *Trypanosoma cruzi* appears at hatching. *Trypanosoma cruzi* infection could be established during embryonic life, but no signs of infection were found in chicks hatched from infected embryos (Nery-Guimarães 1972; Nery-Guimarães & Lage 1972). Although *Trypanosoma cruzi* requires a certain temperature range to survive in the vertebrate host, it appears that other factors are involved in the natural resistance of avians to this protozoan. Kierszenbaum et al. (1976) showed that the resistance of chickens to *Trypanosoma cruzi* infection and the capacity of their sera to lyse the trypomastigote forms of the parasite are complement-dependent.

The complement system has been defined as a group of 9 serum β globulins (C_1, C_4, C_2, C_3, C_5, C_6, C_7, C_8, C_9) that may be activated by two physiologically different pathways. The classic pathway is initiated by the interaction of antigen-antibody complexes with C_1, C_4, and C_2, in the presence of calcium ions. The alternate pathway bypasses these early components and enters the classic pathway with the reaction of C_3, activated in the presence of magnesium ions. The *in vitro* lysis of trypomastigotes by normal chicken serum occurred in the absence of calcium ions, but required magnesium ions, indicating that the complement was activated via the alternate pathway. The role of the complement system in the lysis of trypomastigote forms by normal chicken serum is not dependent on other serum factors.

Decomplemented chickens retained parasites in the blood for 24 hours, whereas immunosuppression did not affect the lytic activity. Further, the *in vitro* lysis of trypomastigotes occurred in the absence of calcium ions, but required magnesium ions, indicating that the alternate pathway of complement activation was involved.

By contrast, it appears that mammals have little natural immunity against *Trypanosoma cruzi* infection (Chagas 1909; Muniz 1962). Muniz & Borriello (1945) studied the lytic effect of sera on culture and blood stages of *Trypanosoma cruzi* and showed that normal human and guinea pig sera have complement-related lytic effects on epimastigote forms. However, amastigotes and trypomastigotes, the stages found in the vertebrate host, were not lysed by normal sera. Rubio (1956) showed that sera from sheep, rat, guinea pig, and hamster can lyse epimastigote forms from culture within one hour, but mouse serum did not show the lytic action.

Sera of lower vertebrates contain substances lytic to culture forms of *Trypanosoma cruzi,* but their main natural defense mechanism against the infective trypomastigotes is probably phagocytosis by macropages. Dias (1933) observed phagocytosis of trypomastigotes adhering to red cells of a reptile (*Ameiva surinamensis*). Rubio (1956) showed that when trypomastigotes are inoculated in fowl, frogs, and toads, some parasites reach the bloodstream and are taken up by macrophages. Pizzi et al. (1954) showed that when *Trypanosoma cruzi* forms of low virulence are injected into nonimmune mice the parasites are largely destroyed by macrophages at the site of inoculation. On the other hand, highly virulent forms multiply in macrophages by binary fission and, although many are destroyed in the phagocytic cell, some become trypomastigotes that escape to infect other cells.

Acquired Immunity

Humoral Immunity

Trypanosoma cruzi antigens stimulate immunocompetent bone-marrow-derived lymphocytes (B cells) that produce antibody. Humoral antibodies may function alone or in conjunction with other serum factors and cells (such as complement and macrophages) to destroy invading organisms.

Trypanosoma cruzi is a strongly immunogenic parasite. High titers of complement-fixing, hemagglutinating, and precipitating antibodies occur in Chagas' disease. The highest titers of antibodies are detected in the serum during the acute phase of Chagas' disease, when large numbers of parasites are circulating in the blood (Muniz & Freitas 1946; Hauschka et al. 1950; Pizzi 1961; Cerisola et al. 1969; Gonzalez-Cappa et al. 1973). These antibodies are mainly of the IgM type. Later, when the parasitemia becomes subpatent (i.e., parasites are not found in the peripheral blood), smaller numbers of specific antibodies are still present in the serum. During the latent and chronic phases of Chagas' disease these antibodies are in the immunoglobulin classes IgG and IgA (Teixeira & Santos-Buch 1974). Seah et al. (1974) reported a curious double peak of IgM in acute experimental Chagas' disease of rhesus monkeys. Marsden, P.D., (personal communication 1975) believes that this second peak of IgM might be regarded as one antigenic variation of *Trypanosoma cruzi* in infected monkeys. Yet the absence of IgM in the latent and chronic phase of Chagas' disease has been reported by many investigators (Alarcón Segovia et al. 1974). Thus, American trypanosomiasis probably differs from African trypanosomiasis in that it does not show repeated antigenic variation, a mechanism that enables African trypanosomes (*Trypanosoma brucei rhodesiense, Trypanosoma brucei gambiense,* and *Trypanosoma brucei brucei*) to evade the host immune response (Vickerman & Luckins 1969; Vickerman 1974).

The role of humoral antibodies in Chagas' disease has been studied *in vitro* and *in vivo* by many investigators (Muniz & Borriello 1945; Muniz & Freitas 1946; Pizzi & Knierim 1955; Adler 1958; Gonzalez-Cappa et al. 1974). Immune sera from a large variety of mammals lyse epimastigote forms in culture, whereas blood trypomastigotes and intracellular amastigotes do not show lytic change in the presence of specific immune sera. Teixeira & Santos-Buch (1974) reported changes in free-swimming trypomastigotes derived from tissue culture after incubation with sera of rabbits and humans with chronic Chagas' disease. In the first 24 to 48 hours there was a continuous change from slender tryposmastigotes to round amastigotes, which form clumps by continuous multiplication. In the ensuing 48 to 72 hours many amastigotes became epimastigotes, which were then identified in the culture medium. The addition of 50 $C'H_{50}$ units per ml of fresh guinea pig complement had no noticeable effect. These data strongly suggest that humoral antibodies have no direct lytic effect on trypomastigotes of *Trypanosoma cruzi* in the presence or absence of serum complement factors. It has also been observed that splenectomy of mice, although decreasing the humoral antibody response, did not change the course of *Trypanosoma cruzi* infection (Galliard 1930; Dias 1934; Goble 1970; Pizzi & Knierim 1955; Pizzi 1961).

Transfer of immune serum from animals that recovered from acute Chagas' disease to normal recipients did not confer resistance to virulent *Trypanosoma cruzi* strains (Dias 1934; Hauschka et al. 1950; Pizzi 1961; Voller & Shaw 1965). However, some investigators (Culbertson & Kolodny 1938; Kolodny 1939; Roberson et al. 1973) have reported protective circulating antibodies that can be transferred. Kagan & Norman (1962) observed that 28% of mice treated by intraperitoneal administration of homologous immune serum were protected.

Other experiments have shown that humoral factors can influence *Trypanosoma cruzi* infection. *Trypanosoma cruzi* previously incubated with immune serum produced less severe parasitemia and fewer deaths in inoculated mice than did *Trypanosoma cruzi* that had not been incubated with immune serum (Pizzi et al. 1954; Pizzi & Rubio 1955). Krettli & Brener (1976) showed that trypomastigotes of the Y strain of *Trypanosoma cruzi* were agglutinated by the immune sera of mice. The infectivity of the agglutinated parasites was reduced when injected into normal mice. However, trypomastigotes of the CL strain neither agglutinated nor declined in infectivity after incubation with immune sera. These results suggest that humoral immunity might play a role in the immune response of mice to some strains of *Trypanosoma cruzi.*

Cell-Mediated Immunity

The primary element in the cellular response is the thymus-dependent lymphocyte (T cell), which becomes immunocompetent during infection. When stimulated with appropriate antigen under adequate conditions, T lymphocytes may become directly cytotoxic; may secrete products that are cytotoxic to either the parasites or the host cells; or may—by their secretions—attract and activate monocytes and macrophages to engulf and kill intracellular parasites.

Man and experimental animals infected with *Trypanosoma cruzi* have reactions resembling cell-mediated immunity that have been observed *in vivo* and *in vitro*. The inflammatory reactions in Chagas' disease, including the reaction at the portal of entry of *Trypanosoma cruzi* to the body, are characterized by lymphocytic infiltrates (Torres 1930; Romaña 1944; Teixeira et al. 1975). Delayed skin response to *Trypanosoma cruzi* antigens (Mazza 1943; Amato Neto et al. 1964; Teixeira & Santos-Buch 1975) and *in vitro* correlates of cell-mediated immunity have also been reported in experimental animals and patients with Chagas' disease. Seah (1970) observed that the spread of macrophages was inhibited when peritoneal exudate cells from immune mice were incubated with *Trypanosoma cruzi* antigens. Yanovsky & Albado (1972) and Lelchuck et al. (1974) observed that the migration of leukocytes taken from patients with Chagas' disease was inhibited in the presence of *Trypanosoma cruzi* antigens. Teixeira & Santos-Buch (1975) showed that migration of blood mononuclear cells from rabbits with chronic Chagas' disease was inhibited when sensitized cells migrated in the presence of *Trypanosoma cruzi* microsomal antigens. On the other hand, Tschudi et al. (1972) showed antigen-specific blast transformation of lymphocytes from patients with Chagas' disease, while Teixeira & Santos-Buch (1975) observed blast transformation and replication of sensitized lymphocytes in the presence of free-swimming trypomastigotes of *Trypanosoma cruzi.*

Taliaferro & Pizzi (1955) pointed out the importance of the lymphocyte-macrophage system in acquired resistance to *Trypanosoma cruzi* infections. These authors compared the noneffective reactions of lymphocytes and macrophages in nonimmunized mice with the effective reactions in immunized mice. Further, Goble & Singer (1960) and Goble & Boyd (1962) showed that blocking the reticuloendothelial system of mice with thorium dioxide or silica particles before challenge with *Trypanosoma cruzi* resulted in higher parasitemia, a prolonged patent period, and higher mortality.

Many investigators have shown that when trypomastigotes of *Trypanosoma cruzi* enter an activated macrophage they can be destroyed in the phagosomes, but that some parasites may remain in the cytoplasm, proliferate, and escape to initiate a new cycle of infection in another cell (Behbehani 1971, 1973; Kierszenbaum et al. 1974; Tanowitz et al. 1975). Nonspecifically activated macrophages behave *in vitro* like macrophages from immune animals. However, Hoff (1975) showed that mice immunized with Bacillus Calmette-Guerin (BCG) or *Listeria monocytogenes,* whose peritoneal macrophages strongly resisted *Trypanosoma cruzi* infection *in vitro,* were not protected *in vivo.* This suggests that specifically sensitized lymphocytes are required to call forth and focus the macrophage reaction on the parasite in the immune host.

Evidence of cell-mediated immunity is also drawn from experiments showing that administration of antilymphocyte sera, along with neonatal thymectomy, results in greater parasitemia and mortality to treated than to control animals. Moreover, the thymectomized mice produced a normal quantity of humoral antibody. This suggests that the lack of cell-mediated immunity was responsible for exacerbated *Trypanosoma cruzi* infection. Cell-mediated immunity has been transferred from animals with Chagas' disease to normal recipients by lymphoid cells (Santos 1973; Roberson & Hanson 1974; Teixeira & Santos-Buch 1975). Furthermore, Santos (1973) reported mice that had received homologous lymphocytes from chagasic donors were resistant to the virulent Y strains of *Trypanosoma cruzi.*

There is abundant laboratory evidence that cell-mediated immunity plays an important role in resistance to *Trypanosoma cruzi.* Unfortunately, the cell-mediated immune mechanisms seem to have a secondary effect: under conditions not yet clear they may harm the host organism. This toxic (or "allergic") component of the cell-mediated immune system appears to be responsible for the tissue damage in chronic Chagas' disease.

AUTOIMMUNITY IN CHAGAS' DISEASE

In acute Chagas' disease many lesions seen in various organs and tissues are probably related to the presence of parasites (Vianna 1911; Crowell 1923; Teixeira et al. 1970). However, some lesions of acute Chagas' disease might not be produced directly by the parasites. For instance, there are quiescent parasitisms of tissue cells (Vianna 1911), contrasting with inflammatory lesions in which parasites are not seen (Mayer & Rocha Lima 1914). It is very likely, therefore, that the latter type of lesion is produced by immunologic means such as those described in the chronic phase of the disease.

In chronic Chagas' disease the lesions seen in the heart and digestive tract are characterized by diffuse lymphocytic infiltrates; there are no parasites *in situ* (Torres 1930; Teixeira et al. 1975). Many authors consider these lesions to be the result of an altered allergic state of the host (Torres 1930; Chagas 1934; Mazza & Jörg 1936; Mazza 1943; Muniz & Penna Azevedo 1947; Jaffe 1959). Kozma et al. (1960) found antiheart antibodies in the sera of patients and experimental animals with Chagas' disease. They postulated that these antibodies play a role in the pathogenesis of Chagas' disease. Others indicate that antiheart antibodies are the consequence rather than the cause of heart cell destruction (Gery & Davies 1961). Recently, Cossio et al. (1974) reported the presence of a circulating antibody that reacted with plasma membrane of striated muscle fibers and endothelial cells in 95% of patients with Chagas' heart disease. Their absorption experiments suggest there are antigen determinants common to mammalian tissues and *Trypanosoma cruzi*. However, the role of these antibodies in the pathogenesis of the disease is not clear.

Santos-Buch & Teixeira (1974) cultivated fetal rabbit heart cells in the presence of rabbit anti-*Trypanosoma cruzi* serum and observed no toxic effect on the cultured heart cells. In addition, when *Trypanosoma cruzi*-sensitized lymphocytes from rabbits with chronic Chagas' disease were incubated with allogeneic fetal rabbit heart cells, destruction of the normal heart cells was observed. The authors showed that a heart cell microsomal antigen inhibits the migration of *Trypanosoma cruzi*-sensitized mononuclear cells. This indicates the presence of an antigenic determinant common to both heart cells and *Trypanosoma cruzi*. Santos-Buch & Teixeria (1974) believe that an antigen of host cells that is cross-reactive with *Trypanosoma cruzi*-sensitized lymphocytes may be the pathogenic basis for subsequent host cell injury in chronic Chagas' disease.

ANTIGENIC STRUCTURE OF *TRYPANOSOMA CRUZI*

Many techniques have been used to identify antigens from various strains of *Trypanosoma cruzi*. Muniz & Freitas (1944) isolated a polysaccharide from cultured *Trypanosoma cruzi* that showed immunologic activity and produced humoral antibodies. Seneca & Peer (1963) extracted nine antigens from sonic lysates of culture forms of *Trypanosoma cruzi*. These gave a distinct line of precipitation with hyperimmune serum by diffusion in agar gel. Tarrant et al. (1965) described the general chemical nature of the *in vitro* exoantigens of *Trypanosoma cruzi*, which they considered to be a glycoprotein with antigenic activity. Goncalves & Yamaha (1969) gave the composition of the polysaccharide obtained from aqueous *Trypanosoma cruzi* extracts. A soluble extract of the Tehuantepec strain of *Trypanosoma cruzi* was shown to give 19 lines of precipitation by diffusion in immunoelectrophoretic plates against antiserum (Afchain & Capron 1971).

Subcellular fractions of *Trypanosoma cruzi* have been tested for their antigenic properties. Gonzalez-Cappa et al. (1968) ruptured culture forms of *Trypanosoma cruzi* by pressure and observed that the soluble extracts produced high titers of complement-fixing antibodies. By contrast, the insoluble portion of the extracts did not produce high titers of humoral antibodies, but was capable of eliciting strong skin response. A detailed study of *Trypanosoma cruzi* subcellular fractions was made by Teixeira & Santos-Buch (1974) using trypomastigotes and amastigotes derived from tissue culture. These were fragmented in a high-rotation tissue homogenizer. Subcellular fractions were obtained by differential centrifugation and their antigenicity characterized in rabbits (Table 1). In general, the soluble supernatant of the homogenates (cytosol) was capable of raising high titers of humoral antibodies as well as an immediate type of skin response. By contrast, the particulate antigens in the subcellular microsomal fractions reacted with lymphocytes from rabbits with chronic Chagas' disease and elicited strong delayed-type hypersensitivity reactions. These observations suggest that soluble substances of *Trypanosoma cruzi* are responsible for the humoral antibody response, whereas the intracytoplasmic particles are involved in eliciting cell-mediated immunity.

Antigenic determinants common to different strains of *Trypanosoma cruzi* have been shown in many laboratories. Hauschka et al. (1950) tested two virulent and five avirulent strains of *Trypanosoma cruzi* (WBH, Brazil, Culbertson, Panama, Monkey, Tatu, and Texas). The strains differed in host background, geographic distribution, virulence, and history of laboratory propagation. Complete antigenic cross-relationship was observed, although there were some quantitative differences in reactivity to agglutination and lysis of culture forms by heterologous serum. Double diffusion techniques have been

Table 1

Humoral and Cell-Mediated Immunity to *T. cruzi* Antigens [a]

T. cruzi [a] antigen's	Skin Response		Hemagglutination Titers	% Inhibition of Monocyte Migration
	Immediate	Delayed		
TH[b]	+++	+++	1:2048	56.7 ± 9.4
F5[c]	+	++	1:4	90.6 ± 12.1
F6[d]	+	++	1:8	76.9 ± 3.9
F7[e]	+++	+	1:2048	48.4 ± 2.3

(a) From Teixeira & Santos-Buch 1974.
(b) TH=initial homogenate of trypomastigote and amastigote forms derived from tissue culture.
(c) F5=microsomal fraction (30,000 g for 35 min) rich in lysosome and membrane.
(d) F6=microsomal fraction (100,000 g for 90 min) rich in ribosomes.
(e) F7=soluble substances, cytosol, derived from TH.

used to establish immunotaxonomic relationships among several strains of *Trypanosoma cruzi* (Nussenzweig et al. 1962, 1963a; Nussenzweig & Goble 1966; Gonzalez-Cappa & Kagan 1969). However, the immunologic types described (A, B, and C) were not clearly associated with either the host species, geographic distribution, or pathogenicity of the strains used. Cross-immunity among these immunologic types is the rule (Nussenzweig et al. 1963b).

Antigenic determinants common to *Trypanosoma cruzi* and other Trypanosomatidae have also been described. Muniz (1930) showed that antigens from *Trypanosoma equiperdum* reacted with sera of Chagas' disease patients in complement fixation tests. Pessoa & Cardoso (1942) showed by complement fixation that *Leishmania donovani* shares a common antigenic determinant with *Trypanosoma cruzi*. Fife & Kent (1960) obtained *Trypanosoma cruzi* antigens that cross-react with antiserum to *Leishmania tropica* and *Leishmania brasiliensis*. Finally, Berrios & Zeledon (1960) showed that an antigen derived from *Strigomonas oncolpeti*, a parasite of plant insects, also reacted with sera of Chagas' disease patients in complement fixation tests.

IMMUNOPROPHYLAXIS IN CHAGAS' DISEASE: LIVE VACCINES

Soon after the discovery of Chagas' disease, it became generally accepted that human and animal survivors of acute Chagas' disease do not undergo the acute phase again. Experimental evidence leaves little doubt that animals which have undergone a primary infection acquire a significant immunity to acute Chagas' disease. This was first reported by Blanchard (1912) and Brumpt (1913), and has been confirmed by many subsequent investigators. Table 2 summarizes the literature on experimental immune protection against acute Chagas' disease.

Immune Protection to Homologous Trypanosoma cruzi Strains

Experiments have been done in many hosts with various *Trypanosoma cruzi* strains (Table 2) whose virulence had been attenuated by drugs (Collier 1931; Fernandes et al. 1966); by serial passage in cultures (Menezes 1968, 1969a, 1969b); or by treatment of the virulent *Trypanosoma cruzi* infection with pharmacological agents such as Bayer 7602 (Hauschka 1949), primaquine (Pizzi 1952), and furaltadone (Brener 1967).

Collier (1931) attenuated a strain of *Trypanosoma cruzi* by subjecting it to trypaflavine. Mice inoculated with the treated *Trypanosoma cruzi* were resistant to a subsequent challenge infection with a virulent, nonattenuated strain. However, parasites persisted in the blood or tissues of 60% of the superinfected animals, indicating that the acquired immunity from the primary infection was nonsterilizing. Collier (1931) concluded that the immunity was the result of continuous antigenic stimulation by parasites that remained in the body (premunition). Fernandes et al. (1966) attenuated virulent *Trypanosoma cruzi* Y strain by treating the cultures with Actinomycin D. The attenuated parasites were inoculated in mice. When these animals were challenged with virulent blood trypomastigotes they all survived, whereas the controls died within 13 days. The parasitemia was also lower in immunized mice than in control mice.

Hauschka et al. (1950) found that mice inoculated with virulent *Trypanosoma cruzi* DBH strain and treated with Bayer 7602 became resistant to challenge infection with the same DBH strain. The challenged animals not only survived, but did not have parasites in the peripheral blood. In similar experiments, Pizzi & Prager (1952) inoculated mice with virulent *Trypanosoma cruzi* Tulahuen strain, but then treated them with primaquine. All survived a challenge infection with the same strain, despite the presence of parasites in the blood. Brener (1967) inoculated mice with two different strains (Berenice and FL) of *Trypanosoma cruzi* and treated them with furaltadone. The survivors were then challenged with the homologous parasites. After 11 days the animals that received the Berenice strain did not show parasites in the blood, whereas those

Table 2
Experimental Immune Protection Against Acute Chagas' Disease: Live Vaccines

Author	Host	Infection (Strain of *T. cruzi)*	Challenge (Strain of *T. cruzi*)	Survival	Parasit-emia
Brumpt (1913)	mouse	Bahia	Chagas	45% after 100 days	+
Collier (1931)	mouse	–	–	100% after 30 days	+
Hauschka et al. (1950)	mouse	WBH	WBH	100% indefinite survival	–
	"	Brazil	WBH	"	+
	"	Culbertson	WBH	"	+
	"	Panama	WBH	"	+
	"	Monkey	WBH	"	+
	"	Tatu	WBH	"	+
	"	Texas	WBH	"	+
Pizzi et al. (1952)	mouse	Tulahuen	Tulahuen	100% after (?)	+
Goble (1959)	dog	Houston	C. Christi	100% after 70 days	–
	"	Houston	Brazil	"	+
	"	C. Christi	Brazil	"	–
	"	Patuxent	Brazil	"	–
Norman & Kagan (1960)	mouse	FH4-opossum	Tulahuen	survived longer than controls	+
	"	FH5-opossum	Tulahuen	"	+
	"	FH6-opossum	Tulahuen	"	+
	"	0R21-opossum	Tulahuen	"	+
	"	FR4-opossum	Tulahuen	"	+
	"	Racoon	Tulahuen	"	+
	"	Skunk	Tulahuen	"	+
	"	C. Christi	Tulahuen	"	+
	"	Brazil	Tulahuen	"	+
	"	Monkey	Tulahuen	survived longer than controls	+

Table 2 *(Continued)*

Author	Host	Infection (Strain of *T. cruzi*)	Challenge (Strain of *T. cruzi*)	Survival	Parasit-emia
Norman & Kagan (1960) (continued)	mouse	*T. duttoni*	Tulahuen	same as controls	+
	"	*T. lewisi*	Tulahuen	same as controls	+
Nussenzweig et al. (1963)	"	Y	Y	survived longer than controls	+
	"	L	Y	"	+
	"	M	Y	"	+
	"	8857	Y	"	+
	"	OPF	Y	"	+
	"	8717	Y	"	+
Fernandes et al. (1966)	mouse	Y	Y	100% after 13 days	+
Brener (1967)	mouse	Berenice	Berenice	100% after 11 days	−
	"	Berenice	FL	"	+
	"	FL	Berenice	"	+
	"	FL	FL	"	+
Menezes (1968, 1969)	mouse	Y[a]	Y	90% after 30 days	+
	"	Y	RC1729	100% after 77 days	+
	"	Y	M1418	"	+
	"	Y	Berenice	"	+
	"	Y	ABC	"	+
	dog	Y	Y	$100 \geqslant$ after 30 days	+
	man	Y	Y	indefinite survival	−
Seah & Marsden (1969)	mouse	Strain 7	Peru	all alive at 3 months	+
Andrade et al. (1970)	mouse	Colombian	Y	survived longer than controls	+
Hungerer et al. (1972)	mouse	D1	D1	80% to 100% after 9 months	+

(a) In the original papers this so-called virulent strain is named PF.

Table 2 *(Continued)*

Author	Host	Infection (Strain of *T. cruzi*)	Challenge (Strain of *T. cruzi*)	Survival	Parasit-emia
Hungerer et al. (1972) (continued)	mouse	Mary	D1	80% to 100% after 9 months	+
	"	CC	D1	"	+
	"	Tulahuen	Brazil	100% after 100 days	+
	"	FH5	"	"	+
	mouse	FH4	Brazil	"	+
	"	CDC	"	"	+
	"	ST-57	"	same as controls	+
	"	ST-58	"	"	+
	"	*T. rangeli*	"	"	+
	"	*T. lewisi*	"	"	+
	"	*L. enrieti*	"	"	+
Souza (1971, 1974)	mouse	*L. Pessoai*	Y	increased survival	+
Deane & Kloetzel (1974)	mouse	*T. lewisi*	Y	same as controls	+

that received the FL strain showed parasitemia. Menezes (1968, 1969a, 1969b, 1971, 1972) inoculated mice and dogs with a so-called avirulent strain of *Trypanosoma cruzi* Y strain kept in cultures for more than 10 years. Later, he challenged the experimental animals with the virulent *Trypanosoma cruzi* Y strain that had been maintained in the laboratory by serial passage in mice. Ninety percent of the mice survived after 30 days, whereas all the dogs were alive 60 days after challenge. Similar limited experiments were also performed in human volunteers. Later, Menezes (1969c) reported on histopathological lesions found in the hearts of "vaccinated" dogs after challenge with the virulent strain. The hearts of the vaccinated animals had mild inflammatory lesions and no parasites, whereas nonvaccinated dogs showed severe inflammatory lesions and many parasitic cysts in cardiac cells. This appears to contrast with the observation of Andrade et al. (1968), who reported that histopathological lesions from multiple infections by a single strain of *Trypanosoma cruzi* were as severe and showed the same features as the lesions resulting from a single infection with the same strain.

In view of the observations mentioned above, it appears that like a primary infection, the course of an infection by rechallenge is unpredictable and varies with the host and strain of the parasite.

Immune Protection to Heterologous *Trypanosoma cruzi* Strains

It was Brumpt (1913) who first showed heterologous immune protection between two distinct strains of *Trypanosoma cruzi*. He observed that mice receiving a primary infection with *Trypanosoma cruzi* Bahia strain became resistant to a challenge with the lethal *Trypanosoma cruzi* Chagas strain. The survivors continued to harbor the parasites in the blood after the challenge. Elegant experiments on this subject were done by Hauschka et al. (1950), Norman & Kagan (1960), and Kagan & Norman (1960, 1961).

Hauschka et al. (1950) tested two lethal and five avirulent strains of *Trypanosoma cruzi* and considered them immunologically related, since primary infection with any of the strains resulted in protection against the otherwise lethal *Trypanosoma cruzi* WBH strain. Furthermore, the protective effect showed no correlation with virulence, since the three least-virulent strains (Tatu, Panama, and Monkey) exhibited the same antigenic efficacy as the lethal WBH and Brazil strains.

Norman & Kagan (1960) reported that mice initially infected with any of the avirulent strains of *Trypanosoma cruzi* isolated from raccoons, skunks, and opossums trapped in Georgia and Florida were protected when challenged with a virulent South American strain, *Trypanosoma cruzi* Tulahuen. This suggests that the North American strains are immunologically related to *Trypanosoma cruzi* from South America. Although immunized mice were protected from death in the acute phase of infection, "challenging" organisms were present in the blood. They persisted in the blood in low numbers for at least 12 months, and were still capable of producing a lethal infection when transferred to normal mice. In further studies, Kagan & Norman (1961) showed that the degree of immune protection in mice was proportional to the time elapsed between primary infection with the avirulent strain and challenge with the virulent parasite. All mice that had been infected one month to one year prior to the challenge survived.

Brener (1967) inoculated mice with two morphologically and biologically distinct strains of *Trypanosoma cruzi*. He observed that both strains—the stout trypomastigotes (FL strain) and the slender trypomastigotes (Berenice strain)— survived in the blood of a group of mice that had received a primary infection with one of the strains and was later challenged with the heterologous strain. A similar observation was made by Andrade et al. (1970), who used other strains of *Trypanosoma cruzi*. These observations show that trypanosomes from a primary infection survive side-by-side with trypanosomes of a second infection in the immune host.

Nussenzweig et al. (1963b) infected mice with *Trypanosoma cruzi* of strains belonging to two distinct immunological groups (see above). Primary infections produced by *Trypanosoma cruzi* of either group A (strains Y, L, and M) or group B (strains 8857, OPF, and 8717) conferred some protection to challenge by the lethal Y strain. Thus, defense mechanisms against acute Chagas' disease may not depend on the antigenic determinants responsible for *in vitro* typing of the strains.

The use of live vaccines against acute Chagas' disease has serious limitations. The avirulent strains theoretically could produce chronic Chagas' disease. The above-mentioned experiments on immune protection, both with homologous and heterologous strains, have shown that attenuated live vaccines can bring forth acquired resistance to acute Chagas' disease. None of these experiments, however, deal with the question of subsequent mortality of vaccinated animals from chronic Chagas' disease.

Immune Protection With Other Trypanosomatidae

Attempts have been made to use parasites of the family Trypanosomatidae in immune protection against *Trypanosoma cruzi*, as shown in Table 2. Trypanosomes of the subgenus *Herpetomonas*, the rodent trypanosomes *Trypanosoma duttoni* and *Trypanosoma lewisi*, and *Trypanosoma rangeli*, which is an apparently harmless parasite of man, were used by Norman & Kagan (1960). Primary infection of mice with these trypanosomes did not protect them against a lethal challenge with *Trypanosoma cruzi* Tulahuen. Hungerer & Enders (1972) used *Leishmania enriettii*, *Trypanosoma lewisi,* and *Trypanosoma rangeli* and observed no immune protection. Two trypanosomes of Asian monkeys (labeled ST-57 and ST-58) also failed to protect mice against challenge with virulent *Trypanosoma cruzi* Brazil strain (Hungerer & Enders 1972). Deane & Kloetzel (1974) observed that mice were not protected against *Trypanosoma cruzi* after multiple injections of *Trypanosoma lewisi.* However, Souza & Roitman (1971) showed that primary infection of mice with *Leptomonas pessoai* induces some degree of immune protection against challenge with lethal *Trypanosoma cruzi* Y strain.

DEAD VACCINES

Immune Protection with Killed *Trypanosoma cruzi* and Its Products

Although various reports show that live *Trypanosoma cruzi* of low virulence induces some resistance to reinfection with virulent strains, the possible influence of vaccination on chronic Chagas' disease is unknown. The theoretical hazards of attenuated live parasites have turned attention to the preparation of vaccines made from killed *Trypanosoma cruzi* and its products. Papers dealing with dead vaccines are summarized in Table 3.

Muniz et al. (1946) injected culture forms of *Trypanosoma cruzi* killed with thimerosal into monkeys. These investigators observed that the animals produced specific humoral antibodies but that immune protection did not ensue. These experiments were repeated later by Kagan & Norman (1961), who also found that mice injected with thimerosal-killed culture forms of *Trypanosoma cruzi* did not become resistant to challenge with virulent *Trypanosoma cruzi* Tulahuen. Hauschka et al. (1950) pretreated mice with three to five subcutaneous injections, spaced 2 to 3 weeks apart, of Formalinized Panama, Texas, and WBH strains of *Trypanosoma cruzi.* They observed no immune protection when these mice were challenged with *Trypanosoma cruzi* WBH one week later. Menezes (1965) used lyophilized culture forms of *Trypanosoma cruzi* Y strain to immunize mice, and observed no immune protection to challenge with virulent parasites of the same strain. The first indication of immune protection by means of dead vaccines was reported by Hauschka et al. (1950). They observed a slight increase in the survival of mice after challenge with the WBH strain of *Trypanosoma cruzi* when the mice had been pretreated with injections of lyophilized spleens heavily parasitized with the same strain.

Encouraging results with killed *Trypanosoma cruzi* were obtained by Rego (1959), who used pulverized culture forms of the Y strain. Mice injected with this material showed increased resistance to challenge with homologous strains.

Table 3
Experimental Immune Protection Against Acute Chagas' Disease: Dead Vaccines

Author	Host	T. cruzi strain (culture forms)	Method of Killing Parasite	Challenge Strain	Results
Muniz & Freitas (1946)	Rhesus monkey	–	thimerosal	–	ineffective
Hauschka et al. (1950)	mouse	WBH	Formalin	WBH	ineffective
		Panama	"	"	ineffective
		Texas	"	"	ineffective
		WBH-spleen	lyophilization	"	little effect
Rego (1959)	mouse	Y	ground-up	Y	survival from 10 to 15 days
Kagan & Norman (1961)	mouse	Tulahuen	thimerosal	Tulahuen	ineffective
Johnson et al. (1963)	mouse	Y	freeze-thawing	Y	greater survival and less parasitemia
	"	C. fasciculata	"	Y	some protection
	"	L. colossoma	"	Y	no protection
	"	T. melophagium	"	Y	no protection
	"	T. mega	"	Y	no protection
Goble (1964)	mouse	Brazil	ultrasonication	Brazil	greater survival from 21 to 42 days
Menezes (1965)	mouse	Y	lyophilization	Y	ineffective
Seneca et al. (1966)	mouse	Tulahuen	sonication	Tulahuen	little effect
	"	"	Formalin-killed	"	ineffective
	"	"	ammonium sulfate	"	greater survival X 2.5
	"	"	phenol	"	100% after 40 days
Gonzalez-Cappa et al. (1968 and 1974)	mouse	–	pressure	–	significant
	"	T	"	T	80% to 100% survival after 4 months

Table 3 *(Continued)*

Author	Host	*T. cruzi* strain (culture forms)	Method of Killing Parasite	Challenge Strain	Results
Gonzalez-Cappa et al. (1968 and 1974) (continued)	mouse	B	pressure	T	80% to 100% survival after 4 months
	"	L	"	G	"
	"	G	"	T	"
Hanson et al. (1974)	mouse	–	irradiation	–	almost complete protection
Souza et al. (1974)	mouse	*L. pessoai*	sonication	Y	no protection

Later, Johnson et al. (1963) used culture forms of *Trypanosoma cruzi* ruptured by quick freezing and thawing. Mice immunized with 0.1 ml of this antigen, emulsified in 0.1 ml of saponin as adjuvant, were found to have significant immune protection against challenge with virulent *Trypanosoma cruzi* Y strain. Further, Goble et al. (1964) and Goble (1970) made experimental vaccines from culture forms of the Brazil strain of *Trypanosoma cruzi* that were ruptured by ultrasonication, pressure, and shaking with glass beads. These vaccines were found to be protective in mice. Homogenates of *Trypanosoma cruzi* prepared by sonication increased the survival time of vaccinated mice from 21 to 42 days. The best preparations were obtained from organisms disintegrated by shaking with glass beads in the cold. The greatest immunity was observed between 3 and 7 weeks after vaccination, but protection persisted as long as 4 months.

Seneca & Peer (1963, 1966) obtained several *Trypanosoma cruzi* antigens by chemical methods after disruption of culture forms by sonication. The protective activity of these antigens was assayed in mice. Seneca et al. (1966) showed that varying degrees of protection were obtained by these antigens. The highest protection was observed when a phenol-extracted lipopolysaccharide antigen (Chagastoxin) was used. They reported that this antigen was present in small quantities in sonic lysates and was very unstable. No further experiments following this line of research are found in the literature.

Gonzalez-Cappa et al. (1968) prepared antigens from culture forms of *Trypanosoma cruzi* in a Ribi Refrigerated Cell Fractionator (RFI—Ivan Sorval, Inc.), with temperature control and in an atmosphere of inert gas. The soluble extract of *Trypanosoma cruzi* prepared at less than 10,000 psi was capable of producing high titers of complement-fixing humoral antibodies and was also very effective in immunization. The survival of mice immunized with this antigen and challenged with a lethal inoculum of *Trypanosoma cruzi* Tulahuen strain varied from 88% to 100%. Some immunized mice showed transient, low parasitemia after challenge infection with *Trypanosoma cruzi* Tulahuen strain.

Recently, Gonzalez-Cappa et al. (1974) used antigens derived from epimastigotes of *Trypanosoma cruzi* belonging to the different immunological groups described earlier. Immune protection was obtained with disrupted epimastigotes of the B, L, and G strains (B, C, and A/C immunological groups, respectively). The survival of the immunized mice after challenge infection with *Trypanosoma cruzi* Tulahuen was as high as 80% to 100% and protection lasted as long as 4 months. Humoral antibodies detected in the sera of all immunized animals were common to antigens of all *Trypanosoma cruzi* strains used. This showed that cross-resistance can be obtained with dead parasites.

Hanson (Chapter 13) reports promising results with a method of vaccination with irradiated parasites. When mice were vaccinated with *Trypanosoma cruzi* tissue culture forms killed by irradiation (150-220 krad), a significant degree of immune protection was observed. From three to five injections of irradiated parasites resulted in almost complete immune protection against a challenge infection with the virulent Brazil strain.

In general, the physical methods for obtaining antigens that give immune protection are superior to the chemical methods so far utilized. The results of many experiments described above suggest that the prospects for vaccination against *Trypanosoma cruzi* infection are promising. Augmentation of the host immune response by means of a potent antigen harmless to the host is desirable. Residual *Trypanosoma cruzi* infection may not be necessary to the development and maintenance of long-lasting resistance against Chagas' disease. Studies should concentrate on possible methods of increasing cell-mediated and/or humoral immune mechanisms for trypanosome inactivation.

Immune Protection With Other Killed Trypanosomatidae

Johnson et al. (1963) used culture forms of *Crithidia fasciculata, Leptomonas collosoma, Trypanosoma melophagium,* and *Trypanosoma mega* killed by quick freezing and thawing. The killed parasites were emulsified with adjuvant and injected subcutaneously in mice. This procedure resulted in some cross-protection against challenge with the virulent Y strain of *Trypanosoma cruzi* when the animals were immunized with killed *Crithidia fasciculata* and *Leptomonas collosoma*. No cross-protection was observed when killed *Trypanosoma melophagium* and *Trypanosoma mega* were used. Souza et al. (1974) used *Leptomonas pessoai* killed by sonication to immunize mice, and showed lack of protection after challenge with virulent *Trypanosoma cruzi* Y strain.

PERSPECTIVES FOR FURTHER STUDIES ON IMMUNOPROPHYLAXIS AGAINST CHAGAS' DISEASE

At present, there is no treatment for Chagas' disease. Countless chemotherapeutic agents have been tested (Goble 1961a; Brener 1966, 1968; Ferreira & Rassi 1972; Haberhorn 1972; Lugones 1972), some of which are effective in eradicating parasites from the blood. The question remains whether or not it is possible to eradicate the intracellular amastigote stages. In this regard, the results achieved with drugs have been disappointing so far.

Studies on vaccination against Chagas' disease described above indicate this to be a promising field for further investigation. Future research work on immunoprophylaxis against Chagas' disease should, however, proceed along two distinct lines: (1) immunoprophylaxis against acute Chagas' disease when parasites are abundant in the host organism; (2) immunoprophylaxis against chronic Chagas' disease when parasites are not usually found in the body.

Immunoprophylaxis Against Acute Chagas' Disease

Vaccination with Living Parasites

Research on cross-immunity between *Trypanosoma cruzi* and other Trypanosomatidae has resulted in obtaining some degree of immune protection to challenge infection with virulent *Trypanosoma cruzi* strains. Further research is needed to investigate cross-protection between *Trypanosoma cruzi* and other cruzi-related trypanosomes of the genus *Schizotrypanum* (Chagas 1909), which are not pathogenic for man or for other mammals.

In view of the possibility that previous infection with these living trypanosomes can give strong immune protection to superinfection with *Trypanosoma cruzi,* they may be safe for prophylactic vaccination. Among these cruzi-like trypanosomes are *Trypanosoma vespertilionis, Trypanosoma phyllostomae,* and *Trypanosoma pipistrelli,* which were considered by Hoare (1972) to be species distinct from *Trypanosoma cruzi.* Of course, other undefined species within the group of cruzi-like trypanosomes, including *Trypanosoma hipposideri, Trypanosoma pteropi,* and the strain derived from *Phyllostomus hastatus* (Barbosa et al. 1973), should also be studied in laboratory animals.

Vaccination With Purified *Trypanosoma cruzi* Antigens

Efforts should be made to obtain *Trypanosoma cruzi* antigen with potent immunogenicity. Previous reports by Gonzalez-Cappa et al. (1968) and Teixeira & Santos-Buch (1974) showed that the soluble substances derived from homogenates of *Trypanosoma cruzi,* the cell sap or cytosol, can induce high titers of humoral antibodies. Gonzalez-Cappa et al. (1968) reported that mice immunized with this antigen showed significant immunity to challenge with virulent *Trypanosoma cruzi.* The augmentation of the immune response elicited by *Trypanosoma cruzi*-soluble antigens and by the other subcellular antigens (Segura et al. 1974) should be further investigated. Studies should concentrate on possible methods of increasing cell-mediated and/or humoral mechanisms for trypanosome inactivation. Although preventive vaccination against bacterial or viral diseases is common in human and veterinary medicine, vaccination against diseases caused by protozoans is still a goal. The possibility of producing a "dead vaccine" effective against *Trypanosoma cruzi* appears to be worth pursuing.

Immunoprophylaxis Against Chronic Chagas' Disease

Acute Chagas' disease is self-limiting. Humans and some experimental animals usually survive acute Chagas' disease but remain with a subpatent infection for life. The parasite persists through cyclic reinfection of cells by parasites that escape the host immune mechanisms. It is not known precisely how the parasite evades the host's immune response.

In chronic Chagas' disease, parasites are not usually present in the blood. Only occasional pseudocysts containing amastigote forms are found in the tissues. These amastigotes seem to be dormant in the nonphagocytic cells and are sheltered from the host's immune mechanisms. Further, there is good evidence that the lesions of chronic Chagas' disease are preceded by delayed-hypersensitivity mechanisms. Here the question seems to be how to prevent the development of lesions that are not directly produced by the parasites.

Cell-mediated immunity plays two distinct roles in Chagas' disease. On the one hand, it is responsible for the host's resistance to *Trypanosoma cruzi.* On the other hand, it is involved in the production of lesions that may lead to death. This toxic or allergic component of cell-mediated immunity might be counteracted by manipulation of the immune system. Thus, the lesions of chronic Chagas' disease might be prevented by specific immune suppression of the toxic component of the cell-mediated immune system. Theoretically this can be done in two distinct ways:

1. Induction of immunological tolerance (unresponsiveness) by antigen-specific dampening of T cells, either by antigenic competition or by the

production of nonspecific factors that might block cytotoxic mechanisms. This concept bears some resemblance to the "desensitization" procedure formerly used in the treatment of tuberculous lesions (Rich 1950).
2. Induction of immunological blockade (enhancement), probably mediated by antibody or immune complexes (Feldman 1972).

There is no indication that humoral immunity parallels cell-mediated immunity in chronic Chagas' disease. It would be of interest to know whether humoral antibodies could block antigenic sites on the surface of sensitized T cells and therefore prevent *Trypanosoma cruzi*-sensitized lymphocyte toxicity to normal target host cells. Immunosuppressive drugs decrease the intensity of tissue lesions (Andrade & Andrade 1966; Brener 1967) but aggravate *Trypanosoma cruzi* infection. Caution is therefore necessary in approaching this problem.

Antigenic variation probably does not occur within strains of *Trypanosoma cruzi*. Moreover, cross-immunity between heterologous strains of the parasite is the rule. These observations point toward an immunoprophylactic approach to the treatment of the disease. However, vaccination has conferred only partial protection to superinfection, and the parasites continue to survive in immunized hosts. Clarification of the mechanisms whereby *Trypanosoma cruzi* evades the host's immune response is clearly essential to further progress in prophylaxis against Chagas' disease.

BIBLIOGRAPHY

Adler, S. 1958. The action of specific serum on a strain of *Trypanosoma cruzi*. *Ann. Trop. Med. Parasitol.* 52: 282-301.

Afchain, D. & Capron, A. 1971. Analyse immunoelectrophorétique des antigens solubles de *Trypanosoma cruzi*. Applications à la trypanosomiase expérimentale de la souris. *Gaz. Med. Bahia* 71: 7-15.

Alarcón Segovia, S., Andrade, Z.A., Bloom, B.R. et al. 1974. Immunology of Chagas' disease. *Bull. WHO* 50: 459-472.

Amato Neto, V., Magalde, C. & Pessoa, S.B. 1964. Intradermoreação para diagnóstico de doença de Chagas com antigeno de *Trypanosoma cruzi* obtido de cultura de tecido. *Rev. Goiana Med.* 10: 121-126.

Amato Neto, V. 1968. Doença de Chagas e transfusão de sangue. *In* Doença de Chagas, J.R. Cançado, Ed.: 130-142. Official Press of Minas Gerais. Belo Horizonte, Brazil.

Andrade, S.G. & Andrade, Z.A. 1966. Doença de Chagas e alterações neuronais no plexo de Auerbach (Estudo experimental em camundongos). *Rev. Inst. Med. Trop. São Paulo* 8: 219-224.

Andrade, S.G., Carvalho, M.L., Figueira, R.M. & Andrade, Z.A. 1970. Recuparação e caracterização de tripanosomas inoculados em animais imunes (Reinoculação com diferentes cepas do *Trypanosoma cruzi). Rev. Inst. Med. Trop. São Paulo* 12: 395-402.

Andrade, S.G., Figueira, R.M. & Andrade, Z.A. 1968. Influência de infecções repetidas no quadro histopatológico da doença de Chagas experimental. *Gaz. Med. Bahia* 68: 115-123.

Andrade, Z.A. 1958. Anatomia patológica da doença de Chagas. *Rev. Goiana Med.* 4: 103-119.

Badinez, O.S. 1945. Contribución a la anatomía patológica de la enfermedad de Chagas experimental. *Biologica* 3: 3-52.

Barbosa, W., Martins, S.P. & Oliveira, R.L. 1973. Nota preliminar sobre trypanosoma variedade *hastatus* isolado de *Phyllostomus hastatus* da Gaverna de Fercal-DF Brasil. *Rev. Patol. Trop.* 2: 367-376.

Barretto, M.P. 1967. Aspectos ecológicos da epidemiologia das doenças transmissíveis, com especial referência às zoonoses. *Rev. Bras. Malariol.* 19: 633-654.

Behbehani, M.K. 1971. Multiplication of *Trypanosoma (Schizotripanum) cruzi* in mouse peritoneal macrophages. *Trans. R. Soc. Trop. Med. Hyg.* 65: 15.

Behbehani, M.K. 1973. Developmental cycles of *Trypanosoma (Schizotrypanum) cruzi* (Chagas 1909) in mouse peritoneal macrophages *in vitro. Parasitology* 66: 343-353.

Berrios, A. & Zeledon, R. 1960. Estudio comparativo entre los antigenos de *Schizotrypanum cruzi* y de *Strigomonos oncolpeti* en la reacción de fijacion del complemento para enfermedad de Chagas. *Rev. Biol. Trop. Univ. Costa Rica* 8: 225-231.

Bittencourt, A.L. 1969. The congenital transmission of Chagas' disease as a cause of abortion. *Gaz. Med. Bahia* 69: 118-122.

Blanchard, M. 1912. Marche de l'infection à *Schizotrypanum cruzi* chez le cobaye et à la souris. *Bull. Soc. Pathol. Exot.* 5: 598-599.

Brener, Z. 1965. Comparative studies of different strains of *Trypanosoma cruzi. Ann. Trop. Med. Parasitol.* 59: 19-26.

Brener, Z. 1966. Chemotherapeutic studies in tissue cultures infected with *Trypanosoma cruzi,* the mode of action of some active compounds. *Ann. Trop. Med. Parasitol.* 60: 445-451.

Brener, Z. 1967. Alguns aspectos da imunidade adquirida em camundongos experimentalmente inoculados com *Trypanosoma cruzi. Rev. Inst. Med. Trop. São Paulo* 9: 233-238.

Brener, Z. 1968. Terapêutica experimental da doença de Chagas. *In* Doença de Chagas, J.R. Cançado, Ed.: 501-516. Official Press of Minas Gerais. Belo Horizonte, Brazil.

Brener, Z. & Chiari, E. 1963. Variações morfológicas observadas em diferentes amostras de *Trypanosoma cruzi. Rev. Inst. Med. Trop. São Paulo* 5: 220-224.

Brener, Z. & Chiari, E. 1965. Aspects of early growth of different *Trypanosoma cruzi* strains in culture medium. *J. Parasitol.* 51: 922-926.

Brener, Z. & Chiari, E. 1967. Suscetibilidade de diferentes amostras de *Trypanosoma cruzi* a vários agentes quimioterápicos. *Rev. Inst. Med. Trop. São Paulo* 9: 197-207.

Brener, Z., Chiari, E. & Alvarenga, N.J. 1974. Observations on *Trypanosoma cruzi* strains maintained over an 8-year period in experimentally inoculated mice. *Rev. Inst. Med. Trop. São Paulo* 16: 39-46.

Brumpt, E. 1913. Immunité partielle dans les infections à *Trypanosoma cruzi*, transmission de ce trypanosome par *Cimex rotundus*. Rôle regulateur des hôtes intermédiaires. Passage à travers la peau. *Bull. Soc. Pathol. Exot.* 6: 172-176.

Cerisola, J.A. 1969. Evolución serologica de pacientes con enfermedad de Chagas aguda tratados con Bay 2502. *Bol. Chil. Parasitol.* 24: 54-59.

Chagas, C. 1909. Nova tripanosomiase humana. Estudos sobre a morfologia e o ciclo evolutivo do *Schizotrypanum cruzi*, n.gen., n.sp., agente etiológico de nova entidade mórbida do homem. *Mem. Inst. Oswaldo Cruz Rio de Janeiro* 1: 159-218.

Chagas, C. 1910. Nova entidade mórbida do homem. *Bras.-Med.* 24: 423-428, 433-437, 443-447.

Chagas, C. 1912. Sobre um trypanosomo do tatu, *Tatusia novemcincta*, transmitido pela *Triatoma geniculata*. Possibilidade de ser o tatu um depositário do *Trypanosoma cruzi* no mundo exterior (Nota previa). *Bras.-Med.* 26: 305-306.

Chagas, C. 1916. Trypanosomiase americana. Forma aguda da moléstia. *Mem. Inst. Oswaldo Cruz Rio de Janeiro* 8: 37-60.

Chagas, C. 1934. Estado actual da Trypanosomiase americana. *Rev. Biol. Hyg., São Paulo* 5: 58-64.

Collier, W.A. 1931. Über Immunität bei der Chagas Krankheit der weissen Maus. *Z. Hyg. Infektionskr.* 112: 88-92.

Cossio, P.M., Laguens, R.P., Diez, C., Szarfman, A., Segal, A. & Arana, R.M. 1974. Chagasic cardiopathy. Antibodies reacting with plasma membrane of striated muscle and endothelial cells. *Circulation* 50: 1252-1259.

Crowell, P.C. 1923. The acute form of American trypanosomiasis; notes on its pathology, with autopsy report and observations on trypanosomiasis cruzi in animals. *Am. J. Trop. Med.* 3: 425-454.

Culbertson, J.T. & Kolodny, M.H. 1938. Acquired immunity in rats against *Trypanosoma cruzi. J. Parasitol.* 24: 83-90.

Deane, P.M. & Kloetzel, J.K. 1974. Lack of protection against *Trypanosoma cruzi*, by multiple doses of *Trypanosoma lewisi* culture forms. A discussion of some strains of "lewisi." *Exp. Parasitol.* 35: 406-410.

Dias, E. 1933. Immunité naturelle des animaux à sang froid vis-à-vis de l'infection par le *Trypanosoma cruzi. Compt. R. Soc. Biol.* 112: 1474-1475.

Dias, E. 1934. Estudios sobre o *Schizotrypanum cruzi. Mem. Inst. Oswaldo Cruz Rio de Janeiro* 28: 1-110.

Dias, E. 1944. Não receptividade do pombo doméstico à infecção por Schizotrypanum. *Mem. Inst. Oswaldo Cruz Rio de Janeiro* 40: 181-193.

Dias, E. 1949. Os riscos de propagação da doença de Chagas pelos serviços de transfusão de sangue. *Bol. Of. Sanit. Panam.* 28: 910-911.

Dias, E. 1956. Chagas-Krankheit. Chagas' disease. *In* Welt-Seuchen-Atlas. E. Rodenwaldt, Ed. Vol. 2: 135-140. Falk-Verlag. Hamburg, Federal Republic of Germany.

Feldman, J.D. 1972. Immunological enhancement: a study of blocking antibodies. *Adv. Immunol.* 15: 167-214.

Fernandes, J.F., Castellani, O. & Okumura, M. 1966. Histopathology of the heart and muscles in mice immunized against *Trypanosoma cruzi. Rev. Inst. Med. Trop. São Paulo* 8: 151-156.

Ferreira, H.O. & Rassi, A. 1972. Tratamento da fase aguda da doença de Chagas. *In* International Symposium of Chagas' Disease: 261-269. Buenos Aires, Argentina.

Fife, E.H. & Kent, J.F. 1960. Protein and carbohydrate complement-fixing antibodies of *Trypanosoma cruzi. Am. J. Trop. Med. Hyg.* 9: 512-517.

Galliard, H. 1930. Infections à *Trypanosoma cruzi* chez les animaux splénectomisés. *Bull. Soc. Pathol. Exot.* 23: 188-192.

Gery, I. & Davies, A.M. 1961. Organ specificity of the heart. II. Immunization of rabbits with homologous heart. *J. Immunol.* 87: 351-356.

Goble, F.C. 1961a. Experimental therapeutics of Chagas' disease. Annual International Congress on Chagas' Disease. 2: 613-633. Rio de Janeiro, Brazil.

Goble, F.C. 1961b. Observations on cross-immunity in experimental Chagas' disease in dogs. Annual International Congress on Chagas' Disease. 2: 603-611. Rio de Janeiro, Brazil.

Goble, F.C. 1970. South American trypanosomes. *In* Immunity to Parasitic Animals. G.J. Jackson, R. Herman & I. Singer, Eds. Vol. 2: 597-689. Appleton-Century-Crofts. New York, N.Y.

Goble, F.C. & Boyd, J.L. 1962. Reticuloendothelial blockage in experimental Chagas' disease. *J. Parasitol.* 48: 223-228,

Goble, F.C. Boyd, J.L., Grim, W.M. & Konrath, M. 1964. Vaccination against experimental Chagas' disease with homogenates of culture forms of *Trypanosoma cruzi. J. Parasitol.* 50 (3, Sec. 2):19.

Goble, F.C. & Singer, I. 1960. The reticuloendothelial system in experimental malaria and trypanosomiasis. *Ann. N.Y. Acad. Sci.* 88: 149-171.

Goncalves, J.M. & Yamaha, T. 1969. Immunochemical polysaccharide from *Trypanosoma cruzi. J. Trop. Med. Hyg.* 72: 39-44.

Gonzalez-Cappa, S.M. & Kagan, I.G. 1969. Agar gel and immunoelectrophoretic analysis of several strains of *Trypanosoma cruzi. Exp. Parasitol.* 25: 50-57.

Gonzalez-Cappa, S.M., Pesce, V.J., Cantarella, A.I. & Schmunis, G.A. 1974. *Trypanosoma cruzi:* protection of mice with epimastigote antigens from immunologically different parasite strains. *Exp. Parasitol.* 35: 179-186.

Gonzalez-Cappa, S.M., Schmunis, G.A., Traversa, O.C., Yanovski, J.F. & Parodi, A.S. 1968. Complement-fixation tests, skin tests, and experimental immunization with antigens of *Trypanosoma cruzi* prepared under pressure. *Am. J. Trop. Med. Hyg.* 17: 709-715.

Gonzalez-Cappa, S.M., Vattuone, N.H., Menes, S. & Schmunis, G.A. 1973. Humoral antibody response and Ig characterization of the specific agglutinins in rabbits during experimental American trypanosomiasis. *Exp. Parasitol.* 34: 32-39.

Guimarães, J.P. & Miranda, A. 1961. Megaesôfago em macaco Rhesus com 10 anos de infeccão chagasica. Annual Brazil, International Congress on Chagas' Disease. 2: 657-671. Rio de Janeiro, Brazil.

Haberhorn, A. 1972. Quimioterapia experimental. Respuesta de diferentes cepas de *Trypanosoma cruzi.* International Symposium of Chagas' Disease: 245-254. Buenos Aires, Argentina.

Hauschka, T.S. 1949. Persistence of strain specific behavior in two strains of *Trypanosoma cruzi* after prolonged transfer through inbred mice. *J. Parasitol.* 35: 593-599.

Hauschka, T.S., Godwin, N.B., Palmquist J. & Brown, E. 1950. Immunological relationship between seven strains of *Trypanosoma cruzi* and its application in the diagnosis of Chagas' disease. *Am. J. Trop. Med. Hyg.* 30: 1-16.

Hoare, C.A. 1972. The Trypanosomes of Mammals. Blackwell Scientific Publications. Oxford, England.

Hoff, R. 1975. Killing *in vitro* of *Trypanosoma cruzi* by macrophages from mice immunized with *Trypanosoma cruzi* or BCG, and absence of cross-immunity on challenge *in vivo J. Exp. Med.* 142: 299-311.

Howard, J.E. & Rubio, M. 1968. Enfermedad de Chagas congenita. I. Estudio clinico y epidemiologico de 30 casos. *Bol. Chil. Parasitol.* 23: 107-112.

Hungerer, K.D. & Enders, B. 1972. Vaccination against Chagas' disease. Mimeographed paper.

Jaffe, R. 1959. Autoallergische Herzveränderungen. *Arzneim-Forsch.* 9: 657.

Johnson, P., Neal, R.A. & Gall, D. 1963. Protective effect of killed trypanosome vaccines with incorporated adjuvants. *Nature* (Lond.). 200: 83.

Kagan, I.G. & Norman, L. 1960. Immunologic studies of *Trypanosoma cruzi* I. Susceptibility of CFW stock mice for the Tulahuen strain of *Trypanosoma cruzi. J. Infect. Dis.* 107: 165-167.

Kagan, I.G. & Norman, L. 1961. Immunologic studies of *Trypanosoma cruzi.* III. Duration of acquired immunity in mice initially infected with a North American strain of *Trypanosoma cruzi. J. Infect. Dis.* 108: 213-217.

Kagan, I.G. & Norman, L. 1962. Immunologic studies of *Trypanosoma cruzi.* IV. Serial transfer of *Trypanosoma cruzi* organisms from immune to non-immune mice. *J. Parasitol.* 48: 584-588.

Kierszenbaum, F., Ivanyi, J. & Budzko, D. 1976. Mechanisms of natural resistance to trypanosomal infection. Role of complement in avian resistance to *Trypanosoma cruzi* infection. *Immunology* 30: 1-6.

Kierszenbaum, F., Knecht, E., Budzko, D. & Pizzimenti, M.C. 1974. Phago-cytosis: a defense mechanism against infection with *Trypanosoma cruzi. J. Immunol.* 112: 1839-1844.

Kilgour, V. & Godfrey, D.G. 1973. Species-characteristic isoenzymes of two aminotransferases in trypanosomes. *Nat. New Biol.* 244: 69-70.

Köberle, F. 1957. Patogenia da moléstia de Chagas. Estudio dos orgãos musculares ocos. *Rev. Goiana Med.* 3: 155-180.

Köberle, F. 1959. El mal de Chagas. Enfermedad del sistema nervioso. *Rev. Med. Cordoba* 47: 105-133.

Köberle, F. 1968. Chagas' disease and Chagas syndromes: the pathology of American trypanosomiasis. *Adv. Parasitol.* 6: 63-116.

Köberle, F. & Nador, E. 1955. Etiologia e patogenia do megaesôfago no Brasil. *Rev. Paul. Med.* 47: 643-661.

Kolodny, M.H. 1939. The transmission of immunity in experimental trypanoso-miasis *(Trypanosoma cruzi)* from mother rats to their offspring. *Am. J. Hyg.* 30: 19-39.

Kozma, C., Jaffe, R. & Jaffe, W.F. 1960. Estudo experimental sobre a pato-genia das miocardites. *Arq. Bras. Cardiol.* 13: 155-161.

Krettli, A.V. & Brener, Z. 1976. Protective effects of specific antibodies in *Trypanosoma cruzi* infections. *J. Immunol.* 116: 755-760.

Laranja, F.S., Dias, E., Nobrega, G. & Miranda, A. 1956. Chagas' disease. A clinical, epidemiological and pathologic study. *Circulation* 14: 1035-1060.

Lelchuck, R.A., Patrucco, A. & Manni, J.A. 1974. Studies of cellular immunity in Chagas disease: effect of glutaraldehyde-treated specific antigen on inhibition of leukocyte migration. *J. Immunol.* 112: 1578-1581.

Lugones, H.S. 1972. Tratamiento de la enfermedad aguda. Experiencia Santiago del Estero. International Symposium of Chagas' Disease: 255-259. Buenos Aires, Argentina.

Marsden, P.D. 1971. South American trypanosomiasis (Chagas' disease). *Int. Rev. Trop. Med.* 4: 97-121.

Mayer, M. & Rocha-Lima, H. 1914. Zum Verhalten von *Schizotrypanum cruzi* in Warm Blutern und Arthropoden. *Arch. Schiffs-Tropenhyg.* 18: 101-106.

Mazza, S. 1943. Naturaleza histopatológica de reacciones alérgicas cutáneas, provocadas en chagásicos con lisados de cultivos de *Schizotrypanum cruzi*. *Univ. Buenos Aires, Mision Estud. Pat. Reg. Argent.* 64: 3-143.

Mazza, S. & Jörg, M.E. 1936. Infección natural mortal por *Schizotrypanum cruzi* en cachorro de perro "Pila" de Jujuy. *9. Reunión de Sociedad Argentina de Patología Regional:* Mendoza, Argentina. 1: 365-411.

Menezes, H. 1965. The use of adjuvants in the vaccination of mice with lyophilized *Trypanosoma cruzi. Hospital* (Rio de Janeiro) 68: 1341-1346.

Menezes, H. 1968. Protective effect of an avirulent (cultivated) strain of *Trypanosoma cruzi* against experimental infection in mice. *Rev. Inst. Med. Trop. São Paulo* 10: 1-4.

Menezes, H. 1969a. Active immunization of dogs with a non-virulent strain of *Trypanosoma cruzi. Rev. Inst. Med. Trop. São Paulo* 11: 258-263.

Menezes, H. 1969b. Active immunization of mice with the avirulent Y strain of *Trypanosoma cruzi* against heterologous virulent strains of the same parasite. *Rev. Inst. Med. Trop. São Paulo* 11: 335-342.

Menezes, H. 1969c. Lesões histológicas do coração em caes "vacinados" com uma cepa avirulenta de *Trypanosoma cruzi. Rev. Bras. Med.* 26: 281-283.

Menezes, H. 1971. Aplicação de vacina viva avirulenta de *Trypanosoma cruzi* em séres humanos (nota prévia). *Rev. Inst. Med. Trop. São Paulo* 13: 144-154.

Menezes, H. 1972. Imunização ativa contra a trypanosomose americana. *Med. Rev. Cent. Acad. Rocha Lima (CARL) Hosp. Clin. Fac. Med. Ribeirao Preto Univ. São Paulo* 5: 85-93.

Moore, D.V. 1957. Antigen relationship of certain hemoflagellates as determined by the Ouchterlony gel diffusion technique. *J. Parasitol.* 43 (Suppl.):16

Mott, K.E. 1972. *American trypanosomiasis. In* Infectious Diseases, Hoeprich, P.D. Ed.: 1065-1072 Harper & Row. New York, N.Y.

Muniz, J. 1930. Del uso del antígeno Watson, *Trypanosoma equiperdum,* en la reacción de desviación del complemento en la enfermedad de Chagas. *5. Reunión de la Sociedad Argentina de Patología Regional del Norte:* Jujuy, Argentina. 2: 897-901.

Muniz, J. 1962. Imunidade na Doença de Chagas (Trypanosomiasis Americana). *Mem. Inst. Oswaldo Cruz Rio de Janeiro* 60: 103-147.

Muniz, J. 1968. Da importância das reações de âmbito imunológico na patogenia da doença de Chagas. *Rev. Goiana Med.* 14: 185-191.

Muniz, J. & Borriello, A. 1945. Estudio sobre a ação litica de diferrentes sôros sobre as formas de cultura e sanguícolas do *"Schizotrypanum cruzi." Rev. Bras. Biol.* 5: 563-576.

Muniz, J. & Freitas, G. 1944. Contribuição para o diagnóstico da doença de Chagas. II. Isolamento de polisacardieos de *Schizotrypanum cruzi* e de outros tripanosomideos, seu comportamento nas reações de precipitação, de fixação de complemento e de hipersensibilidade. Os testes de floculação. (Sublimado e formol-gel.) *Rev. Bras. Biol.* 4: 421-438.

Muniz, J. & Freitas, G. 1946. Estudios sobra a imunidade humoral na doença de Chagas. *Bras-Med.* 60: 337-341.

Muniz, J., Nobrega, G. & da Cunha, M. 1946. Ensaios de vacinação preventiva e curativa nas infecções pelo *Schizotrypanum cruzi. Mem. Inst. Oswaldo Cruz Rio de Janeiro* 44: 529-541.

Muniz, J. & Penna Azevedo, A. 1947. Novo conceito da patogenia de "doença de Chagas" *trypanosomiasis americana;* inflamação alérgica granulomatoide (a), e miocardite hiperergica (b), produzida em "rhesus" *(Macaca mullata)* inoculados com formas mortas de cultivo de *Schizotrypanum cruzi* (Nota previa). *Hospital* (Rio de Janeiro) 32: 165-183.

Nery-Guimarães, F. 1972. A refratariedade das aves ao *Trypanosoma (S.) cruzi*. I. Ausência de passagem para o sangue; duração da viabilidade e destruição dos parasitas na pele. *Mem. Inst. Oswaldo Cruz Rio de Janeiro* 70: 37-48.

Nery-Guimarães, F. & Lage, H.A. 1972. A refratariedade das aves ao *Trypanosoma (S.) cruzi*. II. Refratariedade das galinhas desde o nascimento; persistência da refratariedade após bursectomia; infecções em ovos embrionados. *Mem. Inst. Oswaldo Cruz Rio de Janeiro* 70: 97-107.

Norman, L. & Kagan, I.G. 1960. Immunologic studies on *Trypanosoma cruzi*. II. Acquired immunity in mice infected with avirulent American strains of *Trypanosoma cruzi. J. Infect. Dis.* 107: 168-174.

Nussenzweig, V., Deane, L.M. & Kloetzel, J. 1962. Diversidade na constituição antigênica de amostras de *Trypanosoma cruzi* isoladas do homem e de gambás. (Nota preliminar.) *Rev. Inst. Med. Trop. São Paulo* 4: 409-410.

Nussenzweig, V., Deane, L.M. & Kloetzel, J. 1963a. Differences in antigenic constitution of strains of *Trypanosoma cruzi. Exp. Parasitol.* 14: 221-232.

Nussenzweig, V. & Goble, F.C. 1966. Further studies on the antigenic constitution of strains of *Trypanosoma (Schizotrypanum) cruzi. Exp. Parasitol.* 18: 224-230.

Nussenzweig, V., Kloetzel, J. & Deane, L.M. 1963b. Acquired immunity in mice infected with strains of immunological types A and B of *Trypanosoma cruzi. Exp. Parasitol.* 14: 233-239.

Pan American Health Organization. 1970. Report of a study group on Chagas' disease. *Pan Am. Health Organ. Sci. Publ.* no. 195.

Pessoa, S.B. 1958. Hospedeiros vertebrados (não humanos) do *Trypanosoma cruzi. Rev. Goiana Med.* 4: 83-101.

Pessoa, S.B. & Cardoso, C.A. 1942. Nota sobre a imunidade cruzada na leishmaniose tegumentar e na moléstia de Chagas. *Hospital* (Rio de Janeiro) 21: 187-193.

Phillips, N.R. 1960. Experimental studies on the quantitative transmission of *Trypanosoma cruzi:* Considerations regarding the standardization of materials. *Ann. Trop. Med. Parasitol.* 54: 60-70.

Pizzi, T. 1961. Inmunologia de la enfermedad de Chagas: Estado actual del problema. *Bol. Of. Sanit. Panam.* 51: 450-464.

Pizzi, T. & Knierim, F. 1955. Modificaciones del bazo en relacion con la tasa de anticuerpos circulantes en ratones experimentalmente infectados con *Trypanosoma cruzi. Bol. Chil. Parasitol.* 10: 42-49.

Pizzi, T. & Prager, R. 1952. Inmunidad a la sobreinfeccion inducida mediante cultivos de *Trypanosoma cruzi* de virulencia atenuada. *Bol. Inform. Parasitol. Chil.* 7: 20-21.

Pizzi, T. & Rubio, M. 1955. Aspectos celulares de la inmunidad en la enfermedad de Chagas. *Bol. Chil. Parasitol.* 10: 5-9.

Pizzi, T., Rubio, M. & Knierim, F. 1954. Inmunologia de la enfermedad de Chagas. *Bol. Chil. Parasitol.* 9: 35-47.

Prado, A.A. 1945. Mal de engasgo ou doença de Chagas? (Bloqueio auriculo-ventricular total.) *São Paulo Med.* 18: 95-112.

Prath, A.R. 1968. Formas clinicas da doença de Chagas. *In* Doença de Chagas, Cançado, J.R., Ed.: 344-358. Impr. Ofic. Estado de Minas Gerais. Belo Horizonte, Brazil.

Prath, A.R. 1973. Implicações epidemiológicas e socio-econômicas da doença de Chagas. *Bras.-Med.* 9: 69-71.

Rego, S.F.M. 1959. Estado das lesões provacadas pelo *Trypanosoma cruzi* Chagas, 1909, no baco e no fígado do camundongo branco ("mus musculis"), com diversos graus de resistência. *J. Bras. Med.* 1: 599-674.

Rich, A. 1950. Pathogenesis of Tuberculosis. 2nd ed.: 439-450. C. C Thomas. Springfield, Ill.

Roberson, E.L. & Hanson, W.L. 1974. Transfer of immunity to *Trypanosoma cruzi. Trans. R. Soc. Trop. Med. Hyg.* 68: 338.

Roberson, E.L., Hanson, W.L. & Chapman, W.L. 1973. *Trypanosoma cruzi:* effects of anti-lymphocyte serum in mice and neonatal thymectomy in rats. *Exp. Parasitol.* 34: 168-180

Romaña, O. 1944. Contribuição ao conhecimento da patogenia da trypano-somiase americana (Período inicial da infecção). *Mem. Inst. Oswaldo Cruz Rio de Janeiro.* 39: 253-264.

Rubio, M. 1954. Estudio de los factores que intervienen en la virulencia de una cepa de *Trypanosoma cruzi.* Acción de la cortisona en la capacidad de invasión y multiplicación de parasito. *Biologica* 20: 89-125.

Rubio, M. 1956. Actividad litica de sueros normales sobre formas de cultivo e sanguineas de *Trypanosoma cruzi. Bol. Chil. Parasitol.* 11: 62-69.

Salgado, J.A., Garcez, P.N., Oliveira, C.A. & Galizzi, J. 1962. Revisão clínica atual do primeiro caso humano descrito de doença de Chagas. *Rev. Inst. Med. Trop. São Paulo* 4: 330-337.

Santos, R.R. 1973. Contribuicão ao estudo da imunidade na fase aguda da doença de Chagas experimental. *Rev. Patol. Trop.* 2: 433-463.

Santos-Buch, C.A. & Teixeira, A.R.L. 1974. The immunology of experimental Chagas' disease. 3. Rejection of allogeneic heart cells *in vitro. J. Exp. Med.* 140: 38-53.

Seah, S. 1970. Delayed hypersensitivity in *Trypanosoma cruzi* infection. *Nature* (Lond.) 225: 1256-1257.

Seah, S. & Marsden, P.D. 1969. The protection of mice against a virulent strain of Trypanosoma cruzi by previous inoculation with an avirulent strain. *Ann. Trop. Med. Parasitol.* 63: 211-214.

Seah, S.K., Marsden, P.D., Voller, A. & Pettit, L.E. 1974. Experimental *Trypanosoma cruzi* infection in rhesus monkeys—the acute phase. *Trans. R. Soc. Trop. Med. Hyg.* 68: 63-69.

Segura, E.L., Cura, E.N., Paulone, I, Vasquez, C. & Cerisola, J.A. 1974. Antigenic makeup of subcellular fractions of *Trypanosoma cruzi. J. Protozool.* 21: 571-574.

Seneca, H. & Peer, P. 1963. Immunochemistry of *Trypanosoma cruzi* and immunochemotherapy of experimental Chagas' disease. *Antimicrob. Agents Chemother.* 3: 560-565.

Seneca, H. & Peer, P. 1966. Immuno-biological properties of chagastoxin (lipopolysaccharide). *Trans. R. Soc. Trop. Med. Hyg.* 60: 610-620.

Seneca, H., Peer, P. & Hampar, B. 1966. Active immunization of mice with chagastoxin. *Nature* (Lond.) 209: 309-310.

Souza, M. doC., Reis, A.P., Da Silva, W.D. & Brener, Z. 1974. Mechanism of acquired immunity induced by *Leptomonas pessoai* against *Trypanosoma cruzi* in mice. *J. Protozool.* 21: 579-584.

Souza, M. doC. & Roitman, I. 1971. Protective effect of *Leptomonas pessoai* against the infection of mice by *Trypanosoma cruzi. Rev. Microbiol.* 2: 187-189.

Souza Campos, E. 1927. Estudos sobre uma raça neurotrópica de *Trypanosoma cruzi. An. Fac. Med. Univ. São Paulo* 2: 197-201.

Taliaferro, W.H. & Pizzi, T. 1955. Connective tissue reaction in normal and immunized mice to a reticulotropic strain of *Trypanosoma cruzi. J. Infect. Dis.* 96: 199-226.

Tanowitz, H., Wittner, M., Kress, Y. & Bloom, B. 1975. Studies of *in vitro* infection by *Trypanosoma cruzi*, I. Ultrastructural studies on the invasion of macrophages and L-cells. *Am. J. Trop. Med. Hyg.* 24: 25-33.

Tarrant, C.J., Fife Jr., E.H. & Anderson, R.I. 1965. Serological characteristics and general chemical nature of the *in vitro* exoantigens of *Trypanosoma cruzi*. *J. Parasitol.* 51: 277-285.

Teixeira, A.R.L., Roters, F.A. & Mott, K.F. 1970. Acute Chagas' disease. *Gaz. Med. Bahia* 3: 176-186.

Teixeira, A.R.L. & Santos-Buch, C.A. 1974. The immunology of experimental Chagas' disease. I. Preparations of *Trypanosoma cruzi* antigens and humoral antibody response to these antigens. *J. Immunol.* 113: 859-869.

Teixeira, A.R.L. & Santos-Buch, C.A. 1975. The immunology of experimental Chagas' disease. II. Delayed hypersensitivity to *Trypanosoma cruzi* antigens. *Immunology* 28: 401-410.

Teixeira, A.R.L., Teixeira, M.L. & Santos-Buch, C.A. 1975. The immunology of experimental Chagas' disease in man. IV. The production of lesions in rabbits like those of chronic Chagas' disease in man. *Am. J. Pathol.* 80: 163-180.

Torres, C.B.M. 1930. Patogénia de la miocarditis crónica en la enfermedad de Chagas. 5. Reunión de la Sociedad Argentina de Patologia Regional del Norté Jujuy, Argentina. 2: 902-916.

Torres, C.B.M. & Tavares, B.M. 1958. Miocardite no macaco Cebus após inoculaçôes repetidas com *Schizotrypanum cruzi*. *Mem. Inst. Oswaldo Cruz Rio de Janeiro* 56: 85-152.

Tschudi, E.I., Anziano, D.F. & Dalmasso, A.P. 1972. Lymphocyte transformation in Chagas disease. *Infect. Immun.* 6: 905-908.

Vampré, E. 1923. Terceira contribuição ao estudo do "mal de engasgo." *Bol. Soc. Med. Cir. São Paulo* 6: 75-88.

Vianna, G.O. 1911. Contribuição para o estudo da Anatomia Patólogica da "moléstia de Carlos Chagas." *Mem. Inst. Oswaldo Cruz Rio de Janeiro* 3: 276-294.

Vickerman, K. 1974. Antigenic variation in African trypanosomes. *In* Parasites in the Immunized Host: Mechanisms of Survival. Ciba Foundation Symposium 25 (new series), Porter, R., & Knights, J. Eds.: 53-80. Associated Scientific Publishers. Amsterdam, The Netherlands.

Vickerman, K. & Luckins, A.G. 1969. Localization of variable antigens in the surface coat of *Trypanosoma brucei* using ferritin-conjugated antibody. *Nature* (Lond.) 224: 1125-1126.

Villela, E. 1925. Variação do poder patogênico do *"Trypanosoma cruzi"* (raça neurotropica). *Sci. Med.* 3: 147-148.

Voller, A. & Shaw, J.J. 1965. Immunological observations on an antiserum to *Trypanosoma cruzi*. *Z. Tropenmed. Parasitol.* 16: 181-187.

von Brand, T., Tobie, E.J., Kissling, R.E. & Adams, G. 1949. Physiological and pathological observations on four strains of *Trypanosoma cruzi. J. Infect. Dis.* 85: 5-16.

Yanovsky, J.F. & Albado, E. 1972. Humoral and cellular response to *Trypanosoma cruzi* infection. *J. Immunol.* 109: 1159-1161.

13

EXPERIMENTS ON IMMUNOPROPHYLAXIS AGAINST CHAGAS' DISEASE

William L. Hanson

Department of Parasitology
College of Veterinary Medicine
University of Georgia
Athens, Georgia 30602

It is apparent from Dr. Teixeira's chapter that attempts to immunize experimental animals against acute infections with *Trypanosoma cruzi* have met with only limited success, and virtually nothing is known regarding the possibility of immunoprophylaxis against chronic Chagas' disease. Nevertheless, the limited success achieved thus far offers some encouragement that the development of effective immunizing agents for use against *T. cruzi* is feasible.

The importance of selection of the proper antigen in immunization studies cannot be emphasized too much. Since *T. cruzi* has a relatively complex life cycle and occurs in several morphological stages depending on the environment, the selection of those morphological stages which predominate in the vertebrate host (i.e., trypomastigote and amastigote) for antigen preparation and immunization studies appears highly desirable. The lack of success in many previous studies has possibly resulted, in part, from the fact that many of the studies have been done with antigen preparations obtained from the epimastigote stage of *T. cruzi,* which is not the stage of the parasite that occurs frequently in the vertebrate host.

Experiments were initiated in our laboratory a number of years ago to study the relative efficacy of crude subcellular antigen preparations from epimastigotes and mixtures of trypomastigotes and amastigotes in the stimulation of protective immunity to challenge with virulent *T. cruzi* in mice. In addition, living epimastigotes and mixtures of living trypomastigotes and amastigotes were made apparently noninfective by exposure to high levels of gamma irradiation and compared for efficacy in the immunization of CF_1 mice against virulent *T. cruzi.* While crude antigen preparations obtained from several stages of the parasite by ultrasonication or pressure disintegration were noted to stimulate very little protective immunity against *T. cruzi* in recipient mice, considerably greater protection was obtained in mice receiving a mixture of irradiated trypomastigotes and amastigotes than was observed in mice receiving an equivalent number of irradiated epimastigotes. For example, mice receiving irradiated epimastigotes and challenged with virulent *T. cruzi* developed maximum mean parasitemias of 1.0 to 2.0 X 10^6 organisms per ml blood, whereas those mice immunized with an equivalent number of irradiated trypomastigotes and amastigotes had maximum mean parasitemias of generally less than 50,000 per ml blood. This difference in parasitemia was also reflected in reduced mortality in the mice immunized with irradiated trypomastigotes and amastigotes as well as reduced signs of clinical disease.

Encouraged by markedly better results with irradiated trypomastigotes and amastigotes than were obtained with a variety of subcellular preparations as well as irradiated epimastigotes, several experiments were conducted with irradiated trypomastigotes and amastigotes that are relevant to several points discussed by Dr. Teixeira. Certain of these will be considered subsequently.

Results indicating the persistence of protective immunity against *T. cruzi* in mice following immunization with irradiated *T. cruzi* have been obtained from a series of recent experiments in our laboratory. Following immunization these mice, along with appropriate controls, were challenged with virulent *T. cruzi* at 1, 4, 8, 16, and 24 weeks. All immunized mice were significantly protected to approximately the same extent. Maximum mean parasitemia of the control groups ranged from approximately 2.0 to 4.0 X 10^6 per ml blood, whereas that of the immunized mice did not exceed 52.0 X 10^3 per ml blood. Furthermore, the blood of 20% to 50% of the immunized mice remained microscopically negative for *T. cruzi* following challenge with virulent parasites. This lowered parasitemia was reflected in lower mortality and lessened clinical signs of disease in the immunized mice. The persistence of protective immunity in mice for at least 6 months following immunization with mixtures of irradiated trypomastigotes and amastigotes provides additional encouragement for the feasibility of the development of an effective vaccine for Chagas' disease.

The question of "sterile" immunity in Chagas' disease following acute infections remains unsettled at this time. Current evidence indicates that animals that have recovered from acute infections of *T. cruzi* maintain low-level infections for the remainder of their lives. During the past several years, we have studied several hundred mice for up to one year after recovery from acute disease and have found no evidence for complete eradication of the infection by even a single mouse. On the other hand, the results of immunization studies in several laboratories suggest that protective immunity persists in experimental animals in the absence of a low-level infection. For example, in the immunization studies with irradiated *T. cruzi* in our laboratory mentioned above, the irradiated parasites were not capable of infecting Vero cell cultures or highly susceptible strains of mice but were capable of stimulating a significant protective immunity in immunized mice, which persisted for at least 6 months. No evidence of infection was seen in the immunized mice prior to challenge with virulent *T. cruzi*. It is obvious that one cannot give absolute assurance that no infections were produced in immunized mice in these experiments. However, considerable effort was made to show that the levels of irradiation used made the parasite incapable of infecting the recipients. These precautions included inoculation into Vero cell cultures and inoculation into highly susceptible intact and splenectomized C_3H inbred mice. These procedures are capable of detecting a single living parasite.

The immune mechanisms responsible for the protective immunity seen in mice immunized with irradiated *T. cruzi* remain to be elucidated as do those functioning in acquired immunity in acute infections. We have observed that mice receiving irradiated parasites form detectable antibody. Furthermore, antibody titers rise more rapidly in immunized mice than in nonimmunized controls following challenge with virulent parasites. Spleen cells from immunized animals confer adoptive protection to syngeneic recipients and the extent of the protection is similar to that obtained in similar experiments with spleen cells from donors that have recovered from acute infections with virulent *T. cruzi*. Preliminary experiments failed to demonstrate passive transfer of protection with serum from immunized mice, although serum from experimentally infected mice confers passive protection to recipient mice.

Finally, one cannot overemphasize the need for additional information concerning the fate of immunized animals in regard to chronic Chagas' disease. It is apparent that until much more information is available regarding the immune mechanisms functioning in acquired immunity against *T. cruzi*, as well as the pathogenic mechanisms responsible for chronic Chagas' disease, immunization will be extremely hazardous. Some information currently available suggests that cellular sensitivity may be involved in both acquired resistance to *T. cruzi* and in the pathogenesis of chronic Chagas' disease. Verification of these findings along with extended studies regarding the basic immunologic and pathogenic mechanisms functioning in Chagas' disease are greatly needed to serve as guides in further attempts to develop immunoprophylactic procedures for use in this important disease.

A

PARTICIPANTS IN THE CONFERENCE ON IMMUNOPROPHYLAXIS AGAINST HEMOPARASITIC DISEASES

September 10-13, 1975
Bellagio Study and Conference Center
Bellagio, Italy

Dr. Barry R. Bloom
Department of Microbiology and Immunology
Albert Einstein College of Medicine
Yeshiva University
1300 Morris Park Avenue
Bronx, New York   10461

Dr. K.N. Brown
Department of Parasitology
National Institute for Medical Research
Mill Hill Laboratories
The Ridgeway
London NW7, England

Dr. L.L. Callow
Officer-in-Charge
Tick Fever Research Centre
Department of Primary Industries
Wacol, Queensland, 4076, Australia

Dr. Sydney Cohen
Department of Chemical Pathology
Guy's Hospital Medical School
London SE1 9RT, England

Dr. M.P. Cunningham
Project Manager
Immunological Research on Tick-Borne Diseases
c/o East African Veterinary Research Organization
Muguga, P.O. Box 32 Kikuyu, Kenya

Dr. John J. Doyle
W.H.O. Immunology Research and Training Centre
21, rue du Bugnon
1011 Lausanne, Switzerland

Dr. Howard C. Goodman
World Health Organization
1211 Geneva 27, Switzerland

Dr. William L. Hanson
Head, Department of Parasitology
College of Veterinary Medicine
The University of Georgia
Athens, Georgia   30602

Dr. J.B. Henson
Director
International Laboratory for Research on Animal
    Diseases (ILRAD)
P.O. Box 30709
Nairobi, Kenya

Dr. W.F.H. Jarrett
Department of Veterinary Pathology
University of Glasgow
Veterinary School
Bearsden Road, Bearsden
Glasgow G61 1QH, Scotland

Dr. Elvin A. Kabat
Department of Microbiology
College of Physicians and Surgeons
Columbia University
630 West 168th Street
New York, New York   10032

Dr. W.H.R. Lumsden
Department of Medical Protozoology
London School of Hygiene and Tropical Medicine
Keppel Street (Gower Street)
London WC1E 7HT, England

Dr. Ian McIntyre
Department of Veterinary Medicine
University of Glasgow
Veterinary School
Bearsden Road, Bearsden
Glasgow G61 1QH, Scotland

Dr. John J. McKelvey, Jr.
Associate Director for Agricultural Sciences
The Rockefeller Foundation
1133 Avenue of the Americas
New York, New York   10036

Dr. George B. Mackaness
Trudeau Institute, Inc.
P.O. Box 59
Saranac Lake, New York   12983

Dr. Louis H. Miller
Head, Malaria Section
Laboratory of Parasitic Diseases
National Institute of Allergy and Infectious Diseases
Bethesda, Maryland   20014

Dr. Max Murray
Division d'Hématologie
Hôpital Cantonal
25, rue Micheli-du-Crest
1205 Geneva, Switzerland

Dr. Ruth S. Nussenzweig
Department of Preventive Medicine
School of Medicine
New York University Medical Center
550 First Avenue
New York, New York   10016

Dr. John A. Pino
Director for Agricultural Sciences
The Rockefeller Foundation
1133 Avenue of the Americas
New York, New York   10036

Dr. Miodrag Ristic
Department of Pathology and Hygiene
College of Veterinary Medicine
University of Illinois at Urbana-Champaign
Urbana, Illinois 61801

Dr. Antonio R.L. Teixeira
Departamento de Patologia
Faculdade de Ciencias da Saude
Universidade de Brasilia
70.000 Brasilia, D. Federal, Brasil

Dr. G.M. Urquhart
The Wellcome Laboratories for Experimental Parasitology
University of Glasgow
Bearsden Road, Bearsden
Glasgow G61 1QH, Scotland

B

JOURNAL ABBREVIATIONS

Acta Trop. — Acta Tropica
Acta Vet. Scand. — Acta Veterinaria Scandinavica
Adv. Immunol. — Advances in Immunology
Adv. Microb. Physiol. — Advances in Microbial Physiology
Adv. Parasitol. — Advances in Parasitology
Adv. Vet. Sci. — Advances in Veterinary Science
Am. J. Hyg. — American Journal of Hygiene
Am. J. Med. Sci. — American Journal of the Medical Sciences
Am. J. Ophthalmol. — American Journal of Ophthalmology
Am. J. Pathol. — American Journal of Pathology
Am. J. Trop. Med. — American Journal of Tropical Medicine
Am. J. Trop. Med. Hyg. — American Journal of Tropical Medicine and Hygiene
Am. J. Vet. Res. — American Journal of Veterinary Research
An. Fac. Med. Univ. São Paulo — Anais da Faculdade de Medicina da Universidade do São Paulo
An. Cong. Internac. Doença de Chagas — Anais do Congresso Internacional sobre Doença de Chagas, Rio de Janeiro, 1959
Ann. Soc. Belge Méd. Trop. — Annales de la Société Belge de Médecine Tropicale
Ann. Inst. Pasteur (Paris) — Annales de l'Institut Pasteur (Paris)
Ann. Parasitol. Hum. Comp. — Annales de Parasitologie Humaine et Comparée
Ann. N.Y. Acad. Sci. — Annals of the New York Academy of Sciences
Ann. Trop. Med. Parasitol. — Annals of Tropical Medicine and Parasitology
Antimicrob. Agents Chemother. — Antimicrobial Agents and Chemotherapy
Arch. Schiffs.-Tropenhyg. — Archiv fuer Schiffs- und Tropen-Hygiene, Pathologie und Therapie exotischer Krankheiten
Arch. Inst. Pasteur Alger. — Archives de l'Institut Pasteur d'Algérie
Arq. Bras. Cardiol. — Arquivos Brasileiros de Cardiologia
Arzneim-Forsch. — Arzneimittel-Forschung
Aust. J. Agric. Res. — Australian Journal of Agricultural Research
Aust. J. Sci. — Australian Journal of Science
Aust. Meat Res. Comm. Rev. — Australian Meat Research Committee Review
Aust. Vet. J. — Australian Veterinary Journal
Biken J. — Biken Journal
Biologica — Biologica
Bol. Chil. Parasitol. — Boletín Chileno de Parasitologia

Bol. Soc. Med. Cir. São Paulo — Boletim da Sociedade de Medicina e Cirurgia de São Paulo

Bol. Inf. Parasit. Chil. — Boletín de Informaciones Parasitarias Chilenas

Bol. Of. Sanit. Panam. — Boletín de la Oficina Sanitaria Panamericana

Bras.-Med. — Brasil-Medico

Br. J. Exp. Pathol. — British Journal of Experimental Pathology

Br. Med. Bull. — British Medical Bulletin

Br. Vet. J. — British Veterinary Journal

Bull. Soc. Path. Exot. — Bulletin de la Société de Pathologie Exotique

Bull. Inf. Inst. Agron. Congo Belge — Bulletin d'Information. Institut National pour l'Étude Agronomique du Congo Belge

Bull. Epizoot. Dis. Afr. — Bulletin of Epizootic Diseases of Africa

Bull. WHO — Bulletin of the World Health Organization

Can. J. Microbiol. — Canadian Journal of Microbiology

Cancer Res. — Cancer Research

Cell. Immunol. — Cellular Immunology

Circulation — Circulation

Clin. Exp. Immunol. — Clinical and Experimental Immunology

Compt. R. Soc. Biol. — Comptes Rendus de la Société Biologique

Dtsch. Kolonialbl. — Deutsches Kolonialblatt

E. Afr. Agric. J. — East African Agricultural Journal

E. Afr. Med. J. — East African Medical Journal

E. Afr. Trypanosomiasis Res. Organ. Annu. Rep. — East African Trypanosomiasis Research Organization Annual Report

Exp. Parasitol. — Experimental Parasitology

Gaz. Med. Bahia — Gazeta Medica da Bahia

Indian J. Med. Res. — Indian Journal of Medical Research

Indian Med. Res. Mem. — Indian Medical Research Memoirs

Infect. Immun. — Infection and Immunity

Int. J. Parasitol. — International Journal for Parasitology

Int. Rev. Trop. Med. — International Review of Tropical Medicine

Jap. J. Parasitol. — Japanese Journal of Parasitology

J. Agric. Res. — Journal of Agricultural Research

J. Bras. Med. — Journal Brasileiro de Medicina

J. Cell Sci. — Journal of Cell Science

J. Clin. Invest. — Journal of Clinical Investigation

J. Comp. Pathol. — Journal of Comparative Pathology

J. Comp. Pathol. Ther. — Journal of Comparative Pathology and Therapeutics

J. Exp. Med. — Journal of Experimental Medicine

J. Gen. Microbiol. — Journal of General Microbiology

J. Hyg. — Journal of Hygiene

J. Immunol. — Journal of Immunology

J. Infect. Dis. — Journal of Infectious Diseases

J. Med. Microbiol. — Journal of Medical Microbiology

J. Parasitol. — Journal of Parasitology

J. Pathol. Bacteriol. — Journal of Pathology and Bacteriology

J. Protozool. — Journal of Protozoology

J. Am. Vet. Med. Assoc. — Journal of the American Veterinary Medical Association

J. Malar. Inst. India — Journal of the Malaria Institute of India

J. Nat. Cancer Inst. — Journal of the National Cancer Institute

J. Reticuloendothel. Soc. — Journal of the Reticuloendothelial Society

J. Trop. Med. Hyg. — Journal of Tropical Medicine and Hygiene

Kajian Vet. — Kajian Veterinaire

Med. J. Osaka Univ. — Medical Journal of Osaka University

Med. Rev. Cent. Acad. Rocha Lima (CARL) Hosp. Clin. Fac. Med. Ribeirao Preto Univ. São Paulo — Medicina Revista do Centro Academico Rocha Lima (CARL) do Hospital das Clinicas da Faculdade de Medicina de Ribeirao Preto da Universidade de São Paulo

Medicine (Balt.) — Medicine (Baltimore)

Mem. Inst. Oswaldo Cruz Rio de Janeiro — Memorias do Instituto Oswaldo Cruz, Rio de Janeiro

Mil. Med. — Military Medicine

Mo. Agric. Exp. Stn. Bull. — Missouri Agricultural Experiment Station Bulletin

Nature (Lond.) — Nature (London)

Nat. New Biol. — Nature. New Biology

N. Engl. J. Med. — New England Journal of Medicine

New Sci. — New Scientist

Onderstepoort J. Vet. Res. — Onderstepoort Journal of Veterinary Research

Pan Am. Health Organ. Sci. Publ. — Pan American Health Organization Scientific Publication

Proc. Helminthol. Soc. Wash. — Proceedings of the Helminthological Society of Washington

Proc. Nat. Acad. Sci. U.S.A. — Proceedings of the National Academy of Sciences of the United States of America

Proc. 19th World Vet. Congr. — Proceedings of the 19th World Veterinary Congress

Proc. R. Soc. Med. — Proceedings of the Royal Society of Medicine

Proc. Soc. Exp. Biol. Med. — Proceedings of the Society for Experimental Biology and Medicine

Proc. 3rd Int. Congr. Parasitol. — Proceedings of the 3rd International Congress of Parasitology

Proc. U.S. Anim. Health Assoc. — Proceedings of the United States Animal Health Association

Proc. U.S. Livestock Sanit. Assoc. — Proceedings of the United States Livestock Sanitary Association

Queensl. Agric. J. — Queensland Agricultural Journal

Refu. Vet. — Refuah Veterinarith

Res. Vet. Sci. — Research in Veterinary Science

Rev. Biol. Hig., São Paulo — Revista de Biologia e Higiene, São Paulo

Rev. Biol. Trop., Univ. Costa Rica — Revista de Biologia Tropical, Universidad de Costa Rica

Rev. Bras. Biol. — Revista Brasileira de Biologia

Rev. Bras. Malariol. — Revista Brasileira de Malariologia

Rev. Bras. Med. — Revista Brasileira de Medicina

Rev. Goiana Med. — Revista Goiana de Medicina

Rev. Inst. Zoonosis Invest. Pecu., Lima — Revista del Instituto de Zoonosis y Investigaciones Pecuarias, Lima

Rev. Microbiol. — Revista de Microbiologia

Rev. Med. Cordoba — Revista Médica de Cordoba

Rev. Paul. Med. — Revista Paulista de Medicina

Rev. Inst. Med. Trop. São Paulo — Revista do Instituto de Medicina Tropical de São Paulo

Rev. Patol. Trop. — Revista do Patologia Tropica

Rev. Élevage Méd. Vét. Pays Trop. — Revue d'Élevage et de Médecine Vétérinaire des Pays Tropicaux

São Paulo Med. — São Paulo Medico

Scand. J. Immunol. — Scandinavian Journal of Immunology

Science — Science (Washington, D.C.)

Sci. Med. — Sciencia Medica

Tijdschr. Diergeneeskd. — Tijdschrift voor Diergeneeskunde

Trans. Am. Microsc. Soc. — Transactions of the American Microscopical Society

Trans. R. Soc. Trop. Med. Hyg. — Transactions of the Royal Society of Tropical Medicine and Hygiene

Transplant. Rev. — Transplantation Reviews
Tropenmed. Parasitol. — Tropenmedizin und Parasitologie
Trop. Anim. Health Prod. — Tropical Animal Health and Production
U.S. Dept. Agric. Bur. Anim. Ind. Bull. — United States Department of
    Agriculture, Bureau of Animal Industry Bulletin
Univ. Buenos Aires, Misión Estud. Pat. Reg. Argent. — Universidad de Buenos
    Aires, Misión de Estúdios de Patología Regional Argentina, Jujuy
Vet. Med. Small Anim. Clin. — Veterinary Medicine and Small Animal Clinician
Vet. Parasitol. — Veterinary Parasitology
Vet. Pathol. — Veterinary Pathology
Vet. Rec. — Veterinary Record
World Anim. Rev. — World Animal Review
Z. Hyg. Infektionskr. — Zeitschrift fuer Hygiene und Infektionskrankheiten
Z. Immunitaetsforsch. — Zeitschrift fuer Immunitaetsforschung
Z. Tropenmed. Parasitol. — Zeitschrift fuer Tropenmedizin und Parasitologie
Zentralbl. Veterinaermed. — Zentralblatt fuer Veterinaermedizin

AUTHOR INDEX

SUBJECT INDEX

Abortion
    babesiosis vaccine as cause of, 137
    trypanosomiasis as cause of, 212
Acaricides, 189
Acetaldehyde, 98
Acetic acid, 217
Acquired resistance, 3, 65, 69
    to babesiosis, 124-25
    to Chagas' disease, 250-53
    to malaria, 72, 93-102
    reticuloendothelial changes and, 67
Actinomycin D., 257
Adenosine triphosphate (ATP), 92
Adjuvants, 3 (*See also* Freund's
        complete adjuvant; Freund's
        incomplete adjuvant)
    in anaplasmosis vaccine, 152, 160,
        163, 173
    in babesiosis vaccine, 131
    cell-mediated immunity induction
        by, 70
    in malaria vaccine, 107-8, 114-15
    in trypanosomiasis vaccine, 216,
        219, 220, 228, 231, 265, 266
Africa, 1, 2, 28, 89, 152, 160, 183, 189
African buffalo, 189, 223
African trypanosomes (*See* Salivarian
        trypanosomes)
Agar gel precipitation test, 157
Agglutination, 31 (*See also*
        Capillary tube
        agglutination test;
        Schizont-infected cell
        agglutination test)
    in malaria, 14
    of merozoites, 10, 102

Agglutination (cont.)
    of trypanosomes, 34, 35, 39-41,
        47, 49
    reciprocal, 42
    trypomastigotes, 252
Aitong (Kenya), 194
Algeria, 128
Allergic hypersensitivity, 66
Allergy, bacterial, 70
Alsever's solution, 133
Aluminum hydroxide, 216, 219
Aluminum hydrogel, 107
Ameiva surinamensis, 249, 250
American trypanosomiasis (*See*
        Chagas' disease)
Amphibians, 249
Anaplasma
    food intake among, 157
    inclusion bodies, 152
    persistence in immunologically
        hostile host of, 158
    centrale, 139, 152
        serologic studies of, 158
        vaccination against *A. marginale*
        with, 159-60
    marginale, 135, 151-84
        antigens of, 157-58
        attenuated vaccine of, 3, 161-62,
        168-84
        biological properties of, 152-57
        inactivated vaccine of, 160,
        162-68
        naturally occurring immunogens
        to, 159-60
        serology and kinetics of humoral
        response in, 158, 168